T0226874

Interstitial Lung Disease

Guest Editors

TALMADGE E. KING Jr, MD
HAROLD R. COLLARD, MD
LUCA RICHELDI, MD, PhD

CLINICS IN CHEST MEDICINE

www.chestmed.theclinics.com

March 2012 • Volume 33 • Number 1

SAUNDERS an imprint of ELSEVIER, Inc.

W.B. SAUNDERS COMPANY

A Division of Elsevier Inc.

1600 John F. Kennedy Boulevard • Suite 1800 • Philadelphia, Pennsylvania 19103

http://www.thcclinics.com

CLINICS IN CHEST MEDICINE Volume 33, Number 1
March 2012 ISSN 0272-5231, ISBN-13: 978-1-4557-3842-7

Editor: Katie Hartner
Developmental Editor: Donald E. Mumford

Clinics in Chest Medicine (ISSN 0272-5231) is published quarterly by Elsevier Inc., 360 Park Avenue South, New York, NY 10010-1710. Months of issue are March, June, September, and December. Periodicals postage paid at New York, NY and additional mailing offices. Subscription prices are $316.00 per year (domestic individuals), $506.00 per year (domestic institutions), $151.00 per year (domestic students/residents), $347.00 per year (Canadian individuals), $621.00 per year (Canadian institutions), $431.00 per year (international individuals), $621.00 per year (international institutions), and $211.00 per year (international and Canadian students/residents). International air speed delivery is included in all Clinics subscription prices. All prices are subject to change without notice. **POSTMASTER:** Send address changes to Clinics in Chest Medicine, Elsevier Health Sciences Division, Subscription Customer Service, 3251 Riverport Lane, Maryland Heights, MO 63043. **Customer Service: Telephone: 1-800-654-2452** (U.S. and Canada); **1-314-447-8871** (outside U.S. and Canada). **Fax: 1-314-447-8029. E-mail: journalscustomerservice-usa@elsevier.com** (for print support); **journalsonlinesupport-usa@elsevier.com** (for online support).

Reprints. For copies of 100 or more of articles in this publication, please contact the Commercial Reprints Department, Elsevier Inc., 360 Park Avenue South, New York, NY 10010-1710. Tel.: 212-633-3812; Fax: 212-462-1935; E-mail: reprints@elsevier.com.

Clinics in Chest Medicine is covered in *MEDLINE/PubMed (Index Medicus), Current Contents/Clinical Medicine, EMBASE/ Excerpta Medica, Science Citation Index,* and *ISI/BIOMED.*

Printed and bound by CPI Group (UK) Ltd, Croydon, CR0 4YY

Transferred to Digital Print 2012

Contributors

GUEST EDITORS

TALMADGE E. KING Jr, MD
Julius R. Krevans Distinguished Professorship
in Internal Medicine, Chair, Department
of Medicine, University of California
San Francisco, San Francisco, California

HAROLD R. COLLARD, MD
Associate Professor of Medicine, Director,
Interstitial Lung Disease Program, Division
of Pulmonary and Critical Care Medicine,
Department of Medicine, University of
California San Francisco, San Francisco,
California

LUCA RICHELDI, MD, PhD
Director, Center for Rare Lung Diseases,
Department of Oncology, Hematology and
Respiratory Diseases, University Hospital
Policlinico of Modena, Modena, Italy

AUTHORS

DANIELLE ANTIN-OZERKIS, MD
Assistant Professor of Medicine, Director,
Yale Interstitial Lung Disease Program,
Pulmonary & Critical Care Medicine
Section, Department of Internal Medicine,
Yale University School of Medicine,
New Haven, Connecticut

JÜRGEN BEHR, MD
Professor of Medicine, Director, Department
of Internal Medicine III, University Hospital
Bergmannsheil, Ruhr-University Bochum,
Bochum, Germany

FRANCESCO BONELLA, MD
Department of Pneumology/Allergy,
Ruhrlandklinik, University Hospital,
Essen, Germany

STEFANIA CERRI, MD, PhD
Center for Rare Lung Diseases, Department
of Oncology, Hematology and Respiratory
Diseases, University Hospital Policlinico of
Modena, Modena, Italy

JONATHAN H. CHUNG, MD
Assistant Professor, Division of Radiology,
National Jewish Health, Denver, Colorado

ULRICH COSTABEL, MD, FCCP
Professor of Medicine, Department of
Pneumology/Allergy, Ruhrlandklinik,
University Hospital, Essen, Germany

MEGAN STUEBNER DEVINE, MD
Pulmonary Fellow, Division of Pulmonary and
Critical Care Medicine, Department of Internal
Medicine, Eugene McDermott Center for
Human Growth and Development, University
of Texas Southwestern Medical Center,
Dallas, Texas

JANINE EVANS, MD
Associate Professor of Diagnostic Radiology,
Rheumatology Section, Department of Internal
Medicine, Yale University School of Medicine,
New Haven, Connecticut

CHARLENE D. FELL, MD, MSc, FRCPC
Clinical Assistant Professor of Medicine,
Division of Respirology, University of Calgary,
and Peter Lougheed Hospital, Calgary,
Alberta, Canada

CHRISTINE KIM GARCIA, MD, PhD
Associate Professor, Division of Pulmonary
and Critical Care Medicine, Department of
Internal Medicine, Eugene McDermott Center
for Human Growth and Development,
University of Texas Southwestern Medical
Center, Dallas, Texas

JOSUNE GUZMAN, MD
Professor of General and Experimental
Pathology, Pathologisches Institut der
Ruhr-Universität Bochum, Bochum, Germany

ROBERT J. HOMER, MD, PhD
Professor of Pathology and Medicine
(Pulmonary), Yale University School of
Medicine, New Haven, Connecticut

HAMZA JAWAD, MD
Affiliate, Division of Radiology, National
Jewish Health, Denver, Colorado

KIRK D. JONES, MD
Professor, Department of Pathology, University
of California San Francisco, San Francisco,
California

DONG SOON KIM, MD, PhD
Professor, Department of Pulmonary and
Critical Care Medicine, Asan Medical Center,
University of Ulsan, Seoul, Korea

BRENT WAYNE KINDER, MD, MS
Mercy Health Physicians, Batavia, Ohio;
Mercy Health Partners, Cincinnati, Ohio

FABRIZIO LUPPI, MD, PhD
Center for Rare Lung Diseases, Department
of Oncology, Hematology and Respiratory
Diseases, University Hospital Policlinico of
Modena, Modena, Italy

DAVID A. LYNCH, MD
Professor, Division of Radiology, National
Jewish Health, Denver, Colorado

TOBY M. MAHER, MB, MSc, PhD, MRCP
Consultant Respiratory Physician and
Honorary Senior Lecturer, Interstitial Lung

Disease Unit, Royal Brompton Hospital;
National Heart and Lung Institute, Imperial
College London; Centre for Respiratory
Research, University College London,
London, United Kingdom

RICHARD A. MATTHAY, MD
Boehringer Ingelheim Emeritus Professor
of Medicine and Senior Research Scientist,
Pulmonary & Critical Care Medicine Section,
Department of Internal Medicine, Yale
University School of Medicine, New Haven,
Connecticut

JOHN D. NEWELL Jr, MD, FACR
Professor of Radiology, Department of
Radiology, University of Iowa, Iowa City, Iowa

AMY L. OLSON, MD, MSPH
Assistant Professor, Interstitial Lung Disease
Program, Division of Pulmonary and Critical
Care Medicine, Autoimmune Lung Center,
National Jewish Health, Denver, Colorado

LUCA RICHELDI, MD, PhD
Director, Center for Rare Lung Diseases,
Department of Oncology, Hematology and
Respiratory Diseases, University Hospital
Policlinico of Modena, Modena, Italy

AMI RUBINOWITZ, MD
Associate Professor of Medicine, Department
of Diagnostic Radiology, Yale University
School of Medicine, New Haven, Connecticut

JAY H. RYU, MD
Division of Pulmonary and Critical Care
Medicine, Mayo Clinic, Rochester, Minnesota

PAOLO SPAGNOLO, MD, PhD
Center for Rare Lung Diseases, Department
of Oncology, Hematology and Respiratory
Diseases, University Hospital Policlinico of
Modena, Modena, Italy

JEFFREY J. SWIGRIS, DO, MS
Associate Professor, Interstitial Lung Disease
Program, Division of Pulmonary and Critical
Care Medicine, Autoimmune Lung Center,
National Jewish Health, Denver, Colorado

ANATOLY URISMAN, MD, PhD
Clinical Instructor, Department of Pathology,
University of California San Francisco,
San Francisco, California

ROBERT VASSALLO, MD
Division of Pulmonary and Critical Care
Medicine; Department of Physiology and

Biomedical Engineering, Mayo Clinic,
Rochester, Minnesota

TIMOTHY P.M. WHELAN, MD
Associate Professor of Medicine, Division
of Pulmonary, Allergy, Critical Care, and
Sleep Medicine; Medical Director of Lung
Transplantation, Medical University of South
Carolina, Charleston, South Carolina

Contents

> Interstitial lung diseases (ILDs) encompass a wide range of diffuse pulmonary disor-
> ders, characterized by a variable degree of inflammatory and fibrotic changes of the
> alveolar wall and eventually the distal bronchiolar airspaces. ILDs may occur in iso-
> lation or in association with systemic diseases. The clinical evaluation of a patient
> with ILD includes a thorough medical history and detailed physical examination;
> obligatory diagnostic testing includes laboratory testing, chest radiography, and
> high-resolution computed tomography and comprehensive pulmonary function test-
> ing and blood gas analysis. To optimize the diagnostic yield, a dynamic interaction
> between the pulmonologist, radiologist, and pathologist is mandatory.

> Articles in the past have described the radiological appearances of different interstitial
> lung diseases (ILDs) in varying levels of detail. However, these articles have generally
> been written for radiologists with a background in basic chest computed tomography
> (CT) interpretation. This article summarizes a basic approach for diagnosing ILDs on
> high-resolution CT (HRCT) for the nonradiologist clinician and discusses the most
> common HRCT features of common ILDs.

> Interpretation of lung biopsy specimens is an integral part in the diagnosis of interstitial
> lung disease (ILD). The process of evaluating a surgical lung biopsy for disease involves
> answering several questions. Unlike much of surgical pathology of neoplastic lung dis-
> ease, arriving at the correct diagnosis in nonneoplastic lung disease often requires
> correlation with clinical and radiologic findings. The topic of ILD or diffuse infiltrative
> lung disease covers several hundred entities. This article is meant to be a launching
> point in the clinician's approach to the histologic evaluation of lung disease.

> In 2000, the American Thoracic Society and European Respiratory Society published
> the first consensus statement providing guidelines on the diagnosis and treatment of
> idiopathic pulmonary fibrosis (IPF). This statement presented, for the first time, diag-
> nostic criteria for IPF and recommendations for treatment. Results from several
> studies have reshaped the thinking on IPF, and as a result, the guidelines have
> been recently revised using an evidence-based approach. Meanwhile, several
> epidemiologic studies have yielded data that identify potential risk factors and
> that better define the societal burden of IPF. This article summarizes the approach
> to diagnosing IPF and reviews epidemiologic data on IPF.

tissue and spaces surrounding the alveoli. Patients affected by ILD usually present with shortness of breath or cough; for many, there is evidence of pulmonary restriction, decreased diffusion capacity, and radiographic appearance of alveolar and/or reticulonodular infiltrates. This article reviews the inherited ILDs, with a focus on the diseases that may be seen by pulmonologists caring for adult patients. The authors conclude by briefly discussing the utility of genetic testing in this population.

Traditionally, a subset of patients diagnosed as having idiopathic pulmonary fibrosis had positive results on cellular biopsies (prominent lymphoplasmacytic inflammation), bronchoalveolar lavage lymphocytosis, a clinical response to steroids, and a better long-term prognosis. On review of the lung histopathology, the lesion was characterized by varying degrees of inflammation and fibrosis. This entity is now recognized as a distinct entity among idiopathic interstitial pneumonias.

The connective tissue diseases (CTDs) are inflammatory, immune-mediated disorders in which interstitial lung disease (ILD) is common and clinically important. Interstitial lung disease may be the first manifestation of a CTD in a previously healthy patient. CTD-associated ILD frequently presents with the gradual onset of cough and dyspnea, although rarely may present with fulminant respiratory failure. Infection and drug reaction should always be ruled out. A diagnosis of idiopathic ILD should never be made without a careful search for subtle evidence of underlying CTD. Treatment of CTD-ILD typically includes corticosteroids and immunosuppressive agents.

Hypersensitivity pneumonitis (HP) is a complex syndrome caused by the inhalation of environmental antigens. Chronic HP may mimic other fibrotic lung diseases, such as idiopathic pulmonary fibrosis. Recognition of the antigen is important for diagnosis; avoidance of further exposure is critical for treatment. Fibrosis on biopsy or high-resolution computed tomography is a predictor of increased mortality. Additional research is needed to understand why the disease develops only in a minority of exposed individuals and why cases of chronic HP may progress without further antigen exposure.

Cigarette smoke, a toxic collection of thousands of chemicals generated from combustion of tobacco, is recognized as the primary causative agent of certain diffuse interstitial and bronchiolar lung diseases. Most patients afflicted with these disorders are cigarette smokers, and smoking cessation has been shown to be capable of inducing disease remission and should occupy a pivotal role in the management of all smokers with these diffuse lung diseases. The role of pharmacotherapy with corticosteroids or other immunomodulating agents is not well established but may be considered in patients with progressive forms of smoking-related interstitial lung diseases.

For selected parenchymal lung disease patients who fail to respond to medical therapy and demonstrate declines in function that place them at increased risk for mortality, lung transplantation should be considered. Lung transplantation remains a complex medical intervention that requires a dedicated recipient and medical team. Despite the challenges, lung transplantation affords appropriate patients a reasonable chance at increased survival and improved quality of life. Lung transplantation remains an appropriate therapeutic option for selected patients with parenchymal lung disease.

Clinics in Chest Medicine

RELATED INTEREST

Critical Care Clinics of North America, Volume 26, Issue 1 (January 2010)
Intensive Care of the Cancer Patient
Stephen M. Pastores, and Neil A. Halpern, *Guest Editors*

THE CLINICS ARE NOW AVAILABLE ONLINE!

Access your subscription at:
www.theclinics.com

Preface

The interstitial lung diseases (ILDs) are a large and heterogeneous group of disease entities that differ significantly with respect to presentation, cause, prevention, therapy, and prognosis. Many of them have no clear etiology. However, over the past 10 years, considerable progress has been made in our understanding of these entities. In this issue of *Clinics in Chest Medicine*, we discuss the most important of the ILDs and update the reader about their management.

Arriving at the correct diagnosis often requires correlation with clinical, radiologic, and pathologic findings. The diagnostic strategy that should be employed when faced with a patient with ILD is described. Given the important role of high-resolution computed tomography (HRCT) in the diagnosis of ILD, we introduce pulmonologists and clinicians to the imaging appearances of ILDs by providing a pattern approach to the evaluation of HRCT. In addition, a focused discussion of the HRCT findings in the common ILDs is presented. Although the frequency of lung biopsy is declining, histopathological assessment remains an integral part in the diagnosis of interstitial lung disease.

Idiopathic pulmonary fibrosis (IPF) is the most important of the idiopathic interstitial pneumonias. Over the past decade, our thinking about IPF has been reshaped and guidelines have been revised using an evidence-based approach. A number of epidemiologic studies have identified potential risk factors for IPF. We summarize the approach to diagnosing IPF and review its epidemiology. With improved understanding of IPF, we now recognize that there may also be distinct phenotypes among this group of patients. Further, we describe how the identification and management of comorbidities may improve the overall quality of life and well being of these patients. It has become clear that the clinical course of individual patients with IPF is highly variable and that the sudden deterioration of a patient's respiratory condition during a relatively stable course is not uncommon. This deterioration can result from well-known causes such as infection, pulmonary embolism, congestive heart failure, pneumothorax, or drugs. However, in many cases the etiology is not certain despite rigorous searches. These idiopathic episodes of rapid deterioration have been called acute exacerbation of IPF. The current state of our understanding of this important manifestation of IPF is discussed. Also, the mechanisms of action of potential IPF therapies are reviewed, with particular reference to current disease understanding and to highlight areas of IPF disease biology that afford attractive targets for the development of the new treatments. Given that no specific treatment exists for IPF, the general management of a patient with IPF is described, especially the management of important comorbidities (eg, pulmonary hypertension and gastroesophageal reflux) and symptoms (eg, dyspnea, exercise limitation, fatigue, anxiety, mood disturbance, sleep disorders) that dramatically affect IPF patients' lives. Furthermore, the increasingly important role of lung transplantation in the treatment of patients with ILD is discussed, especially the evidence suggesting that patients with pulmonary fibrosis undergoing lung transplantation have a favorable long-term survival compared with other disease indications.

Finally, several articles review important individual ILD entities, including inherited fibrotic lung diseases, nonspecific interstitial pneumonia, ILD associated with connective tissue diseases, chronic hypersensitivity pneumonitis, and smoking-related ILDs.

Talmadge E. King Jr, MD
Department of Medicine
University of California San Francisco
505 Parnassus Avenue, Box 0120
San Francisco, CA 94143-0120, USA

Harold R. Collard, MD
Division of Pulmonary and Critical Care Medicine
Department of Medicine
University of California San Franciscio
505 Parnassus Avenue
San Francisco, CA 94143, USA

Luca Richeldi, MD, PhD
Center for Rare Lung Diseases
Department of Oncology
Hematology and Respiratory Diseases
University Hospital Policlinico of Modena
Via del Pozzo 71, 41124 Modena, Italy

E-mail addresses:
tking@medicine.ucsf.edu (T.E. King)
Hal.Collard@ucsf.edu (H.R. Collard)
luca.richeldi@unimore.it (L. Richeldi)

Clin Chest Med 33 (2012) xiii
doi:10.1016/j.ccm.2012.01.005

Approach to the Diagnosis of Interstitial Lung Disease

Jürgen Behr, MD

KEYWORDS

- Interstitial lung disease • Idiopathic interstitial pneumonia
- Diagnosis

Interstitial lung diseases (ILDs) are a heterogeneous group of more than 150 disease entities that differ significantly with respect to prevention, therapy, and prognosis. The current classification scheme of ILDs is shown in **Fig. 1**.[1]

The diagnostic strategy in a patient with ILD is based on considerations regarding the dynamic time course (acute, subacute, chronic), the cause (known or unknown), and the context of the disease at presentation (presence of extrapulmonary/systemic disease manifestations). **Fig. 2** summarizes the main disease categories that have to be differentiated during the diagnostic process.[1–3]

Once an interstitial disease process has been recognized in a patient, there are 3 crucial questions that have to be addressed in the diagnostic workup:

1. Is there a discernible cause for the disease?
2. If no cause is identifiable, is it idiopathic pulmonary fibrosis (IPF)?
3. If there is no cause of the disease and if it is not IPF, should surgical lung biopsy be recommended?

After a diagnosis has been established, the severity and dynamics of the disease have to be assessed and monitored, with or without therapy. Diagnosis and disease severity/dynamics are fundamental for treatment decisions and to predict prognosis. The diagnostic approach to ILD may have to be adapted to different clinical scenarios that eventually lead to presentation of a patient:

1. Patient presents with clinical symptoms (eg, dry cough, dyspnea).
2. Patient is at risk of ILD due to known exposures (eg, amiodarone, asbestos).
3. Patient is at risk of ILD due to family history.
4. Patient is asymptomatic but presents with chance finding on chest radiography or computed tomography.
5. Patient is asymptomatic but presents with chance finding on pulmonary functioning test (eg, restrictive pattern, reduced gas transfer).

This article deals with diagnostic approaches suitable for patients presenting with clinical symptoms of ILD in the first place.

CLINICAL EVALUATION
History Taking

A comprehensive patient history taking is of crucial importance for the diagnosis of ILD. There are 4 main questions to be answered: (1) when did respiratory symptoms start, (2) how did the disease develop over time to the present, (3) are there or have there been any exposures to

Disclosures: J.B. has received fees for speaking from Actelion, Altana, Bayer-Schering, Boehringer-Ingelheim, GSK, InterMune, PARI Pharma, Pfizer, Lilly, Novartis, and Nycomed. He has served as consultant/advisor for Actelion, Bayer-Schering-Pharma, InterMune, Lilly, PARI Pharma, Gilead, GSK, and Pfizer. J.B. has received research grants from Actelion, Bayer-Schering, BMBF, DFG, LMU, and PARI Pharma.
Department of Internal Medicine III, University Hospital Bergmannsheil, Ruhr-University Bochum, Buerkle-de-la-Camp Platz 1, 44789 Bochum, Germany
E-mail address: juergen.behr@bergmannsheil.de

Clin Chest Med 33 (2012) 1–10
doi:10.1016/j.ccm.2011.12.002
0272-5231/12/$ – see front matter

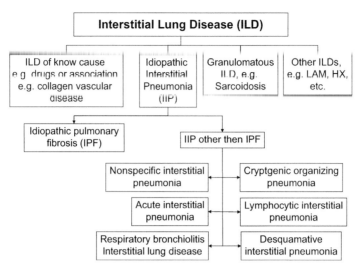

Fig. 1. Classification of ILDs. HX, histiocytosis X; LAM, lymphangiomyomatosis. (*Adopted from* American Thoracic Society/European Respiratory Society international multidisciplinary consensus classification of the idiopathic interstitial pneumonias. Am J Respir Crit Care Med 2002;165:279; with permission.)

etiologic agents known to cause ILD, and (4) what is the severity of symptoms at presentation.[1]

The disease chronology can be subdivided into 4 categories: (1) acute, days up to a few weeks; (2) subacute, 4 to 12 weeks; (3) chronic, longer than 12 weeks; and (4) episodic, ie, symptomatic phases that are followed by asymptomatic phases. In addition, all available radiographs of the lung should be reviewed to characterize the nature and development of the radiologic pattern. Flitting opacities on chest imaging studies may drive the differential diagnosis to focus on eosinophilic pneumonia,

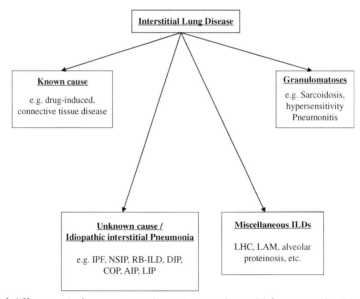

Fig. 2. Overview of different ILD disease categories. AIP, acute interstitial pneumonia; COP, cryptogenic organizing pneumonia; DIP, desquamative interstitial pneumonia; IPF, idiopathic pulmonary fibrosis; LAM, lymphangioleiomyomatosis; LCH, Langerhans cell histiocytosis; LIP, lymphoid interstitial pneumonia; NSIP, nonspecific interstitial pneumonia; RB-ILD, respiratory bronchiolitis and interstitial lung disease. (*Data from* American Thoracic Society/European Respiratory Society international multidisciplinary consensus classification of the idiopathic interstitial pneumonias. Am J Respir Crit Care Med 2002;165:279; with permission.)

hypersensitivity pneumonitis (HP), vasculitis, or organizing pneumonia.[1,3,4]

Assessment of Symptoms

Dyspnea with exertion or at rest is the predominant symptom in most ILDs.[5,6] It is of importance to accurately assess the degree of exercise limitation and dyspnea in a reproducible manner by asking specific questions: after what distance, after how many steps, or after how many stairs or floors does dyspnea occur and for how long has the patient experienced this degree of dyspnea and how fast did it develop or when was the most recent change. The degree of dyspnea is linked to disease severity and prognosis.[5] It is also necessary to exclude nonrespiratory symptoms as a cause of the exercise limitation, for example, joint pains, muscle pains, or weakness.

Cough is the second most frequent symptom in patients with ILD and sometimes becomes really bothersome. Although a dry cough is common in IPF, cough is generally an airway symptom and therefore more indicative of airway-centered diseases such as sarcoidosis, HP, or organizing pneumonia. Increased secretions from ILD-associated bronchitis or bronchiectasis cause productive cough. Wheeze is another airway-associated symptom that is infrequent in ILD but may occur in certain entities such as Churg-Strauss syndrome, HP (eg, pigeon breeder's lung), or airway-stenotic sarcoidosis.[7]

Pleural pain and effusion in the context of an ILD indicate connective tissue disease (eg, systemic lupus erythematosus or rheumatoid arthritis) or drug-induced or asbestos-related disease. Differential diagnoses include complications such as infections or pulmonary embolism. Hemoptysis is always an alarming signal and may indicate manifestation of pulmonary hemorrhagic syndromes, for example, Goodpasture syndrome or granulomatosis with polyangiitis (GPA, previously called Wegener disease). Alternatively, infections, lung cancer, or pulmonary embolism have to be considered.[3] Gastroesophageal reflux is another common symptom in patients with ILD that is suspected of causing or at least exacerbating ILD. A history of acid reflux should, therefore, be taken in all patients with ILD.[8]

Extrapulmonary features of associated diseases may provide important hints to the correct diagnosis. Therefore, joint pain and swelling (rheumatoid arthritis), cutaneous thickening, Raynaud phenomenon and dysphagia (systemic sclerosis), oculocutaneous albinism and colitis (Hermansky-Pudlak syndrome), chronic granulomatous sinusitis (GPA and Churg-Strauss syndrome), renal failure

(Goodpasture syndrome), renal angiomyolipoma (lymphangioleiomyomatosis), and Crohn disease should be carefully asked and sought for.[2,3,7]

Next Step is a Comprehensive Investigation of Possible Causes for ILDs

Causative agents

A comprehensive history taking of all respiratory risk factors and exposures in the past and present is of utmost importance. Because history taking is a very complex and time-consuming task, it is often helpful to use a standardized questionnaire, as that available from the American College of Chest Physicians.[9] The following items have to be checked: (1) smoking history, (2) hobbies, (3) travel, (4) occupations, and (5) drug history and treatments (eg, radiation therapy).[3,10,11] Of special interest in this context is the family history as it becomes more and more clear that a considerable subset of patients and diseases do have hereditary traits.[2,3,12]

Comorbid diseases

There are several diseases that mimic or that are associated with ILDs: (1) Infectious agents such as mycobacteria, cytomegalovirus, *Pneumocystis jiroveci*, and human immunodeficiency virus (HIV) and parasite infestations are able to cause an ILD-like condition. (2) Connective tissue diseases are frequently associated with ILDs. This is especially the case for systemic sclerosis and rheumatoid arthritis. (3) Vasculitides, for example, GPA, Churg-Strauss syndrome, and microscopic polyangiitis, are able to manifest in the lungs as ILD.[3,7]

PHYSICAL EXAMINATION

On physical examination, inspection of the integument may reveal valuable findings: skin thickening and acral necrosis (scleroderma), oculocutaneous albinism (Hermansky-Pudlak syndrome), clubbing (up to 40% in all ILDs, up to 66% in IPF), livedo racemosa (systemic lupus erythematosus), cutaneous vasculitis (Churg-Strauss syndrome), and edematous-cyanotic skin (dermatomyositis, "disease lilac").[2,3,7] Palpation may reveal lymphadenopathy, hepatosplenomegaly pointing at sarcoidosis, HIV infection, or connective tissue disease.

On auscultation of the lungs, symmetric fine "Velcro-like" inspiratory crackles are found in more than 90% of patients with IPF and in about 60% of patients with connective tissue disease–associated ILD. Crackles are less frequent in HP and rare in sarcoidosis. Wheezing and inspiratory squeaks reflect bronchiolitis and/or bronchial obstruction and are associated with

Churg-Strauss syndrome, HP, and rarely nonspecific interstitial pneumonia.[1-3] Cyanosis may be present and should be confirmed by pulse oximetry, which can be easily performed in clinic.[2,3,7]

LABORATORY TESTING

There are no specific laboratory tests that allow for the diagnosis of an ILD, but, in an appropriate clinical setting, laboratory test results may be strongly supportive of a specific diagnosis. Routine laboratory testing should include a complete blood cell count; leukocyte differential; platelet count; erythrocyte sedimentation rate; determination of serum electrolyte levels, including calcium, serum urea nitrogen, and creatinine; liver function tests; and urinary sediment.[7] These laboratory values allow the exclusion or suggestion of an associated hematologic, liver, or kidney disease in a potential context of systemic disease (eg, sarcoidosis, vasculitis, amyloidosis), malignancy (eg, lymphoma), or infection (eg, tuberculosis, HIV). To further evaluate the presence of connective tissue disease, systemic disease (eg, sarcoidosis,

connective tissue disease) or HP additional measures may be appropriate as summarized in **Table 1**

There have been multiple attempts to find biomarkers to monitor disease activity or to predict prognosis in different ILDs. Intraindividual changes of serum angiotensin-converting enzyme activity or of serum concentration of the soluble interleukin 2 receptor are to some extent helpful in monitoring disease activity in sarcoidosis.[13] The serum lactate dehydrogenase activity is to some extent predictive of prognosis in IPF. Limited data are available for serum levels of Krebs von der Lungen 6, a high-molecular-weight glycoprotein representing human MUC1 mucin, surfactant proteins A and D, matrix metalloproteinases, and CCL-18.[3,14] However, none of these biomarkers have been validated sufficiently to be recommended for the routine use in the monitoring and follow-up of patients with ILD.

PULMONARY FUNCTION TESTING

Patients with ILD should undergo comprehensive pulmonary function testing, which includes arterial

Table 1
Useful laboratory tests for patients with ILD, beyond routine laboratory testing

Laboratory Test	Indication	Interpretation
ANA; rheumatoid factor; ANA differentiation, including Jo-1 or ScL-70 antibodies	Suspected CTD or idiopathic ILD for which CTD cannot be excluded	Low titers occur in up to 20% of patients with IPF, high titers suggest underlying CTD
Creatine kinase activity, myoglobin, aldolase	Suspected myositis	Elevated values support a diagnosis of dermatomyositis
Immunoglobulins	Suspicion of immunodeficiency	Decreased serum immunoglobulins suggest common variable immunodeficiency syndrome or LIP
c-ANCA, p-ANCA	Suspected vasculitis	c-ANCA suggestive of GPA (Wegener syndrome), microscopic polyangiitis p-ANCA suggestive of CSS or MPA
Antiglomerular basement membrane antibody	Hemoptysis due to DAH, renal failure	Positive result is diagnostic of Goodpasture syndrome
Serum angiotensin-converting enzyme activity, serum-soluble interleukin 2 receptor	Sarcoidosis	Low sensitivity and specificity
Specific serum IgG antibodies	Exposure to antigens that cause HP	Valid only within an appropriate clinical context

Abbreviations: ANA, antinuclear antibody; c-ANCA, cytoplasmic antineutrophil cytoplasmic antibody (antiproteinase 3); CSS, Churg-Strauss syndrome; CTD, connective tissue disease; DAH, diffuse alveolar hemorrhage; LIP, lymphocytic interstitial pneumonia; MPA, microscopic polyangiitis; p-ANCA, perinuclear antineutrophil cytoplasmic antibody (antimyeloperoxidase).

or capillary blood gas analysis at rest and eventually under exertion, spirometry and body plethysmography, as well as measurement of the diffusion capacity using carbon monoxide as a tracer in the single-breath method (DLco).[1,3,4,15] In addition, measurement of compliance may be helpful in objectifying the elevated stiffness of the lung.[15] Pulmonary function tests are in general not able to support a specific ILD diagnosis, but they are necessary to assess the respiratory limitations and to monitor the disease during follow-up.[2,3]

Lung function abnormalities generally reflect the effects of interstitial inflammation and scarring resulting in a restrictive ventilatory deficit and impaired gas exchange as well as reduced compliance. Airway obstruction and emphysema are not features of ILD, however, may be present when bronchial asthma or chronic obstructive pulmonary disease coexist in the patient. Moreover, some diseases such as lymphangioleiomyomatosis, Langerhans cell histiocytosis, sarcoidosis, and HP may present with airway obstruction and/or hyperinflation as part of the underlying disease process or associated bronchiolitis.[3,7] A disproportionate decrease of the DLco in comparison with the restrictive ventilatory deficit should prompt suspicion of emphysema or pulmonary hypertension (PH).[16]

During follow-up, changes in lung function parameters are widely used and helpful for disease monitoring.[2,3,15] Especially in IPF, a small decrease of only 5% to 10% of forced vital capacity during an observation period of 6 months is already indicative of increased mortality.[17] Less well established are changes of DLco and blood gases as prognostic predictors, but these parameters may well be used to support the clinical relevance of marginal changes in forced vital capacity. Calculated lung function indices may also be helpful to objectify the course and prognosis of the disease. The composite physiologic index (CPI) is such a calculated index that reflects the extent of fibrosis on high-resolution computed tomography (HRCT) and corrects for coexisting emphysema.[18] An increase in CPI indicates progression of fibrosis and is associated with increased mortality.[18–20]

RADIOLOGIC ASSESSMENT

An abnormal chest radiograph is often the initial finding in patients with ILD. A diffuse reticulonodular pattern, ground-glass opacities, or both are the most common findings on a chest radiograph in patients with ILD. The pattern and distribution of radiologic appearances contribute to initial diagnostic considerations as summarized in **Table 2**.[1–3,7]

For a more subtle diagnosis, HRCT is the key diagnostic procedure and is sufficient for diagnosis in a significant number of patients with IPF.[2] The criteria that aid in making a confident diagnosis of IPF are presented in **Table 3**.[3] HRCT findings suggestive of an alternative diagnosis other than IPF are shown in **Tables 4** and **5**.

Interpretation of chest radiographs and HRCTs should always include a complete review of all images available for a specific patient and should be done in direct communication between the pulmonologist and the radiologist to optimize the diagnostic yield.

BRONCHOSCOPY

In patients with ILD, bronchoscopy can be performed to obtain materials for microbiological, cytologic, and histologic analyses. The applied techniques encompass bronchoalveolar lavage (BAL), transbronchial lung biopsy (TBLB), and transbronchial needle aspiration (TBNA) for cytologic or histologic (Wang needle) analyses. However, bronchoscopy is associated with some morbidity and even a very low rate of mortality and therefore is not an obligatory diagnostic procedure for all patients with ILD.[2,3] Moreover, to make bronchoscopy and BAL/TBLB a valuable tool in the workup of patients with ILD, each clinical site must establish routine methods for handling and analysis of the materials.[2] Best use of this BAL/TBLB requires that the clinician identify very clear questions that are to be addressed with the biological materials obtained and that it is reasonable these questions can be answered with these materials before the procedure is performed. If these obligatory prerequisites are fulfilled, bronchoscopy and BAL with or without TBLB are valuable tools in the diagnostic workup of patients with ILD.[21]

With the use of BAL, TBLB, and/or TBNA (eventually endobronchial ultrasonography guided), a diagnosis of sarcoidosis, lymphangitis carcinomatosa, eosinophilic pneumonia, alveolar proteinosis, Langerhans cell histiocytosis, lymphoid interstitial pneumonia, and several bacterial, viral, and fungal infections can be confirmed, thus avoiding more invasive procedures such as mediastinoscopy, video-assisted thoracoscopic (VATS) biopsy, or open surgical lung biopsy. In several patients with probable or possible IPF, bronchoscopic techniques may be used to rule out alternative diagnoses, such as HP in selected patients,[21] especially if VATS biopsy seems too risky or has to be performed in elderly patients.

Table 2
Diagnostic considerations based on a chest radiograph

Low lung volumes	IPF; CTD-related ILD; chronic HP; asbestosis; chronic drug-induced fibrosis; chronic COP, CEP, or DIP
Preserved/increased lung volumes	RB-ILD, IPF plus emphysema, LCH, LAM, sarcoidosis, tuberous sclerosis, neurofibromatosis, bronchiolitis
Upper zone predominance	Sarcoidosis, silicosis, coal workers' pneumoconiosis, HP, LCH, berylliosis, CEP, Caplan syndrome, nodular rheumatoid arthritis
Lower zone predominance	IPF, CTD-associated ILD, asbestosis, DIP, chronic HP
Peripheral predominance	IPF, COP, CEP
Micronodular	Infection, sarcoidosis, HP, malignancy
Septa thickening	Malignancy, chronic left heart failure, infection, pulmonary veno-occlusive disease
Honeycombing	IPF, asbestosis, CTD-associated ILD, chronic HP, sarcoidosis
Migratory opacities	Löffler disease, COP, HP, ABPA
Kerley B lines	Chronic left heart failure, lymphangitic carcinomatosa
Pleural disease	CTD-associated ILD, asbestosis, malignancy, radiation-induced ILD, sarcoidosis
Pneumothorax	LCH, LAM, tuberous sclerosis, neurofibromatosis
Mediastinal/hilar lymphadenopathy	Sarcoidosis, malignancy, silicosis, berylliosis, CTD-associated ILD, infection
Normal (about 10%)	HP, NSIP, CTD-associated ILD, RB-ILD, bronchiolitis, sarcoidosis

Abbreviations: ABPA, allergic bronchopulmonary aspergillosis; CEP, chronic eosinophilic pneumonia; COP, cryptogenic organizing pneumonia; CTD, connective tissue disease; DIP, desquamative interstitial pneumonia; LAM, lymphangioleiomyomatosis; LCH, Langerhans cell histiocytosis; NSIP, nonspecific interstitial pneumonia; RB-ILD, respiratory bronchiolitis and ILD.

Table 3
Criteria diagnostic for IPF

UIP Pattern (All 4 Features)	Possible UIP Pattern (All 3 Features)	Inconsistent with UIP Pattern (Any of the 7 Features)
• Subpleural basal predominance • Reticular abnormality • Honeycombing with or without traction bronchiectasis • Absence of features listed as inconsistent with UIP pattern (see third column)	• Subpleural basal predominance • Reticular abnormality • Absence of features listed as inconsistent with UIP pattern (see third column)	• Upper lung or midlung predominance • Peribronchovascular predominance • Extensive ground-glass abnormality (extent>reticular abnormality) • Profuse micronodules (bilateral, predominantly upper lobes) • Discrete cysts (multiple, bilateral, away from areas of honeycombing) • Diffuse mosaic attenuation/air trapping (bilateral, in ≥3 lobes) • Consolidation in bronchopulmonary segments/lobes

From Raghu G, Collard HR, Egan JJ, et al. An Official ATS/ERS/JRS/ALAT statement: idiopathic pulmonary fibrosis: evidence-based guidelines for diagnosis and management. Am J Respir Crit Care Med 2011;183:794; with permission.

Table 4
HRCT findings suggesting specific alternative diagnoses other than IPF

HRCT Features Atypical for IPF	Probable Diagnosis
Centrilobular nodules, air trapping, ground-glass opacities, relative sparing of bases	HP
Pleural effusion, pleural thickening, esophageal dilation	Collagen vascular disease
Pleural plaques, pleural thickening	Asbestosis
Focal abnormality	Localized scar

However, especially in patients with IPF, bronchoscopy and BAL have the potential of triggering acute exacerbation of IPF, so that the indication for bronchoscopic evaluation should be discussed critically in every individual patient.[2]

SURGICAL LUNG BIOPSY

Surgical lung biopsy, nowadays preferentially performed during VATS, is the most invasive diagnostic procedure used for diagnosis of ILD. It is associated with significant morbidity and mortality and should be reserved for those patients in whom the management and treatment could change depending on the result of biopsy.[2,3,22,23] In IPF, histologic analysis from a surgical lung biopsy is no longer the gold standard of diagnosis because it has become clear that because of sampling error and uniformity of disease pattern in patients with advanced disease, histologic examination will not provide the diagnostic clue in many patients.[2]

Consequently, in IPF, the multidisciplinary discussion (MDD) involving the pulmonologist, radiologist, and pathologist has become the gold standard for diagnosis. This also seems the appropriate approach to diagnosis for the vast majority of patients with ILD. Because IPF is one if not the most important differential diagnosis in most patients with ILD, an MDD seems to be the most promising approach to reach a confident diagnosis.[2,24]

ASSESSMENT OF PH

PH is frequently associated with ILD. Among patients with advanced disease on the waiting list for lung transplantation, 40% to 80% have PH. In patients with less-advanced disease, still 10% have significant PH. Moreover, PH in ILD is clinically relevant because it is associated with an excess exercise intolerance and mortality. Consequently, this condition is of clinical relevance

Table 5
Diagnostic considerations based on HRCT patterns

Specific Computed Tomographic Findings	Entity
Cysts	Langerhans cell histiocytosis Lymphangioleiomyomatosis Lymphoid interstitial pneumonia Birt-Hogg-Dube syndrome
Perilymphatic nodules	Sarcoidosis Chronic beryllium disease Lymphangitic carcinoma Lymphoma
Centrilobular nodules	HP Respiratory bronchiolitis
Tree-in-bud pattern	Infection Aspiration Other forms of bronchiolitis
Mosaic attenuation	HP Obliterative bronchiolitis Pulmonary thromboembolism

for the general management of patients with ILD to diagnose PH, even though no targeted therapy is yet approved for this condition. In patients with ILD, the diagnosis of associated PH may avoid overtreatment with immunosuppressive agents and provide early indication for the initiation of long-term oxygen therapy or listing for lung transplantation. In addition, identification of PH may support the diagnosis of other treatable conditions, such as left heart disease.[16,25]

To find PH in patients with ILD, clinical symptoms are rather unspecific. Lung function showing a disproportionate reduction in DLco and very low oxygen partial pressures in arterial or capillary blood at rest and/or during mild exercise may indicate the presence of PH. Doppler echocardiography is suitable as a screening tool to support a clinical suspicion of PH, but about one-third of the patients will have a technically insufficient result. Brain natriuretic peptide may be used as a biomarker but is per se not sufficient to prove or exclude PH.[16,25–27] In patients with signs and symptoms of PH associated with ILD, in whom a therapeutic consequence is feasible, a right

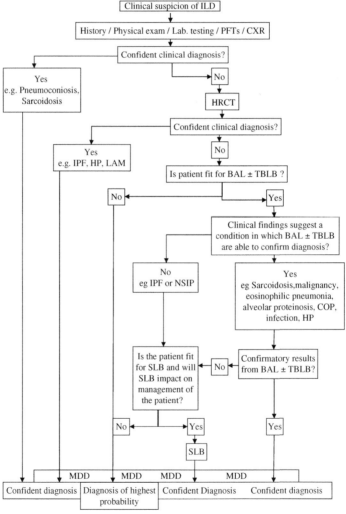

Fig. 3. Algorithm for the diagnosis of ILD. COP, cryptogenic organizing pneumonia; CXR, chest radiography; HP, hypersensitivity pneumonitis; LAM, lymphangioleiomyomatosis; MDD, multidisciplinary discussion; NSIP, nonspecific interstitial pneumonia; PFT, pulmonary function testing; SLB, surgical lung biopsy. (*Data from* Raghu G, Mageto YN, Lockhart D, et al. The accuracy of the clinical diagnosis of new-onset idiopathic pulmonary fibrosis and other interstitial lung disease: a prospective study. Chest 1999;116:1168–74; with permission; and Bradley B, Branley HM, Egan JJ, et al. British Thoracic Society Interstitial Lung Disease Guideline Group, British Thoracic Society Standard of Care Committee; Thoracic Society of Australia; New Zealand Thoracic Society; Irish Thoracic Society. Interstitial lung disease guideline. Thorax 2008;63(Suppl 5):v57.)

Table 6
Characterization of different disease patterns as a guide to treatment approach and monitoring strategy

Pattern of Disease	Broad Treatment Approach	Monitoring Strategy
Self-limited inflammation	Remove cause/observe or treat (usually with steroid therapy) in short term	Short-term monitoring to confirm disease regression
Major inflammation with risk of progression to fibrosis	Antiinflammatory therapy (eventually high dose) for a response, then rationalize lower-dose therapy to maintain response	Monitor in short term to quantify the response to high-dose treatment. Monitor less frequently in long term to ensure that gains are preserved
Stable fibrosis	Observation alone (in treatment-naive patients, a treatment trial may be considered)	Long-term monitoring to ensure ongoing stability
Progressive fibrosis with stabilization realistic	Treat with steroid or immunosuppressive therapy, high dose if necessary to stabilize; consider antifibrotic drugs	Long-term monitoring to confirm absence of progression
Inexorably progressive fibrosis	Consider therapy to slow progression but avoid toxic agents	Long-term monitoring to quantify rapidity of progression with a view to transplant or for effective palliation

Data from Wells AU. Diffuse parenchymal lung disease: an introduction. In: Warrell DA, Cox TM, Firth JD, editors. Oxford textbook of medicine. Vol 2. 5th edition. Oxford (United Kingdom): Oxford University Press; 2010. p. 3365–75.

heart catheterization should be performed to make a firm diagnosis of PH and to differentiate precapillary and postcapillary PH.[16] Right heart catheterization may prompt the performance of left heart catheterization and coronary angiography in addition to show or rule out treatable left heart disease.

DIAGNOSTIC ALGORITHM

A diagnostic algorithm for patients with ILD is shown in **Fig. 3**. After differentiating ILDs with known causes from those with unknown causes, HRCT is the crucial diagnostic procedure that loads to a final diagnosis, for example, IPF, or that prompts further diagnostic steps, which eventually include bronchoscopic techniques such as BAL and TBLB or VATS lung biopsy. The evolution of the prognostic process may vary depending on the clinical presentation or setting, that is, symptomatic patients or asymptomatic patients with risk factors for ILD or chance findings of ILD. In all cases, a multidisciplinary discussion involving pulmonologists, radiologists, and pathologists should be used to establish a confident diagnosis.[2]

CLASSIFICATION OF DISEASE BEHAVIOR

In addition to a diagnosis based on nosology, it is of critical importance to also stratify a particular patient with ILD according to the disease behavior, which may have a more profound impact on management and therapy of an individual patient than the specific ILD diagnosis by itself. In **Table 0**, a classification scheme for the disease behavior is proposed that will guide the choice of treatment options. Obviously, there is an interaction between the underlying diagnosis and the prevalence of one or another pattern of disease behavior. Nonetheless, it seems very helpful to select the broad treatment approach in an individual patient by applying the patterns of disease behavior characterized in **Table 6**.

REFERENCES

1. American Thoracic Society/European Respiratory Society international multidisciplinary consensus classification of the idiopathic interstitial pneumonias. Am J Respir Crit Care Med 2002;165: 277–304.

2. Raghu G, Collard HR, Egan JJ, et al. An official ATS/ERS/JRS/ALAT statement: idiopathic pulmonary fibrosis: evidence-based guidelines for diagnosis and management. Am J Respir Crit Care Med 2011;183:788–824.

3. Bradley B, Branley HM, Egan JJ, et al. British Thoracic Society Interstitial Lung Disease Guideline Group, British Thoracic Society Standard of Care Committee; Thoracic Society of Australia; New Zealand Thoracic Society; Irish Thoracic Society. Interstitial lung disease guideline. Thorax 2008; 63(Suppl 5):v1–58.

4. Raghu G, Mageto YN, Lockhart D, et al. The accuracy of the clinical diagnosis of new-onset idiopathic pulmonary fibrosis and other interstitial lung disease: a prospective study. Chest 1999;116: 1168–74.

5. King TE Jr, Tooze JA, Schwarz MI, et al. Predicting survival in idiopathic pulmonary fibrosis: scoring system and survival model. Am J Respir Crit Care Med 2001;164:1171–81.

6. Gribbin J, Hubbard RB, Le Jeune I, et al. Incidence and mortality of idiopathic pulmonary fibrosis and sarcoidosis in the UK. Thorax 2006;61:980–5.

7. Yang S, Raghu G. Clinical evaluation. In: Costabel U, duBois RM, Egan MM, editors. Diffuse parenchymal lung disease. Basel (Switzerland): Karger; 2007. p. 22–8.

8. Raghu G, Freudenberger TD, Yang S, et al. High prevalence of abnormal acid gastro-oesophageal reflux in idiopathic pulmonary fibrosis. Eur Respir J 2006;27:136–42.

9. Diffuse Lung Disease Questionnaire for Patients. Available at: www.chestnet.org/accp/patient-guides/interstitial-diffuse-lung-disease-questionnaire-accp-members.

10. Cooper JA Jr, White DA, Matthay RA. Drug-induced pulmonary disease. Part 1: cytotoxic drugs. Am Rev Respir Dis 1986;133:321–40.

11. Cooper JA Jr, White DA, Matthay RA. Drug-induced pulmonary disease. Part 2: noncytotoxic drugs. Am Rev Respir Dis 1986;133:488–505.

12. Steele MP, Speer MC, Loyd JE, et al. Clinical and pathologic features of familial interstitial pneumonia. Am J Respir Crit Care Med 2005;172:1146–52.

13. Costabel U, Hunninghake GW. ATS/ERS/WASOG statement on sarcoidosis. Sarcoidosis Statement Committee. American Thoracic Society. European Respiratory Society. World Association for Sarcoidosis and Other Granulomatous Disorders. Eur Respir J 1999;14:735–7.

14. Prasse A, Probst C, Bargagli E, et al. Serum CC-chemokine ligand 18 concentration predicts outcome in idiopathic pulmonary fibrosis. Am J Respir Crit Care Med 2009;179:717–23.

15. Behr J, Furst DE. Pulmonary function tests. Rheumatology 2008;47(Suppl 5):v65–7.

16. Hoeper MM, Andreas S, Bastian A, et al. Pulmonary hypertension due to chronic lung disease. Recommendations of the Cologne Consensus Conference 2010. Dtsch Med Wochenschr 2010;135(Suppl 3): S115–24 [in German].

17. Zappala CJ, Latsi PI, Nicholson AG, et al. Marginal decline in forced vital capacity is associated with a poor outcome in idiopathic pulmonary fibrosis. Eur Respir J 2010;35:830–5.

18. Wells AU, Desai SR, Rubens MB, et al. Idiopathic pulmonary fibrosis: a composite physiologic index derived from disease extent observed by computed tomography. Am J Respir Crit Care Med 2003;167: 962–9.

19. Latsi PI, du Bois RM, Nicholson AG, et al. Fibrotic idiopathic interstitial pneumonia: the prognostic value of longitudinal functional trends. Am J Respir Crit Care Med 2003;168:531–7.

20. Behr J, Demedts M, Buhl R, et al, IFIGENIA study group. Lung function in idiopathic pulmonary fibrosis—extended analyses of the IFIGENIA trial. Respir Res 2009;10:101.

21. Ohshimo S, Bonella F, Cui A, et al. Significance of bronchoalveolar lavage for the diagnosis of idiopathic pulmonary fibrosis. Am J Respir Crit Care Med 2009;179:1043–7.

22. Chechani V, Landreneau RJ, Shaikh SS. Open lung biopsy for diffuse infiltrative lung disease. Ann Thorac Surg 1992;54:296–300.

23. Kreider M, Hansen-Flaschen J, Ahmad N, et al. Complications of video-assisted thoracoscopic lung biopsy in patients with interstitial lung disease. Ann Thorac Surg 2007;83(3):1140–4.

24. Flaherty KR, King TE Jr, Raghu G, et al. Idiopathic interstitial pneumonia: what is the effect of a multidisciplinary approach to diagnosis? Am J Respir Crit Care Med 2004;170:904–10.

25. Galiè N, Hoeper MM, Humbert M, et al. Guidelines for the diagnosis and treatment of pulmonary hypertension. The Task Force for the Diagnosis and Treatment of Pulmonary Hypertension of the European Society of Cardiology (ESC) and the European Respiratory Society (ERS), endorsed by the International Society of Heart and Lung Transplantation (ISHLT). Eur Respir J 2009;34:1219–63.

26. Leuchte HH, Neurohr C, Baumgartner R, et al. Brain natriuretic peptide and exercise capacity in lung fibrosis and pulmonary hypertension. Am J Respir Crit Care Med 2004;170:360–5.

27. Leuchte HH, Baumgartner RA, Nounou ME, et al. Brain natriuretic peptide is a prognostic parameter in chronic lung disease. Am J Respir Crit Care Med 2006;173:744–50.

Radiological Approach to Interstitial Lung Disease: A Guide for the Nonradiologist

Hamza Jawad, MD[a], Jonathan H. Chung, MD[a],
David A. Lynch, MD[a], John D. Newell Jr, MD[b],*

KEYWORDS

- Interstitial lung disease
- High-resolution computed tomography • Nonradiologist

The term interstitial lung disease (ILD) comprises more than 200 separate disease entities, each having its separate and often unique radiological manifestations. Because the clinical presentation of most of these diseases is similar (dyspnea and cough) high-resolution computed tomography (HRCT) becomes a valuable tool in narrowing the differential diagnosis. The importance of HRCT is further underlined by the fact that there is no gold-standard diagnostic test for ILD; rather, a multidisciplinary approach, with integration of radiological, pathologic, and clinical data, is generally the best approach.

Multiple studies have described the HRCT patterns of specific ILDs; however, these have generally been written for the radiologist who already has a strong background in imaging. The purpose of this review is to introduce pulmonologists and clinicians to the imaging appearances of ILDs on HRCT, using a pattern approach in addition to focused discussion of the common ILDs.

BASIC ARCHITECTURE OF THE LUNG INTERSTITIUM

The lung interstitium is made up of 3 components, as described originally by Weibel[1]; these include the axial interstitium, the peripheral interstitium, and the septal interstitium. The axial interstitium is the connective tissue surrounding bronchovascular bundles as they emerge from the pulmonary hila and extend peripherally to the level of respiratory bronchioles. The septal interstitium consists of a fine network of connective tissue inside the secondary pulmonary lobule that supports the structure of the entire lobule. The peripheral interstitium originates from the undersurface of the visceral pleura, extending into the lung parenchyma; the venules and lymphatics that drain the visceral pleura and peripheral parts of the lung traverse the peripheral interstitium.

Lung tissue has a limited and predictable response to injury; therefore, a variety of disease processes may lead to similar alterations in the pulmonary anatomy, resulting in overlapping imaging findings. The pattern and distribution of these lung findings are what may suggest a specific diagnosis.

APPROACH TO HRCT

Having an organized approach is essential for efficient and accurate interpretation of HRCT studies. An example of this approach is a sequential analysis of the airways (the main bronchi as well as the smaller bronchioles), followed by the lung parenchyma (with separate attention to each lobe), the pleura itself, and the mediastinum. Each finding should be further described concerning size, shape, location within the lungs, and relationship to any normal surrounding structures. This approach is a sample approach describing the

[a] Division of Radiology, National Jewish Health, 1400 Jackson Street, Denver, CO 80206, USA
[b] Department of Radiology, University of Iowa, 200 Hawkins Drive, CC701GH, Iowa City, IA 52242, USA
* Corresponding author.
E-mail address: john-newell@uiowa.edu

Clin Chest Med 33 (2012) 11–26
doi:10.1016/j.ccm.2012.01.002
0272-5231/12/$ – see front matter © 2012 Elsevier Inc. All rights reserved.

components that need to be addressed and can be tailored and reorganized according to one's own style.

Lung parenchymal abnormalities can be grossly divided into those with increased attenuation or decreased attenuation. It is important to take note of both lobar and individual lung volumes because as a general trend (not absolute) the lung volumes are increased with processes that produce decreased attenuation, like air trapping and emphysema, and are decreased with processes that produce reticulations and honeycombing. The most common abnormal findings seen on HRCT are described later.

INCREASED ATTENUATION
Reticulation/Reticular Opacities

Reticulation refers to a netlike pattern. This pattern is most commonly the result of thickened interlobular and intralobular septa, connecting and interbridging with one another at different angles. On HRCT, this pattern is most frequently seen in the peripheral and basal lung zones (**Fig. 1**). The diseases that can cause this pattern are summarized in **Table 1**.

Ground-glass Pattern

Ground-glass opacities are defined as areas of increased attenuation that are not dense enough to obscure the underlying bronchovascular markings (**Fig. 2**). A wide variety of pathologic mechanisms can give rise to a ground-glass pattern on HRCT, including airspace disease, alveolar collapse, interstitial thickening, and increased vascularity of the alveoli.[2] In cases of pulmonary fibrosis, ground-glass opacity can also represent very fine interstitial fibrosis beyond the spatial resolution of the scan obtained. The common ILDs that can

present with ground-glass opacities on HRCT are summarized in **Table 1**.

Ground-glass opacities often signify a reversible disease process. However, about one-third of these cases may be associated with fibrosis. In the absence of any signs of fibrosis such as traction bronchiectasis and honeycombing, ground-glass opacity should be presumed to represent a reversible disease process.[3]

Consolidation

Consolidation appears as an area of increased attenuation, but it can be differentiated from ground-glass opacities by the inability to visualize bronchovascular markings in the affected areas. Air bronchograms are a common finding because of the resultant interface between the consolidated (high attenuation) lung parenchyma and the air-filled airways (low attenuation). This situation typically results from filling of the airspaces with fluid such as edema, blood, or pus. A large list of ILDs that can produce consolidation on HRCT is summarized in **Table 1**.

Nodules

Nodules are focal areas of increased attenuation, usually with discrete borders. They can vary in size from a few millimeters to up to 3 cm. Greater than 3 cm is referred to as a mass. Once shown on computed tomography (CT), they need to be further analyzed with respect to their size, density, borders, number, and location. The initial approach should focus on categorizing them into 1 of 3 categories (based on their relation with the secondary pulmonary lobule): centrilobular, perilymphatic, and random (**Table 2**).

Centrilobular nodules are characterized by their central location in the secondary pulmonary lobules; their base of origin can be either the pulmonary artery or the bronchiole, both of which traverse the center of the secondary pulmonary lobule. On HRCT, the features that can help in their recognition include their even-spaced distribution with respect to one another, central location in the secondary pulmonary lobule, lung parenchyma surrounding the nodule, and the absence of contact with the visceral pleural surface. Centrilobular nodules can be further subcategorized based on presence or absence of an associated tree-in-bud pattern, which appears as centrilobular nodules with a V-shaped or Y-shaped configuration. The tree-in-bud pattern is believed to be secondary to pus or mucus impaction within the centrilobular bronchioles, resulting in bronchial impaction and peribronchial inflammation. Tree-in-bud opacities are most often caused by

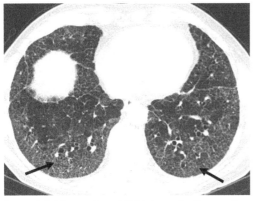

Fig. 1. Axial image from HRCT shows basilar predominant reticulation (*arrows*) in this patient with nonspecific interstitial pneumonia.

Table 1
Common abnormal findings found on HRCT and associated diseases

Abnormal HRCT Pattern		
Reticular Opacities	**Ground-Glass Opacities**	**Consolidation**
• UIP	• NSIP	• COP
• NSIP	• AIP (acute, subacute)	• Polymyositis/dermatomyositis
• Collagen vascular disease	• DIP	• Acute exacerbation of ILD
• Asbestosis	• RB-ILD	• AIP
• Drug-related pulmonary fibrosis	• LIP	• Acute HP
	• COP	• Drugs
	• Subacute HP	• Sarcoidosis
	• Acute exacerbation of ILD	

Abbreviations: AIP, acute interstitial pneumonia; COP, cryptogenic organizing pneumonia; DIP, desquamative interstitial pneumonia; HP, hypersensitivity pneumonitis; LIP, lymphoid interstitial pneumonia; NSIP, nonspecific interstitial pneumonia; RB-ILD, respiratory bronchiolitis-ILD; UIP, usual interstitial pneumonia.

infection or aspiration. In the absence of tree-in-bud, the differential diagnosis is broad.

Perilymphatic nodules are found where the lymphatics are most concentrated, including the areas adjacent to the visceral pleura, interlobular septa, and adjacent to the bronchovascular bundles. The diseases that can present with perilymphatic nodular pattern are presented in **Table 2**.

Random nodules are found diffusely throughout the lung parenchyma and do not show a predominant distribution within either the secondary pulmonary lobules or the lymphatics. There is the additional finding that random nodules may be seen at the termination of small pulmonary arterial vessels. These nodules (**Fig. 3**) usually imply a hematogenous route of entry into the lungs; hematogenous spread of infection and metastases are the most common conditions that produce randomly distributed nodules. The conditions that can present with such a pattern are listed in **Table 2**.

An established algorithm for nodule characterization on HRCT is presented in **Fig. 4**.[4]

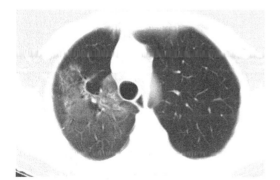

Fig. 2. Axial image shows central ground-glass opacity in the right upper lung parenchyma in this patient with organizing pneumonia.

Linear Opacities

There are several different patterns of linear opacities on the HRCT scan. The common ones include interlobular septal thickening, parenchymal bands, subpleural curvilinear densities, and intralobular septal thickening or irregular linear opacities.

The normal nonthickened interlobular septa are generally too fine to be detected on standard HRCT, but when abnormally thickened they are detectable on HRCT. They appear as linear opacities extending from and perpendicular to the pleura (**Fig. 5**A). It is common to find a few of them in normal cases; however, the presence of diffuse, multiple thickened interlobular septa should raise the suspicion of an underlying interstitial disease process. They can be classified as either smooth (eg, from hydrostatic edema, lymphatic congestion), irregular (eg, from fibrosis, lymphoma, secondary solid tumor), or nodular (eg, from sarcoid, lymphoma, secondary tumor).

Parenchymal bands are linear opacities in contact with the pleura and generally greater in length compared with interlobular septa (see **Fig. 5**B). These bands usually represent fibrosis or a component of atelectasis. Subpleural lines are curvilinear densities seen adjacent and parallel to the visceral pleura. Like parenchymal bands, these also represent fibrosis or atelectasis and are seen frequently in asbestosis. Intralobular septal thickening or irregular linear opacities are linear densities that cannot be categorized into any of the above 3 categories; they are relatively nonspecific.

DECREASED ATTENUATION
Honeycombing

Honeycombing can be identified on HRCT as subpleural regions of clustered cysts, usually stacked

Table 2
Types of nodules found on HRCT and associated diseases

Types of Nodules		
Centrilobular Nodularity	**Perilymphatic Nodules**	**Random Nodules**
• Subacute hypersensitivity pneumonitis • Respiratory bronchiolitis-ILD • Langerhans cell histiocytosis	• Sarcoidosis • Silicosis • Coal worker pneumoconiosis • Berylliosis • Lymphoid interstitial pneumonia	• Hematogenous metastases • Miliary fungal infection • Miliary tuberculosis • Silicosis (mimic) • Coal worker pneumoconiosis (mimic) • Sarcoidosis (mimic)

together in 1 or more layers (**Fig. 6**). The cysts are generally 3 to 10 mm thick and have a uniform size. Honeycomb cysts can be differentiated from emphysema by their thick, well-defined walls, usually but not always lower lobe predominance, and noncentrilobular distribution. Honeycombing represents areas of destroyed and fibrotic lung tissue on histology, where the architecture has been lost; therefore, it is not uncommon to find associated coarse reticulation, architectural distortion, and traction bronchiectasis on imaging. The diseases that may present with honeycombing on HRCT are shown in **Table 3**.

Cysts

On HRCT, cysts are rounded areas of low attenuation that are well demarcated from normal lung parenchyma by a thin wall; the walls of a cyst are usually less than 2 mm thick. The most common conditions associated with cystic lung changes are listed in **Table 3**.

SPECIFIC DISEASES
Langerhans Cell Histiocytosis

Langerhans cell histiocytosis (LCH) is a granulomatous disease of unknown cause. It has a strong association with smoking, and usually affects young adults. In later stages of the disease process, the granulomas are replaced by fibrosis and may cavitate, leading to cyst formation[5,6]; however, the mechanism of the disease still remains unknown. The prominent findings on HRCT consist of multiple irregular cysts and nodules (**Fig. 7**). In

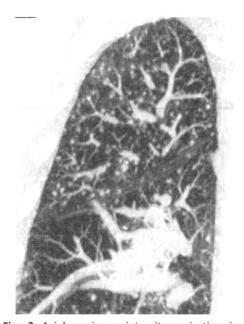

Fig. 3. Axial maximum intensity projection image shows random nodules throughout the left lower lobe in this patient with disseminated mycobacterial infection; nodules are uniformly distributed throughout the lobe without sparing of fissures or subpleural lung.

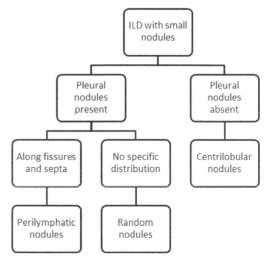

Fig. 4. This flowchart shows an effective approach to recognizing the 3 different patterns of nodules on HRCT.

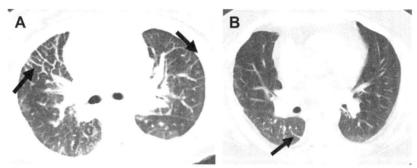

Fig. 5. Linear opacities. (*A*) interlobular (axial image from noncontrast chest CT shows diffuse interlobular septal thickening (*arrows*), which highlights the margins of secondary pulmonary lobules). (*B*) Parenchymal bands (axial image from noncontrast chest CT shows a focal linear opacity (*arrow*) extending orthogonally from the subpleural aspect of the right lower lobe consistent with a focal parenchymal band).

contrast to lymphangioleiomyomatosis (LAM), the cysts of LCH are irregularly shaped; they may have either thick or thin walls. The disease process classically affects the upper lung zones, with sparing of the costophrenic angles.[5,7] Nodules may be the only abnormality in early disease, with cysts developing in the area of the nodules later in the disease course.[5]

LAM

LAM can be an idiopathic disease, but is more commonly seen secondary to tuberous sclerosis.[8] The cystic changes are believed to be a direct result of peribronchial atypical smooth muscle cell proliferation, with resultant air trapping.[9] The cysts of LAM are generally thin-walled, multiple, uniform, and diffuse, without any specific regional distribution or sparing: they are typically 2 to 5 mm in size with a rounded or ovoid shape (**Fig. 8**). The remaining lung parenchyma is generally normal, but rarely there can a few scattered centrilobular nodules; however, they are not so prominent and diffuse as those seen in LCH. Associated findings that may support the diagnosis of

LAM include the presence of pleural effusions (usually chylous as a result of lymphatic obstruction by smooth muscle cells) and pneumothorax.[10] There is some degree of overlap in the appearance of LAM and LCH.

Lymphoid Interstitial Pneumonia

Lymphoid interstitial pneumonia (LIP) is a rare disease. It can be idiopathic, or secondary to lymphoproliferative disorders and immunodeficiency states such as Sjögren syndrome, common variable immune deficiency, and human immunodeficiency virus syndrome. HRCT shows a diffuse or lower lobe predominant involvement, including ground-glass abnormality, septal thickening, centrilobular nodules, and perivascular or subpleural cysts (**Fig. 9**).[11,12] Cysts are the only finding that may be irreversible, and characteristically form in the areas of previous centrilobular nodules.[13] The combination of small bronchovascular and subpleural cysts along with widespread ground-glass abnormality and centrilobular nodules is highly suggestive of LIP.

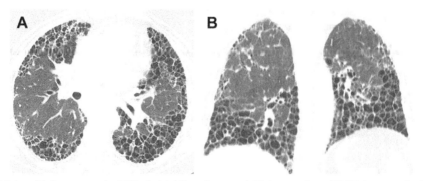

Fig. 6. Usual interstitial pneumonia (UIP). Axial (*A*) and coronal (*B*) images from HRCT show stacked thin-walled cysts that extend to the subpleural portion of the lungs. As in most typical cases of UIP, lung fibrosis is most severe in the basilar and peripheral portions of the lungs.

Table 3
Decreased attenuation found on HRCT and associated diseases

Decreased Attenuation	
Honeycombing	**Cystic Diseases**
• Usual interstitial pneumonia/idiopathic pulmonary fibrosis (most common) • Fibrotic nonspecific interstitial pneumonia • Drugs • Late asbestosis • Sarcoidosis (stage IV) • Chronic hypersensitivity pneumonitis • Collagen vascular disease	• Langerhans cell histiocytosis • Lymphangioleiomyomatosis • Lymphoid interstitial pneumonia • Desquamative interstitial pneumonia • Birt-Hogg-Dubé • Light-chain deposition disease

Light-chain Deposition Disease

Light-chain deposition disease is a rare form of cystic ILD; only a few case series and case reports on the pulmonary manifestations of this disease have been reported. It is most commonly seen in patients with underlying plasma cell dyscrasias, such as multiple myeloma and Waldenström macroglobulinemia, but has also been associated with B-cell lymphomas. The pathogenesis involves deposition of monoclonal immunoglobulin light chains in the lung parenchyma, resulting in parenchymal destruction. The HRCT findings include cystic and, rarely, nodular changes. The nodules can vary in size from 2 mm to 5 cm. The cysts are believed to be a result of small airway dilation.[14]

Birt-Hogg-Dubé Syndrome

Birt-Hogg-Dubé (BHD) syndrome is a rare autosomal-dominant disorder with multisystemic involvement; typical findings include facial fibrofolliculomas, malignant renal tumors, and pulmonary cystic changes. On HRCT, the predominant finding is multiple thin-walled cysts. The size of these cysts can vary from a few millimeters to 2 cm. These cysts can have multiple septations.[15] Differentiation from LAM can be difficult because the cysts are similar in appearance and both conditions can have an associated pneumothorax; however, the cysts of BHD syndrome are characteristically more concentrated in the lower and medial lung zones, whereas those of LAM are more diffuse.[16–18] Cysts along the proximal lower lung pulmonary arteries and veins suggest the diagnosis.[17]

IDIOPATHIC INTERSTITIAL PNEUMONIAS
Idiopathic Pulmonary Fibrosis

Idiopathic pulmonary fibrosis (IPF) is the most common entity in the spectrum of interstitial

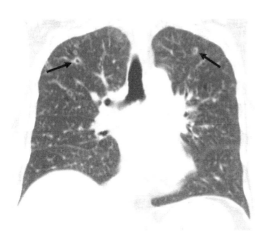

Fig. 7. LCH. Coronal reformation from chest CT shows multiple small mildly thick-walled lung cysts (*arrows*) and multiple centrilobular nodules suggestive of LCH in this smoker.

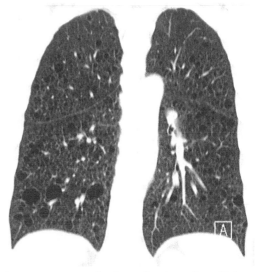

Fig. 8. LAM. Coronal reformation from chest CT shows diffuse thin-walled lung cysts consistent with LAM.

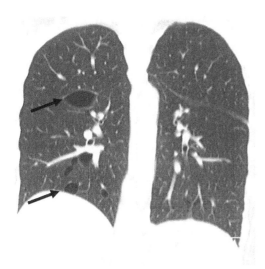

Fig. 9. LIP. Coronal reformation from chest CT shows subpleural and bronchovascular thin-walled lung cysts (*arrows*) consistent with LIP in this patient with Sjögren syndrome.

idiopathic pneumonias (IIPs), accounting for 50% to 60% of cases.[19] The prognosis is usually worse compared with other IIPs, with a median survival time of 2 to 4 years.[20] These patients are also at a higher risk of bronchogenic carcinoma than the general population, there is a predilection for the lower lobes as opposed to smoking-related bronchogenic carcinoma, which most often affects the upper lobes. IPF is characterized by the radiological pattern of usual interstitial pneumonia (UIP). UIP is most often seen in IPF; however, it can occasionally be caused by a multitude of other diseases including collagen vascular disease, chronic hypersensitivity pneumonitis (HP), drugs (eg, bleomycin, amiodarone), and asbestosis. A definite UIP pattern on HRCT in a patient without clinical evidence of an alternative diagnosis is sufficient for a confident diagnosis of IPF and carries an accuracy of 79% to 90%.[21,22] Biopsy is generally reserved for atypical or uncertain cases.[23,24] HRCT findings of UIP pattern include a predominantly subpleural disease pattern, with an apical-basal gradient. The specific features include honeycombing, peripheral reticular opacities, and minimal ground-glass abnormality. Honeycombing, if present, is shown to be the strongest predictor of the diagnosis of IPF,[21] although it may be present in other causes of pulmonary fibrosis. Traction bronchiectasis is commonly associated with the reticular pattern and signifies advanced fibrosis with architectural distortion.[25] Lower lobe volume loss is also a common finding. Ground-glass abnormality is

minimal or absent, never being the predominant pattern. Many patients with IPF may show atypical features of UIP on HRCT, with overlapping features of nonspecific interstitial pneumonia (NSIP), chronic HP, or sarcoidosis; in these patients open lung biopsy is usually necessary to establish a confident diagnosis.[26]

NSIP

NSIP is a common, albeit less prevalent entity than IPF. NSIP can be caused by many different disorders, including connective tissue diseases, HP, and drugs.[27–29] When no associated process can be found in a patient with histologic or radiologic pattern of NSIP, the diagnosis of idiopathic NSIP is established.

On HRCT the predominant abnormality includes widespread, bilateral ground-glass opacities, which may be associated with peripheral irregular linear or reticular opacities (**Fig. 10**).[30] The degree of reticulation and traction bronchiectasis has been shown to correlate with the amount of fibrosis present.[31] The disease distribution is mainly peripheral and basal. Subpleural sparing, if present, is a highly specific feature of NSIP, although seen in only a few cases.[32] In a few cases, there may be additional findings such as micronodules, foci of consolidation, or mild honeycombing. Honeycombing, when present, is usually mild, as opposed to UIP, in which honeycombing tends to be more severe.[31] Differentiation between fibrotic NSIP and UIP requires surgical lung biopsy.[22]

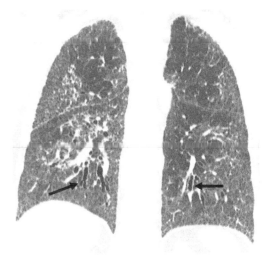

Fig. 10. NSIP. Coronal image from HRCT shows basilar predominant ground-glass opacity, reticulation, and traction bronchiectasis (*arrows*) consistent with fibrotic NSIP.

Cryptogenic organizing pneumonia

Cryptogenic organizing pneumonia (COP), previously known as bronchiolitis obliterans organizing pneumonia, is the idiopathic form of organizing pneumonia. On HRCT, the 2 most frequently seen features include bilateral, multifocal, patchy consolidation (present in up to 90% of cases) and ground-glass abnormalities (**Fig. 11**A).[33,34] The lung volumes are generally preserved. COP tends to preferentially involve the subpleural and bronchovascular regions of the lung parenchyma.[35] There may also be bronchial dilation and air bronchograms associated with regions of consolidation. The imaging findings in these cases can often be mistaken for pneumonic consolidation. The foci of consolidation generally involve the lower lung zones and have a tendency to migrate, especially after therapy. A perilobular pattern of increased attenuation has also been described in COP, which can resemble, and be confused with, interlobular septal thickening.

Other less common findings that may be present in a subset of patients include irregular linear or reticular opacities and large nodules (<20% of cases) that may simulate lung cancer. In some cases, HRCT may also reveal the classic reverse halo/atoll sign, which is defined as a central focus of ground-glass opacity with a surrounding rim of consolidation (see **Fig. 11**B).

Respiratory bronchiolitis-ILD

Respiratory bronchiolitis (RB)-ILD (RB-ILD) is part of the spectrum of smoking-related lung diseases. It is possible that RB-ILD and desquamative interstitial pneumonia (DIP) are similar processes but at the opposite ends of the disease spectrum. RB-ILD is differentiated from simple RB on a clinical basis.

The predominant finding on HRCT is ground-glass abnormality[36]; this is generally more patchy and less extensive than that seen in DIP and preferentially involves the upper lobes. The ground-glass abnormality of RB-ILD has been shown to represent areas of macrophage accumulation in the distal airspaces.[37] An important finding that may help to distinguish RB-ILD form DIP is the presence of centrilobular nodules in the former (**Fig. 12**).[38] Small cyst formation is unusual in RB-ILD. Bronchial wall thickening is another feature that can be present in RB-ILD or DIP. A large proportion of patients with either RB-ILD or DIP may also have concomitant upper lobe emphysema as a result of long smoking history.

DIP

DIP is a rare form of ILD. The usual age of presentation is 40 to 50 years, with men affected more than women (male/female >2:1). The disease predominantly affects smokers (90% cases), but can also be seen secondary to lung infections, organic dust exposure, and marijuana smoke inhalation.

HRCT typically shows a ground-glass pattern, which is caused by diffuse macrophage infiltration of the alveoli along with interstitial septal thickening; this is generally present in all cases of DIP.[39] The ground-glass pattern can either be patchy or diffuse, with a predilection for peripheral and basal lung zones.[40] Some cases may also show fine linear or reticular opacities, also concentrated in the peripheral and basal lung zones. In some cases HRCT may reveal small lung cysts that are generally thin-walled and less than 2 cm (**Fig. 13**); these cysts are believed to represent dilated bronchioles and alveolar ducts distal to the sites of obstruction; some of them may resolve over time.[7,41] Severe honeycombing is unusual.[40]

Acute interstitial pneumonia

Acute interstitial pneumonia (AIP) is notable for its acute presentation. On HRCT, the most common

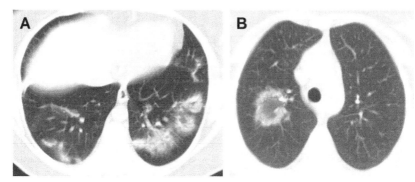

Fig. 11. COP. (*A*) Axial image from chest CT shows bronchovascular consolidation and ground-glass opacity consistent with organizing pneumonia. (*B*) More superiorly in the thorax, there is an example of reversed halo sign in the right upper lobe (central ground-glass focus surrounded by a thin rim of consolidation), which is suggestive of organizing pneumonia.

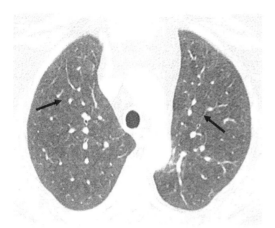

Fig. 12. RB-ILD. Axial image from HRCT shows innumerable centrilobular ground-glass nodules (*arrows*) in the upper lobes, highly suggestive of RB-ILD, in this symptomatic smoker.

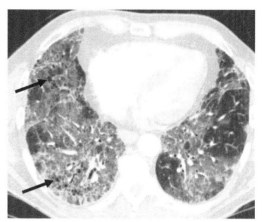

Fig. 14. AIP. Axial image from contrast-enhanced chest CT shows diffuse ground-glass opacity and reticulation with relative sparing of the left lower lobe in this patient with acute interstitial pneumonitis. Mild traction bronchiolectasis (*arrows*) is present in the right lung, probably from underlying pulmonary fibrosis.

findings include ground-glass abnormalities, traction bronchiectasis, and architectural distortion (**Fig. 14**).[42] The ground-glass pattern is patchy in most cases, with areas of lobular sparing; however, some cases may show a more diffuse distribution.[43] Consolidation can be present in some cases and preferentially affects the lower lobes. Traction bronchiectasis can be observed within areas of ground-glass or consolidation and represents fibrotic changes.[44] Although a considerable overlap exists between AIP and acute respiratory distress syndrome (ARDS) in terms of HRCT findings, the presence of symmetric lower lobe abnormalities with honeycombing may be more suggestive of AIP.[45] Among survivors with AIP, most experience marked improvement of the disease. Some may progress to a chronic, fibrotic

phase.[46] Fibrosis in AIP and ARDS typically manifests as reticular abnormalities and traction bronchiectasis in the nondependent portions of the lung (in portions of the lungs more exposed to the deleterious effects of long-term positive pressure ventilation).[42]

Occupational Lung Disease

Asbestosis

Asbestosis refers to interstitial fibrosis caused by inhalation of asbestos fibers. The average latent period for the appearance of ILD is 20 years.[47] Asbestosis must be differentiated from asbestos-related lung disease, which includes noninterstitial manifestation such as pleural plaques, pleural thickening, pleural effusions, bronchogenic carcinoma, and malignant mesothelioma.[48]

In the early stages of the disease, HRCT scans typically reveal multiple subpleural nodules, patchy ground-glass opacities, and mild septal thickening along with reticular abnormalities (mostly in the subpleural and basal aspects of the lungs). Parenchymal bands may be noted in a few cases as well. Another early finding is subpleural curvilinear lines, representing peribronchial fibrosis.[49] In advanced disease, asbestosis most closely resembles UIP (**Fig. 15**). However, a basal and subpleural-dominant disease pattern coupled with the presence of pleural plaques favors the diagnosis of asbestosis over UIP.[50]

Silicosis Silicosis is one of the more common occupational ILDs encountered; pathogenesis involves inhalational lung injury secondary to silica

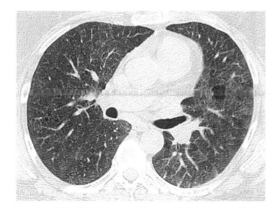

Fig. 13. DIP. Axial image from HRCT shows diffuse ground-glass opacity with superimposed small cysts highly suggestive of desquamative interstitial pneumonitis in this heavy smoker.

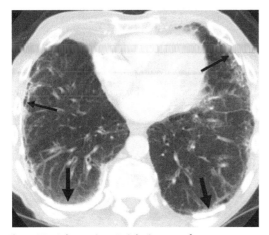

Fig. 15. Asbestosis. Axial image from contrast-enhanced chest CT shows peripheral reticulation and honeycombing (*thin arrows*) as well as calcified pleural plaques (*thick arrows*) consistent with asbestosis. Histologically, the pulmonary fibrosis pattern in asbestosis most often shows a UIP pattern.

dust exposure. Associated occupations include rock mining, sandblasting, drilling, quarrying, foundry working, and ceramic manufacturing.[51] Silicosis can have an acute as well as a chronic form, the latter being the more common ILD pattern. Chronic silicosis can be further subclassified into a simple and a complicated type based on HRCT findings.

Simple silicosis, on HRCT, is characterized by the presence of multiple nodules, which can either be diffuse or concentrated in the centrilobular and subpleural portions of the lungs (**Fig. 16**A).[52] The nodules are generally small, ranging from 2 to 5 mm. Calcifications may be seen within some of the nodules as well. With disease progression, the initial subpleural nodules may coalesce and result in a pseudoplaque appearance, a finding

that should not be confused with asbestos-related plaques. Mediastinal lymphadenopathy is a common feature of silicosis, usually showing intra-nodal calcifications; these may have either a punctuate, diffuse, or a peripheral (egg shell) pattern.[53]

Complicated silicosis, also termed progressive massive fibrosis, results from the confluence of the earlier nodules.[52,54] This lesion manifests as large, soft tissue masses with ill-defined borders; these conglomerate masses are mainly seen in the upper lung zones, and often show areas of calcification and cavitation (see **Fig. 16**B).

Coal worker pneumoconiosis Coal worker pneumoconiosis is caused by inhalation of washed coal that leads to interstitial lung inflammation and fibrosis. A simple and a complicated form of coal worker pneumoconiosis can be recognized on imaging. The imaging appearance of coal worker pneumoconiosis is identical to that of silicosis.[55]

HP HP is a granulomatous disease with an immunologic basis. It can occur in response to a variety of environmental antigens.[56] Classically, it can be separated into 3 phases: an acute, subacute, and a chronic phase, depending on the temporality relative to initial exposure. All 3 stages have a significant overlap, and a large number of patients may present with findings representative of more than 1 stage.[57]

Acute HP generally presents within a few hours of antigen exposure, and is characterized by widespread homogeneous or heterogeneous opacities; these may mimic acute pulmonary edema.[58] Subacute HP occurs in response to intermittent or low-dose antigen exposure, and is characterized by poorly defined widespread centrilobular nodularity and patchy ground-glass opacity (**Fig. 17**A). The ground-glass pattern is generally

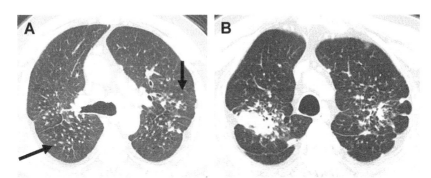

Fig. 16. Silicosis. (*A*) Axial images from HRCT show centrilobular nodules (*arrows*) in the upper lobes and superior segments of the lower lobes; there is mediastinal lymphadenopathy, which is common in silicosis. (*B*) Nodules have coalesced into progressive massive fibrosis in the upper lung zones.

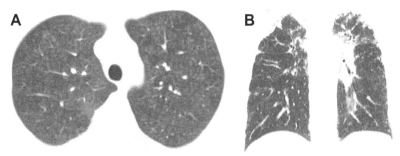

Fig. 17. HP. (*A*) Axial image from chest CT shows innumerable centrilobular ground-glass nodules; in the chronic setting, the differential diagnosis includes HP and RB. History is often helpful in suggesting 1 diagnosis over the other considering that smoking is more common in RB and less common in HP. (*B*) Coronal image from HRCT in a different patient shows upper lobe predominant pulmonary fibrosis characterized by ground-glass opacity, reticulation, traction bronchiectasis, and subpleural consolidation with upper lobe volume loss in this patient with chronic HP.

symmetric and diffuse but can be asymmetric in some cases. There may be concomitant reticulation and bronchiectasis in some cases, which may resemble NSIP. Some cases may show cystic changes as well.[59] Expiratory images generally show mosaic attenuation, corresponding with areas of air trapping. This finding is believed to represent bronchiolitis and the resultant bronchiolar obstruction.[60] Chronic HP classically occurs after a long-term antigen exposure, and usually shows a fibrotic pattern resembling UIP or fibrotic NSIP (see **Fig. 17**B). The imaging findings of chronic HP may be superimposed on a background of subacute HP pattern in some cases. Centrilobular nodules, if present, favor chronic HP over UIP.[61] Also, the fibrosis in chronic HP generally involves the mid and upper lung zones, with sparing of the bases, whereas UIP and fibrotic NSIP tend to affect the lung bases more severely. Open lung biopsy is required to make a confident diagnosis in borderline cases.

Sarcoidosis Sarcoidosis is a multisystem inflammatory disease of unknown cause, characterized histologically by the formation of multiple noncaseating granulomas. The disease is 3 times more prevalent in African Americans than in Whites.[62] Pulmonary involvement is the most common cause of morbidity and mortality in these patients, with up to 90% patients affected, and 20% developing chronic fibrotic lung disease.[63] Based on the findings on standard chest radiograph, the disease is categorized into 5 stages, with increasing stage implying a worse prognosis.[64] The stages of sarcoidosis are summarized in **Table 4**.

Sarcoidosis preferentially involves the upper lung zones: however, it can also have a more diffuse distribution in advanced stages of the disease. The most commonly observed finding on standard HRCT is multiple nodular opacities in a perilymphatic distribution (**Fig. 18**), which correlate with sites of granulomatous inflammation on histology.[65] HRCT becomes indispensable in the management of sarcoidosis when there is a need for differentiating reversible granulomatous inflammation from fibrosis (a direct determinant of patient staging). Early findings, which may improve with treatment, include interstitial septal thickening, reticular or linear opacities, alveolar opacities, ground-glass opacities, foci of consolidation, and nodules.[66] Of these findings, the presence of ground-glass abnormality and consolidation portend a worse prognosis compared with the rest.[67] On the other hand, honeycombing, traction bronchiectasis, architectural distortion, upper lobe volume loss, and hilar retraction suggest an irreversible fibrotic component to the lung disease.[68] Expiratory CT images can show focal air trapping in any stage of the disease.[69]

Berylliosis Berylliosis is an uncommon occupational ILD, caused by exposure to beryllium dust or fumes. It is most frequently seen in people working in the nuclear industry, ceramic manufacture plants, or the aerospace industry. Like most

Table 4
Chest radiographic stages of sarcoidosis

Stage	Chest Radiograph
0	Normal
1	Hilar adenopathy alone
2	Hilar adenopathy with lung parenchymal abnormalities
3	Lung parenchymal abnormalities alone
4	Lung fibrosis

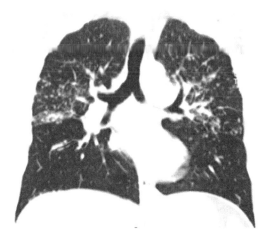

Fig. 18. Sarcoidosis. Coronal image from noncontrast chest CT shows multiple small nodules primarily in the midlung zone; there is clustering of nodules along interlobular septa, fissures, and bronchovascular structures, diagnostic of a perilymphatic pattern.

occupational diseases, berylliosis has an acute and a chronic stage. The ILD pattern encountered in clinical practice is most often the chronic form. Chronic beryllium disease requires initial sensitization to beryllium before development of overt disease. This sensitivity to beryllium can be easily detected on a lymphocyte transformation test using blood or bronchoalveolar lavage fluid.

On HRCT, chronic berylliosis closely mimics sarcoidosis, with the most common finding being perilymphatic nodules along the bronchovascular bundles and interstitial septa (**Fig. 19**).[70] Other common findings include interstitial septal thickening, ground-glass opacities, and bronchial wall thickening. Mediastinal and hilar lymphadenopathy can be present as well. Ground-glass

opacities, believed to be related to granulomatous changes, are more commonly seen in chronic berylliosis than in sarcoidosis, and therefore, may help in differentiation between the two.[71] With disease progression, a fibrotic pattern may emerge with development of peripheral reticular or linear opacities; honeycombing may be present in some of these cases as well.[70]

COLLAGEN VASCULAR DISEASES
Rheumatoid Arthritis

Rheumatoid arthritis can be associated with a wide variety of possible pulmonary complications, including nodules, fibrosis, airway disease, and pleural disease. The most common findings on HRCT include bronchial wall thickening, bronchiectasis, and nodules; other less common findings are nonseptal thickening, ground-glass opacities, reticular abnormality, honeycombing, and consolidation (**Fig. 20**).[72,73] The most common pattern of ILD in rheumatoid arthritis is UIP, followed by NSIP, and COP. The HRCT findings in early rheumatoid disease (<1 year) include expiratory air trapping, bronchiectasis, and a ground-glass pattern.[74]

Systemic sclerosis
Systemic sclerosis is a type of multisystemic connective tissue disease. The lungs are one of the most commonly affected organs in the diffuse form of the disease, but can be present in more limited forms as well.

The predominant HRCT pattern consists of widespread, confluent ground-glass opacities along with associated reticular abnormalities (**Fig. 21**).[75]

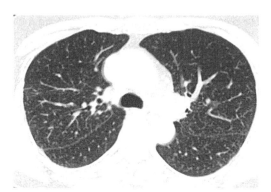

Fig. 19. Berylliosis. Axial image from HRCT shows fine nodularity along the fissures and along interlobular septa (perilymphatic) in this patient with chronic beryllium disease.

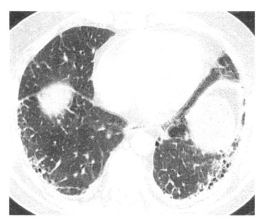

Fig. 20. Rheumatoid arthritis. Axial image from HRCT shows subpleural reticulation, traction bronchiolectasis, ground-glass opacity, and mild honeycombing consistent with a UIP pattern in this patient with rheumatoid arthritis.

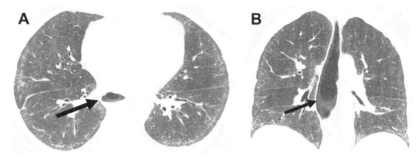

Fig. 21. Scleroderma. (*A*) Axial image showing peripheral predominant ground-glass opacity and mild reticulation with subpleural sparing, highly suggestive of NSIP. (*B*) Coronal image showing the dilated esophagus with gas-fluid level (*arrows in A and B*) is essentially diagnostic of esophageal dysmotility in this patient with scleroderma.

These findings predominantly involve the basal and posterior-lateral lung zones, as well as the subpleural regions.[76] Airways are also commonly affected, showing traction bronchiectasis and bronchiolectasis. Mild honeycombing can be present in up to one-third of cases.[75] The CT findings can be similar to those of idiopathic NSIP in many cases; this is not surprising, because 75% of scleroderma cases show a histologic NSIP pattern.[77]

Systemic lupus erythematosus
Systemic lupus erythematosus (SLE) can present with a variety of different patterns on HRCT, including airway disease, pleuritis, lymphadenopathy, and pulmonary hemorrhage. ILD is present in up to one-third of SLE cases.[78] The most common pattern seen is UIP or NSIP, usually mild. Diaphragmatic dysfunction in these patients may lead to low lung volumes (also known as shrinking lung syndrome).

Mixed connective tissue disease
Mixed connective tissue disease (MCTD) is a connective disorder with overlapping features of other connective tissue diseases such as SLE, PM, diabetes mellitus, rheumatoid arthritis and others. The lungs are commonly affected; in 1 study, up to 67% patients with MCTD had evidence of infiltrative lung disease. The most common HRCT findings include ground-glass opacity, along with subpleural nodules, and reticular or linear opacities, often resulting in an NSIP pattern (**Fig. 22**).[79]

Drug-related ILD Drugs can cause a wide variety of pulmonary manifestations, which may be nonspecific in most cases and can overlap with the disease pattern described earlier (**Fig. 23**). Some of the more common drugs and their HRCT manifestations are shown in **Table 5**.

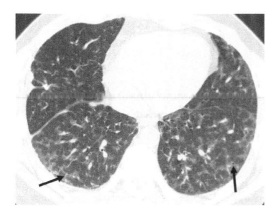

Fig. 22. MCTD. Axial image from HRCT shows patchy bronchovascular ground-glass opacity and mild bronchiolectasis (*arrows*) in this patient with MCTD-related ILD.

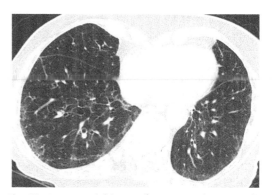

Fig. 23. Drugs. Axial image from HRCT shows patchy ground-glass opacity, interlobular septal thickening, and very mild traction bronchiolectasis in this patient with nitrofurantoin lung.

Table 5
Drug-induced ILD

Drug	HRCT Findings
Amiodarone	NSIP; diffuse ground-glass; multiple areas of organizing pneumonia; diffuse reticular opacities
Bleomycin	Early: reticular or nodular opacities involving the bases and costophrenic angles Late: diffuse fibrosis
Cyclophosphamide	Basal reticular or nodular opacities; pleural thickening
Methotrexate	Hilar lymphadenopathy; basal reticular or nodular opacities
Nitrofurantoin	Early: basal opacities; diffuse ground-glass Late: basal reticular or nodular opacities along with fibrosis
Nitrosoureas	Patchy or diffuse ground-glass abnormalities

SUMMARY

ILD is a broad category of diseases that may present with different but overlapping findings on HRCT. It is important for physicians taking care of patients with ILD to know the important HRCT findings of the lung that are representative of ILD. The different HRCT findings and the location of these findings in the lung often enable a specific diagnosis of ILD to be made in a given patient.

REFERENCES

1. Weibel ER. Fleischner Lecture. Looking into the lung: what can it tell us? AJR Am J Roentgenol 1979;133:1021.
2. Leung AN, Miller RR, Müller NL. Parenchymal opacification in chronic infiltrative lung diseases: CT-pathologic correlation. Radiology 1993;188:209.
3. Remy-Jardin M, Giraud F, Remy J, et al. Importance of ground-glass attenuation in chronic diffuse infiltrative lung disease: pathologic-CT correlation. Radiology 1993;189:693.
4. Gruden JF, Webb WR, Naidich DP, et al. Multinodular disease: anatomic localization at thin-section CT–multireader evaluation of a simple algorithm. Radiology 1999;210:711.
5. Abbott GF, Rosado-de-Christenson ML, Franks TJ, et al. From the archives of the AFIP: pulmonary Langerhans cell histiocytosis. Radiographics 2004; 24:821.
6. Colby TV, Lombard C. Histiocytosis X in the lung. Hum Pathol 1983;14:847.
7. Koyama M, Johkoh T, Honda O, et al. Chronic cystic lung disease: diagnostic accuracy of high-resolution CT in 92 patients. AJR Am J Roentgenol 2003;180: 827.
8. McCormack FX. Lymphangioleiomyomatosis: a clinical update. Chest 2008;133:507.
9. Chu SC, Horiba K, Usuki J, et al. Comprehensive evaluation of 35 patients with lymphangioleiomyomatosis. Chest 1999;115:1041.
10. Kirchner J, Stein A, Viel K, et al. Pulmonary lymphangioleiomyomatosis: high-resolution CT findings. Eur Radiol 1999;9:49.
11. Ichikawa Y, Kinoshita M, Koga T, et al. Lung cyst formation in lymphocytic interstitial pneumonia: CT features. J Comput Assist Tomogr 1994;18:745.
12. Johkoh T, Müller NL, Pickford HA, et al. Lymphocytic interstitial pneumonia: thin-section CT findings in 22 patients. Radiology 1999;212:567.
13. Johkoh T, Ichikado K, Akira M, et al. Lymphocytic interstitial pneumonia: follow-up CT findings in 14 patients. J Thorac Imaging 2000;15:162.
14. Colombat M, Stern M, Groussard O, et al. Pulmonary cystic disorder related to light chain deposition disease. Am J Respir Crit Care Med 2006; 173:777.
15. Agarwal PP, Gross BH, Holloway BJ, et al. Thoracic CT findings in Birt-Hogg-Dube syndrome. AJR Am J Roentgenol 2011;196:349.
16. Ayo DS, Aughenbaugh GL, Yi ES, et al. Cystic lung disease in Birt-Hogg-Dube syndrome. Chest 2007; 132:679.
17. Tobino K, Gunji Y, Kurihara M, et al. Characteristics of pulmonary cysts in Birt-Hogg-Dubé syndrome: thin-section CT findings of the chest in 12 patients. Eur J Radiol 2011;77:403.
18. Tobino K, Hirai T, Johkoh T, et al. Differentiation between Birt-Hogg-Dubé syndrome and lymphangioleiomyomatosis: quantitative analysis of pulmonary cysts on computed tomography of the chest in 66 females. Eur J Radiol 2011. [Epub ahead of print].
19. Travis WD, King TE Jr, Bateman ED, et al. American Thoracic Society/European Respiratory Society international multidisciplinary consensus classification of the idiopathic interstitial pneumonias. Am J Respir Crit Care Med 2002;165:277.

20. Katzenstein AL, Myers JL. Idiopathic pulmonary fibrosis: clinical relevance of pathologic classification. Am J Respir Crit Care Med 1998;157:1301.
21. Sumikawa H, Johkoh T, Ichikado K, et al. Usual interstitial pneumonia and chronic idiopathic interstitial pneumonia: analysis of CT appearance in 92 patients. Radiology 2006;241:258.
22. Tsubamoto M, Müller NL, Johkoh T, et al. Pathologic subgroups of nonspecific interstitial pneumonia: differential diagnosis from other idiopathic interstitial pneumonias on high-resolution computed tomography. J Comput Assist Tomogr 2005;29:793.
23. Hunninghake GW, Zimmerman MB, Schwartz DA, et al. Utility of a lung biopsy for the diagnosis of idiopathic pulmonary fibrosis. Am J Respir Crit Care Med 2001;164:193.
24. Raghu G, Mageto YN, Lockhart D, et al. The accuracy of the clinical diagnosis of new-onset idiopathic pulmonary fibrosis and other interstitial lung disease: a prospective study. Chest 1999; 116:1168.
25. Nishimura K, Kitaichi M, Izumi T, et al. Usual interstitial pneumonia: histologic correlation with high-resolution CT. Radiology 1992;182:337.
26. Sverzellati N, Wells AU, Tomassetti S, et al. Biopsy-proved idiopathic pulmonary fibrosis: spectrum of nondiagnostic thin-section CT diagnoses. Radiology 2010;254:957.
27. Kim EA, Lee KS, Johkoh T, et al. Interstitial lung diseases associated with collagen vascular diseases: radiologic and histopathologic findings. Radiographics 2002;22:S151.
28. Kim JS, Lee KS, Koh EM, et al. Thoracic involvement of systemic lupus erythematosus: clinical, pathologic, and radiologic findings. J Comput Assist Tomogr 2000;24:9.
29. Rossi SE, Erasmus JJ, McAdams HP, et al. Pulmonary drug toxicity: radiologic and pathologic manifestations. Radiographics 2000;20:1245.
30. MacDonald SL, Rubens MB, Hansell DM, et al. Nonspecific interstitial pneumonia and usual interstitial pneumonia: comparative appearances at and diagnostic accuracy of thin-section CT. Radiology 2001;221:600.
31. Johkoh T, Müller NL, Colby TV, et al. Nonspecific interstitial pneumonia: correlation between thin-section CT findings and pathologic subgroups in 55 patients. Radiology 2002;225:199.
32. Silva CI, Müller NL, Lynch DA, et al. Chronic hypersensitivity pneumonitis: differentiation from idiopathic pulmonary fibrosis and nonspecific interstitial pneumonia by using thin-section CT. Radiology 2008; 240:200.
33. Jara-Palomares L, Gomez-Izquierdo L, Gonzalez-Vergara D, et al. Utility of high-resolution computed tomography and BAL in cryptogenic organizing pneumonia. Respir Med 2010;104:1706.
34. Lee JW, Lee KS, Lee HY, et al. Cryptogenic organizing pneumonia: serial high-resolution CT findings in 22 patients. AJR Am J Roentgenol 2010;195:916.
35. Lee KS, Kullnig P, Hartman TE, et al. Cryptogenic organizing pneumonia: CT findings in 43 patients. AJR Am J Roentgenol 1994;162:543.
36. Ryu JH, Myers JL, Capizzi SA, et al. Desquamative interstitial pneumonia and respiratory bronchiolitis-associated interstitial lung disease. Chest 2005; 127:178.
37. Remy-Jardin M, Remy J, Boulenguez C, et al. Morphologic effects of cigarette smoking on airways and pulmonary parenchyma in healthy adult volunteers: CT evaluation and correlation with pulmonary function tests. Radiology 1993;186:107.
38. Heyneman LE, Ward S, Lynch DA, et al. Respiratory bronchiolitis, respiratory bronchiolitis-associated interstitial lung disease, and desquamative interstitial pneumonia: different entities or part of the spectrum of the same disease process? AJR Am J Roentgenol 1999;173:1617.
39. Johkoh T, Müller NL, Cartier Y, et al. Idiopathic interstitial pneumonias: diagnostic accuracy of thin-section CT in 129 patients. Radiology 1999;211:555.
40. Hartman TE, Primack SL, Swensen SJ, et al. Desquamative interstitial pneumonia: thin-section CT findings in 22 patients. Radiology 1993;187:787.
41. Akira M, Yamamoto S, Hara H, et al. Serial computed tomographic evaluation in desquamative interstitial pneumonia. Thorax 1997;52:333.
42. Johkoh T, Müller NL, Taniguchi H, et al. Acute interstitial pneumonia: thin-section CT findings in 36 patients. Radiology 1999;211:859.
43. Primack SL, Hartman TE, Ikezoe J, et al. Acute interstitial pneumonia: radiographic and CT findings in nine patients. Radiology 1993;188:817.
44. Ichikado K, Johkoh T, Ikezoe J, et al. Acute interstitial pneumonia: high-resolution CT findings correlated with pathology. AJR Am J Roentgenol 1997; 168:333.
45. Tomiyama N, Müller NL, Johkoh T, et al. Acute respiratory distress syndrome and acute interstitial pneumonia: comparison of thin-section CT findings. J Comput Assist Tomogr 2001;25:28.
46. Bouros D, Nicholson AC, Polychronopoulos V, et al. Acute interstitial pneumonia. Eur Respir J 2000;15: 412.
47. Akira M. High-resolution CT in the evaluation of occupational and environmental disease. Radiol Clin North Am 2002;40:43.
48. McLoud TC, Woods BO, Carrington CB, et al. Diffuse pleural thickening in an asbestos-exposed population: prevalence and causes. AJR Am J Roentgenol 1985;144:9.
49. Akira M, Yokoyama K, Yamamoto S, et al. Early asbestosis: evaluation with high-resolution CT. Radiology 1991;178:409.

50. Copley SJ, Wells AU, Sivakumaran P, et al. Asbestosis and idiopathic pulmonary fibrosis: comparison of thin-section CT features. Radiology 2003;229:731.

51. Bang KM, Attfield MD, Wood JM, et al. National trends in silicosis mortality in the United States, 1981-2004. Am J Ind Med 2008;51:633.

52. Stark P, Jacobson F, Shaffer K. Standard imaging in silicosis and coal worker's pneumoconiosis. Radiol Clin North Am 1992;30:1147.

53. Antao VC, Pinheiro GA, Terra-Filho M, et al. High-resolution CT in silicosis: correlation with radiographic findings and functional impairment. J Comput Assist Tomogr 2005;29:350.

54. Bégin R, Ostiguy G, Fillion R, et al. Computed tomography scan in the early detection of silicosis. Am Rev Respir Dis 1991;144:697.

55. Remy-Jardin M, Degreef JM, Beuscart R, et al. Coal worker's pneumoconiosis: CT assessment in exposed workers and correlation with radiographic findings. Radiology 1990;177:363.

56. Kim KI, Kim CW, Lee MK, et al. Imaging of occupational lung disease. Radiographics 2001;21:1371.

57. Mohr LC. Hypersensitivity pneumonitis. Curr Opin Pulm Med 2004;10:401.

58. Hansell DM, Wells AU, Padley SP, et al. Hypersensitivity pneumonitis: correlation of individual CT patterns with functional abnormalities. Radiology 1996;199:123.

59. Franquet T, Hansell DM, Senbanjo T, et al. Lung cysts in subacute hypersensitivity pneumonitis. J Comput Assist Tomogr 2003;27:475.

60. Small JH, Flower CD, Traill ZC, et al. Air-trapping in extrinsic allergic alveolitis on computed tomography. Clin Radiol 1996;51:684.

61. Buschman DL, Gamsu G, Waldron JA, et al. Chronic hypersensitivity pneumonitis: use of CT in diagnosis. AJR Am J Roentgenol 1992;159:957.

62. Henke CE, Henke G, Elveback LR. The epidemiology of sarcoidosis in Rochester, Minnesota: a population-based study of incidence and survival. Am J Epidemiol 1986;123:840.

63. Hunninghake GW, Costabel U, Ando M, et al. Statement on sarcoidosis. Am J Respir Crit Care Med 1999;160:736.

64. Siltzbach LE. Sarcoidosis: clinical features and management. Med Clin North Am 1967;51:483.

65. Lynch DA, Webb WR, Gamsu G, et al. Computed tomography in pulmonary sarcoidosis. J Comput Assist Tomogr 1989;13:405.

66. Muller NL, Miller RR. Ground-glass attenuation, nodules, alveolitis, and sarcoid granulomas. Radiology 1993;189:31.

67. Akira M, Kozuka T, Inoue Y, et al. Long-term follow-up CT scan evaluation in patients with pulmonary sarcoidosis. Chest 2005;127:185.

68. Baughman RP, Winget DB, Bowen EH, et al. Predicting respiratory failure in sarcoidosis patients. Sarcoidosis Vasc Diffuse Lung Dis 1997;14:154.

69. Bartz RR, Stern EJ. Airways obstruction in patients with sarcoidosis: expiratory CT scan findings. J Thorac Imaging 2000;15:285.

70. Newman LS, Buschman DL, Newell JD, et al. Beryllium disease: assessment with CT. Radiology 1994;190:835.

71. Naccache JM, Marchand-Adam S, Kambouchner M, et al. Ground-glass computed tomography pattern in chronic beryllium disease: pathologic substratum and evolution. J Comput Assist Tomogr 2003;27:496.

72. Gabbay E, Tarala R, Will R, et al. Interstitial lung disease in recent onset rheumatoid arthritis. Am J Respir Crit Care Med 1997;156:528.

73. Mori S, Cho I, Koga Y, et al. Comparison of pulmonary abnormalities on high-resolution computed tomography in patients with early versus longstanding rheumatoid arthritis. J Rheumatol 2008;35:1513.

74. Metafratzi ZM, Georgiadis AN, Ioannidou CV, et al. Pulmonary involvement in patients with early rheumatoid arthritis. Scand J Rheumatol 2007;36:338.

75. Goldin JG, Lynch DA, Strollo DC, et al. High-resolution CT scan findings in patients with symptomatic scleroderma-related interstitial lung disease. Chest 2008;134:358.

76. Schurawitzki H, Stiglbauer R, Graninger W, et al. Interstitial lung disease in progressive systemic sclerosis: high-resolution CT versus radiography. Radiology 1990;176:755.

77. Desai SR, Veeraraghavan S, Hansell DM, et al. CT features of lung disease in patients with systemic sclerosis: comparison with idiopathic pulmonary fibrosis and nonspecific interstitial pneumonia. Radiology 2004;232:560.

78. Fenlon HM, Doran M, Sant SM, et al. High-resolution chest CT in systemic lupus erythematosus. AJR Am J Roentgenol 1996;166:301.

79. Kozuka T, Johkoh T, Honda O, et al. Pulmonary involvement in mixed connective tissue disease: high-resolution CT findings in 41 patients. J Thorac Imaging 2001;16:94.

Histopathologic Approach to the Surgical Lung Biopsy in Interstitial Lung Disease

Kirk D. Jones, MD*, Anatoly Urisman, MD, PhD

KEYWORDS

- Interstitial lung disease • Biopsy • Fibrosis • Pneumonia

Interpretation of lung biopsy specimens is an integral part in the diagnosis of interstitial lung disease. The process of evaluating a surgical lung biopsy for disease involves answering several questions. Unlike much of surgical pathology of neoplastic lung disease, arriving at the correct diagnosis in nonneoplastic lung disease often requires correlation with clinical and radiologic findings. The topic of interstitial lung disease or diffuse infiltrative lung disease covers several hundred entities, and the pathology of interstitial lung disease has been the topic of several comprehensive textbooks. This article is not meant to be an encyclopedic overview of the topic but is rather meant to be a launching point in the clinician's approach to the histologic evaluation of lung disease.

WHAT DOES NORMAL LOOK LIKE

The first step in evaluating abnormal lung tissue is to understand the normal appearance of the lung. Just as the pulmonologist knows the difference between a healthy and sick patient, so the pathologist must know the difference between normal and diseased tissue when evaluating factors such as inflammation and fibrosis.

The lung can be divided into separate anatomic compartments of alveolar spaces, alveolar interstitium, large airways, small airways, pulmonary vessels, and pleura. When examining the lung, it is important to recognize the possibility of disease in any and all of these components. In addition, the alveolar parenchyma can be divided into various zones that can aid in generation of differential diagnoses. Several definitions are required here. A primary lobule is defined as that portion of the lung supplied by one respiratory bronchiole. A secondary lobule is defined as a region of lung, centered on a respiratory bronchiole, bound on its peripheral margins by fibrous interlobular septa and extending distally to the pleural surface (**Fig. 1**). This histologic construct is more easily recognized microscopically than the primary lobule; therefore, pathologists (and radiologists) often use the term lobule interchangeably with secondary lobule.

Much of the histologic assessment of the lung is performed by evaluation of the structures of the secondary lobule. The central portion of a secondary lobule contains the bronchovascular bundle, consisting of a small airway with associated pulmonary artery. The surrounding tissue consists of alveolar spaces and alveolar septa. The interlobular septa, at the periphery of the lobule, contain the pulmonary veins. The distal boundary of the lobule consists of the visceral pleura. The pulmonary lymphatics are present in the bronchovascular bundles, the interlobular septa, and the subpleural connective tissue. Using the structural unit of the

Disclosures: Dr Jones is a consultant for Actelion Pharmaceuticals.
Department of Pathology, University of California San Francisco, 505 Parnassus Avenue, Room M343, San Francisco, CA 94143-0102, USA
* Corresponding author.
E-mail address: kirk.jones@ucsf.edu

Clin Chest Med 33 (2012) 27–40
doi:10.1016/j.ccm.2012.01.003
0272-5231/12/$ – see front matter © 2012 Elsevier Inc. All rights reserved.

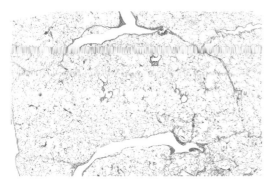

Fig. 1. The secondary lobule. Low magnification image of normal lung parenchyma highlights the pulmonary lobular architecture. Bronchioles and paired branches of pulmonary artery comprise the center of the lobule. The peripheral boundaries are delineated by the interlobular septa containing pulmonary veins and lymphatics and the visceral pleura.

lobule, several patterns of distribution can be described. A diffuse interstitial process involves the majority of the alveolar septa within the lobule. A bronchiolocentric process shows accentuation of the disease in the tissue surrounding the small airways. A peripheral lobular pattern shows accentuation of inflammation or fibrosis in the sub-pleural and paraseptal regions. A lymphatic pattern shows a distribution of disease involving the sub-pleural regions, the interlobular septa, and the bronchovascular bundles. Other patterns of disease include angiocentric and random distribution. Several of these distribution patterns can also describe consolidative processes in which there is alveolar filling.

Once one is familiar with normal tissue, there are a series of questions that can be asked to help define the disease process within the lung biopsy.

IS THIS ACUTE LUNG INJURY

Two common patterns of acute lung injury include diffuse alveolar damage and organizing pneumonia. Because these diseases can mimic other chronic fibrosing diseases, the first question to ask when evaluating a biopsy is if this can all be an acute process.

Diffuse alveolar damage is a histologic pattern of lung injury that results from damage to the endothelial and epithelial component of the alveolus: the alveolar capillary and type 1 pneumocyte. Histologically, the appearance of diffuse alveolar damage varies based on the time from the initial injury.[1,2] In the first hours after injury, the leaky alveolar vascular-epithelial barrier results in an accumulation of proteinaceous fluid within the alveolar spaces. Over the course of 12 to 24 hours, the alveolar septa become thickened by edema

and minimal acute and chronic inflammation. As the injury progresses, the alveolar walls have the appearance of granulation tissue–like fibrosis with proliferating fibroblasts within a myxoid matrix. The alveolar spaces show additional filling by hyaline membranes (Fig. 2). These hyaline membranes appear homogenously eosinophilic with a slight waxy appearance (the term is based on hyalos, Greek for glass). They are present in close apposition to the alveolar surface. Although appearing quite uniform on light microscopy, when viewed ultrastructurally, these hyaline membranes appear to be composed of a porridge of nucleoplasm, cytoplasm, fibrin, and other proteins secondary to the cell death that resulted from the acute injury. Often small vessels (usually pulmonary arteries ≤2 mm) show small luminal fibrin thrombi. This is thought to be secondary to activation of the coagulation cascade due to tissue damage.[3]

Over the course of days to weeks, the lung begins the process of attempted healing. This is termed organization and is characterized histologically by thickened alveolar septa, often with a sparse chronic inflammatory infiltrate, with a loose granulation tissuelike fibrosis. The alveolar walls are lined by type 2 pneumocytes, and there may be an increase in alveolar macrophages (Fig. 3). Often squamous metaplastic changes are observed in the distal bronchioles. The histologic changes of acute lung injury are summarized in Box 1.

The differential diagnosis in cases of acute lung injury includes infection, drug reaction, connective tissue disease, and fume inhalation injury. Many cases are idiopathic. Despite the prominence of neutrophils in alveolar lavage in patients with diffuse alveolar damage, most cases lack marked

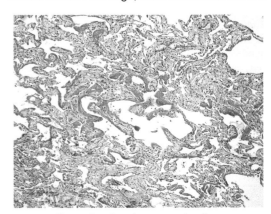

Fig. 2. Diffuse alveolar damage. Alveolar septa are thickened by edema and a sparse lymphocytic infiltrate. Alveolar spaces contain hyaline membranes, brightly eosinophilic filmlike material accumulating along alveolar septa.

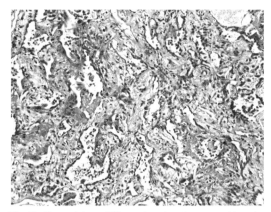

Fig. 3. Organizing diffuse alveolar damage. Alveolar septa are markedly thickened by granulation tissue–like fibrosis and mild chronic inflammation. There is prominent type 2 pneumocyte hyperplasia. The alveolar spaces contain increased alveolar macrophages as well as focal fibrinous material.

histologic neutrophilia. In patients with increased neutrophil levels, the differential diagnosis includes pulmonary infection, sepsis, trauma, and transfusion-related acute lung injury.

Organizing pneumonia is characterized histologically by alveolar filling with polypoid plugs of granulation tissue (**Fig. 4**A).[4,5] These plugs are rounded, often branching, and have a myxoid edematous quality. One can usually identify a separation from the alveolar septa at the periphery of these regions of airspace organization, a feature that differentiates them from interstitial fibroplasia. The term bronchiolitis obliterans organizing pneumonia has been used synonymously with organizing pneumonia, but this has been discouraged because of its confusion with bronchiolitis obliterans (aka constrictive bronchiolitis or cicatricial bronchiolitis), a disease characterized by circumferential

---

Box 1

Features of acute lung injury

Uniform alveolar septal thickening (may occasionally spare adjacent lobules)

Alveolar septal edema

Granulation tissue–like fibrosis

Hyaline membranes (pathognomonic of diffuse alveolar damage)

Fibrin and edema in airspaces

Type 2 pneumocyte hyperplasia

Small vessel thrombi

Squamous metaplasia of distal airways and alveolar ducts

Clinical picture of acute respiratory compromise

---

scarring of small airways and physiologic obstruction.[6,7] In organizing pneumonia, the airspace polyps are often present within the bronchiolar lumens, mimicking bronchiolar obliteration. Often the central portion of the polypoid plug contains the organized contents of the alveolar space. These may be chronic inflammatory cells, macrophages, or aspirated foreign material. Although etiologic clues may sometimes be found within these cores (see **Fig. 4**B), most often the polyps have only the appearance of bland granulation tissue. In these cases, histologic separation of cryptogenic organizing from an organizing infectious pneumonia or some other secondary organizing pneumonia (eg, from connective tissue disease) can be a futile task.

A third pattern of acute lung injury is acute fibrinous organizing pneumonia.[8] This pattern has a hybrid appearance between diffuse alveolar damage and organizing pneumonia and is characterized histologically by polypoid plugs of fibrin within airspaces (**Fig. 5**).

IS THERE FIBROSIS

Lung fibrosis can be simply defined as excess collagen deposition in the lung. This can be in the form of loose edematous granulation tissue–like fibrosis, as in organizing diffuse alveolar damage or organizing pneumonia, or dense collagenous fibrosis, as in fibrosing interstitial pneumonias.

Fibrotic lung disease can be evaluated using a pattern-based system categorized by the distribution within the secondary lobule. Certain diseases tend to follow a characteristic pattern of fibrosis. Whether the disease shows a peripheral lobular pattern, a diffuse pattern, a bronchiolocentric pattern, or a combination of these patterns can help establish a diagnosis or differential diagnosis (**Fig. 6**).

IS THIS USUAL INTERSTITIAL PNEUMONIA

Usual interstitial pneumonia (UIP) is characterized by peripheral lobular fibrosis such that the fibrosis is accentuated subpleurally and along interlobular septa. The histologic diagnosis is more accurately made when evidence of chronic active disease is seen; the chronicity is represented by fibrosis and microscopic honeycombing and the activity is represented by fibroblast foci.[9,10] Microscopic honeycombing really does not look much like honeycomb. Honeycomb, the wax structure made by bees, consists of a series of uniform hexagonal cells with thin partitions. Microscopic honeycombing of the sort observed in UIP is rarely uniform appearing and is characterized by

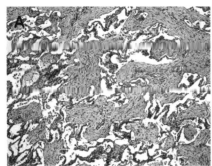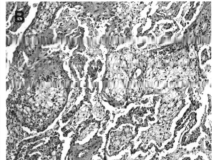

Fig. 4. Organizing pneumonia. (*A*) Cryptogenic organizing pneumonia. Alveolar spaces are consolidated by prominent rounded and branching polypoid plugs of granulation tissue. (*B*) Secondary organizing pneumonia due to amiodarone toxicity. Alveolar spaces are expanded by rounded aggregates of foamy macrophages containing lipid-like material. Focally, the foam cells are being incorporated into the interstitium. Type 2 pneumocyte hyperplasia is prominent.

irregular enlarged airspaces, lined by bronchiolar or cuboidal epithelium, frequently filled with mucin-containing occasional macrophages and neutrophils, surrounded by dense collagenous fibrosis often with interspersed smooth muscle. Fibroblast foci are usually present at the interface between the dense peripheral fibrosis and the central less-involved lung tissue. These foci are composed of fibroblasts within an edematous myxoid matrix. The fibroblasts are often arranged with their spindled nuclei parallel to the alveolar surface. An overlying layer of plump reactive epithelial cells is frequently present at the alveolar border. Fibroblast foci can occasionally be difficult to separate from organizing pneumonia but can be recognized by histologic clues and a clinical history of chronicity (**Table 1**). This variation in the stage of fibrosis from chronic to active within the same biopsy specimen has been termed temporal heterogeneity. This term has to be used with caution, however, for not everything that shows temporal heterogeneity is UIP (eg, a patient with fibrosis from smoking who has an acute pneumonia shows temporal heterogeneity). The temporal heterogeneity of UIP is often stereotypical with the worst fibrosis in subpleural regions, normal lung adjacent to bronchovascular bundles, and fibroblast foci at the interface between the two (**Fig. 7**). When one sees this classical temporal heterogeneity, the diagnosis is UIP and often correlates with the clinical entity idiopathic pulmonary fibrosis (IPF).

There are other diseases that may show similar histology, and it is important to look for clues that might separate them from IPF (**Box 2**).[11] Chronic hypersensitivity pneumonia may show peripheral fibrosis but is often also associated with bronchiolocentric fibrosis and poorly formed granulomas. Connective tissue disease may show a partial UIP pattern, but often the more central tissue is not normal and will have a uniform alveolar septal thickening (combining this UIP pattern with a nonspecific interstitial pneumonia [NSIP] pattern).[12,13] Connective tissue disease may also show pleural inflammation or prominent parenchymal lymphoid aggregates. Other diseases may show similar peripheral lobular fibrosis, but the distribution within the lung may be wrong (eg, apical subpleural fibrosis in a patient with spontaneous pneumothorax). This last point emphasizes why it is important to correlate all histologic findings with the imaging data.

When the biopsy consists of microscopic honeycombing and there is diffuse destructive fibrosis, it is tempting to use the term end-stage fibrotic lung or honeycomb lung. This may be acceptable in cases in which the pathologist knows the extent of disease by computed tomographic scan (and

Fig. 5. Acute fibrinous organizing pneumonia. The alveolar duct shows a rounded branching polypoid plug of organizing fibrin with sparse mixed inflammatory cells.

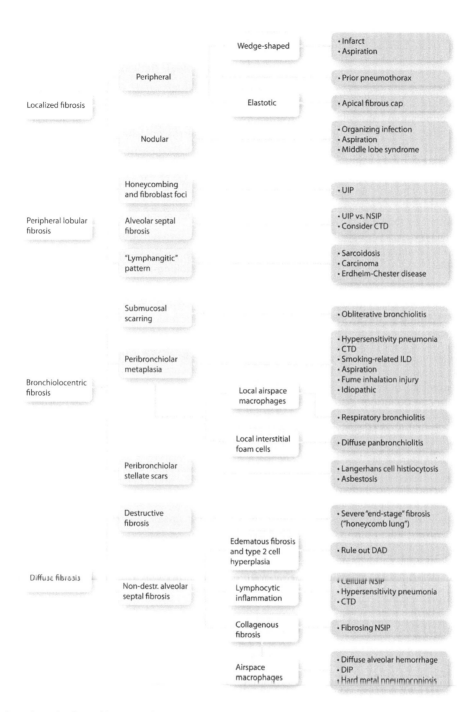

Fig. 6. Flow chart for lung fibrosis evaluation.

there is widespread uniform fibrosis), but occasionally this is not the case, and a biopsy report of end-stage lung is overzealously given to a localized region of scarring. It is preferable to be descriptive in these cases and to make the diagnosis of extensive interstitial fibrosis with a comment explaining that a scarring process is present throughout the biopsy. If clinical and radiologic data are available, it can be stated whether the histologic features are consistent with the clinical diagnosis. In many of these cases, the clinical data support a diagnosis of UIP.

Table 1 Differentiation of organizing pneumonia from fibroblast foci	
Organizing Pneumonia	Fibroblast Foci
Rounded or polypoid appearance	Bulgelike or crescentic
Airspace visible on most surfaces	Dense collagen present along half of surface
Located within airway or airspace	Located within interstitium
Branching common Thin or absent surface epithelial layer	Branching rare Reactive surface epithelial layer
Haphazardly arranged fibroblasts	Fibroblasts often parallel to alveolar surface

IS THIS NONSPECIFIC INTERSTITIAL PNEUMONIA

Diffuse widening of the alveolar septa without significant architectural destruction is referred to as Nonspecific Interstitial Pneumonia (NSIP). NSIP pattern can be further classified as cellular, in which inflammatory cells are the source of alveolar septal thickening, or fibrotic, in which collagen deposition is the cause of alveolar septal thickening.[14] The pattern of fibrosis in NSIP has been described as dusty cobweb fibrosis (**Fig. 8**). This is an easy description to remember, and it effectively describes the uniform alveolar septal thickening that is observed. The alveolar architecture remains relatively intact in this nondestructive type of fibrosis until fairly late in the disease when there is often alveolar simplification. The prognosis in NSIP is related to the extent of fibrosis, with cellular cases having a favorable prognosis and fibrotic cases showing decreased survival (although still somewhat better than UIP).[10,14]

Several pulmonary diseases show an NSIP pattern (**Box 3**). The most common entities with

Box 2 Diagnosis of UIP
Pathologic findings
Basilar and peripheral fibrosis grossly/radiographically
Subpleural and paraseptal fibrosis microscopically
Microscopic honeycombing subpleurally
Fibroblast foci at interface between fibrotic and less-involved lung
Normal appearance of the lung in centrilobular regions
Clues for alternative diagnoses
Bronchiolocentric fibrosis: chronic HP, CTD, smoking-related lung disease
Granulomas: chronic HP
Centrilobular lung shows diffuse NSIP-like thickening: CTD
Pleural inflammation/fibrosis: CTD
Apical distribution: apical fibrous cap, prior pneumothorax, pneumoconiosis
Alveolar macrophage accumulation: smoking-related lung disease, drug reaction
Age <50 years: CTD, familial interstitial fibrosis (surfactant C mutations, telomerase mutations)
Abbreviations: CTD, connective tissue disease; HP, hypersensitivity pneumonia.

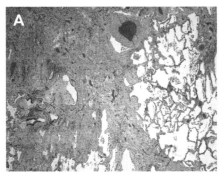
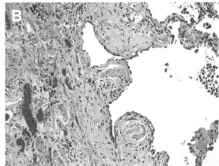

Fig. 7. UIP. (*A*) Low magnification image shows the classical temporal heterogeneity of UIP. Marked interstitial fibrosis with subpleural microscopic honeycombing is present at lower left, while relatively normal-appearing parenchyma is seen more centrally at lower right. (*B*) High magnification view of an area at the interface between fibrotic and less-involved parenchyma shows several fibroblast foci. Note the presence of type 2 cell hyperplasia in the overlying epithelium.

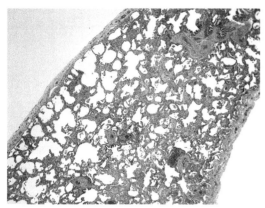

Fig. 8. Fibrotic NSIP. Low magnification view of lung parenchyma shows variable but diffuse alveolar septal thickening by collagenous fibrosis. Patchy chronic interstitial inflammation and peribronchiolar metaplasia is present.

this pattern are connective tissue disease, drug reactions, and hypersensitivity pneumonia. Other diseases that show diffuse alveolar septal widening that can mimic NSIP include acute diseases such as organizing diffuse alveolar damage,[2] fibrotic diseases such as smoking-related interstitial fibrosis,[15] and more unusual diseases such as the alveolar septal pattern of amyloidosis.[16]

IS THE FIBROSIS BRONCHIOLOCENTRIC

There are 2 forms of bronchiolocentric fibrosis. In the first, the fibrosis extends along the alveolar ducts and peribronchiolar alveolar septa without significant architectural destruction. This peribronchiolar fibrosis is often accompanied by a change

in the alveolar lining from type 1 pneumocytes to a cuboidal or respiratory epithelium. This process is known as peribronchiolar metaplasia, bronchiolization of alveolar ducts, or lambertosis (**Fig. 9**). This peribronchiolar metaplasia often results in a lacy appearance in the central portion of the secondary lobule, which can be appreciated at low power. The second type of bronchiolocentric fibrosis, obliterative bronchiolitis, is often more difficult to identify histologically and is described later.

Peribronchiolar fibrosis is present in several conditions, most of which share a common etiology of chronic bronchiolar irritation or inflammation.[17–19] The differential diagnosis includes smoking-related interstitial lung disease (respiratory bronchiolitis (**Fig. 10**), pulmonary Langerhans cell histiocytosis), connective tissue disease, chronic hypersensitivity pneumonia, pneumoconiosis, fume inhalation injury, chronic aspiration, infection, and diffuse panbronchiolitis.

IS THE BIOPSY TOO CELLULAR OR INFLAMED

The normal alveolar septum is a delicate-appearing structure with only a few visible nuclei. Across the length of an alveolar wall, there are distinct spaces between nuclei, and only rare back-to-back nuclei are noted across its width. If nuclear crowding is observed with several nuclei touching each other along the length, or several septa thicker than 2 cells, then the interstitium is too cellular. In the normal septum, the nuclei are derived from capillary endothelial cells and pneumocytes. When the septa are too cellular, the cause is often lymphocytic inflammation. As the inflammatory infiltrate increases within the alveolar

---

Box 3
Diagnosis of nonspecific interstitial pneumonia

Pathologic findings

Uniform alveolar septal thickening (ie, there are similar degrees of inflammation or fibrosis in peripheral, central, and transitional zones within the lobule)

Clues for alternative diagnoses

Bronchiolocentric fibrosis: chronic HP, CTD, smoking-related ILD

Granulomas: chronic HP

Pleural inflammation/fibrosis: CTD

Lymphoid aggregates/germinal centers: CTD, smoking-related ILD

Abbreviations: CTD, connective tissue disease; HP, hypersensitivity pneumonia; ILD, interstitial lung disease.

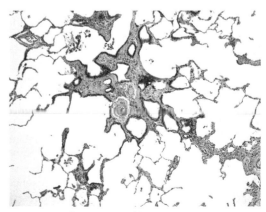

Fig. 9. Bronchiolocentric fibrosis. The alveolar septa surrounding a central bronchiole shows mild thickening by collagenous fibrosis. The fibrosis is associated with prominent peribronchiolar metaplasia. Note the normal delicate alveolar septa more distally.

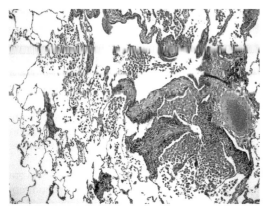

Fig. 10. Respiratory bronchiolitis. Alveolar spaces surrounding an airway are filled with lightly pigmented (smoker's) macrophages. Subtle bronchiolocentric fibrosis with mild chronic inflammation and peribronchiolar metaplasia are also present.

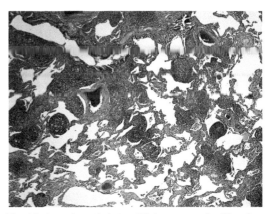

Fig. 11. Lymphocytic interstitial pneumonia. The alveolar septa show prominent diffuse thickening by lymphocytes, occasionally forming rounded lymphoid aggregates with germinal center formation.

septa, the diagnosis moves from cellular nonspecific pneumonia (or cellular interstitial pneumonia) to lymphocytic interstitial pneumonia.[20] If the cellularity is accentuated around bronchioles in lymphoid follicles, the term follicular bronchiolitis is used.

IS THIS CELLULAR NONSPECIFIC INTERSTITIAL PNEUMONIA

Cellular NSIP is characterized by uniform alveolar septal thickening by mild to moderate chronic inflammation composed of lymphocytes and plasma cells.[14] The differential diagnosis in cellular NSIP is similar to that for fibrotic NSIP. When a diagnosis of cellular NSIP is made, connective tissue disease, drug reaction, hypersensitivity pneumonia, and infection should be considered.

As the number of lymphoid aggregates and density of the lymphocytic infiltrate increase, the term lymphocytic interstitial pneumonia may be more appropriate (**Fig. 11**).[20] The question how dense should the infiltrate be tends to be subjective. Most cases tend to show alveolar septa that are at least half as wide as the adjacent alveolar space. The differential diagnosis includes connective tissue disease (eg, Sjögren syndrome, rheumatoid arthritis), immune deficiency states (eg, congenital human immunodeficiency viral infection, common variable immunodeficiency), and lymphoma. Lymphomas are often identified by the presence of a dominant nodule with lymphangitic extension of the inflammatory infiltrate along interlobular septa and subpleural regions. They are also more commonly of B-lymphocytic origin, whereas most cases of lymphocytic interstitial pneumonia are rich in T lymphocytes. Flow cytometric analysis of

lymphocyte surface markers or immunohistochemical staining for B and T lymphocyte markers may be used to separate neoplastic lymphoproliferative disorders from nonneoplastic processes.

ARE THERE GRANULOMAS

Granulomas are aggregates of inflammatory cells (particularly histiocytes) that form as a result of chronic irritation, infection, inflammation, or immune stimulation. Within the lung, solitary localized granulomatous nodules or diffuse granulomatous diseases can be observed.

HOW CAN THE GRANULOMAS BE FURTHER CLASSIFIED

The pathologist assesses several histologic features of the granuloma simultaneously to make a correct diagnosis.[21–24] These features include aspects of distribution (eg, random, lymphangitic), quantity (frequent or rare), and quality of the granulomas (eg, necrosis, coalescence). In practice, most pathologists are familiar with several histologic patterns that characterize granuloma types, including sarcoidal granulomas, necrotizing granulomas, and scattered small granulomas within a background of interstitial inflammation or fibrosis (**Box 4**).

Sarcoidal Granulomas

Sarcoidal granulomas show several classic histologic features. The granulomas are composed of tightly packed histiocytes, many of which show a characteristic boomerang-shaped nucleus. There is little to no lymphocytic inflammatory cuff (thus the designation of naked granuloma) (**Fig. 12**A). Rather the granulomas, as they age,

---

Box 4
Differential diagnosis for granulomatous diseases

Sarcoidal granulomas: characterized by rounded, coalescent, well-defined granulomas with sparse inflammation and no necrosis

  Sarcoidosis

  Metal-related sarcoid reaction (eg, chronic beryllium disease)

  Drug reaction (eg, interferon-α therapy)

  Infection (sarcoidal granulomas are often present at the periphery of necrotic granulomas)

Necrotizing granulomas: Characterized by central necrosis with surrounding histiocytic inflammation

  With granular necrosis (caseation): mycobacterial infection, fungal infection

  With infarctlike necrosis: parasite (eg, *Dirofilaria*), mycobacteria, fungus

  With prominent eosinophils: coccidioidomycosis, parasite

  With prominent neutrophils: blastomycosis, aspiration, actinomycosis, nocardiosis

Interstitial pneumonias with granulomas: characterized by interstitial inflammation or fibrosis with small nonnecrotizing granulomas

  Hypersensitivity pneumonia

  Atypical mycobacteria (eg, hot tub lung, Lady Windermere syndrome)

  Drug reaction (eg, methotrexate)

  Connective tissue disease (especially Sjögren syndrome)

  Inflammatory bowel disease

  Common variable immunodeficiency (granulomatous lymphocytic interstitial lung disease)

Mimics and granuloma-like diseases: characterized by histiocyte-rich inflammation or nodular necrosis

  Wegener granulomatosis

  Rheumatoid nodule

  Lymphomatoid granulomatosis

  Pulmonary venous infarction

  Malakoplakia

---

often obtain a cuff of hyaline collagenous fibrosis. The distribution is characteristically in a lymphangitic pattern, present in bronchovascular bundles, along the pleura, and in interlobular septa (see Fig. 12B). In addition, the granulomas frequently merge into each other, making a coalescent multinodular beading along the routes mentioned earlier. Although the classic description of sarcoidosis is nonnecrotizing, small central areas of fibrinoid necrosis can occasionally be observed, which can mimic caseation.

Sarcoidal granulomas are present in the multisystemic inflammatory disease sarcoidosis. They can also be observed in metal-related sarcoid reactions as in chronic beryllium disease and rare earth metal exposure, drug reactions as in interferon-α or antiretroviral therapy, or in infection. Infectious granulomas often show a prominent dominant necrotic granuloma with satellite sarcoidal granulomas in the adjacent tissue.

Although the granulomas of sarcoidosis have several distinct qualities that make them some of the more easily recognizable granulomatous illnesses, most pathologists and pulmonologists have heard the mantra that sarcoidosis is a diagnosis of exclusion. The pathologist should recognize the features that make a biopsy likely to represent sarcoidosis and then give a descriptive diagnosis, such as nonnecrotizing granulomas. Then the diagnosis can be qualified with the statement "consistent with sarcoidosis" in either the diagnosis line or in a diagnostic comment.

Necrotizing Granulomas

Granulomatous inflammation with (usually central) necrosis is referred to as necrotizing. This term is not precisely synonymous with caseating, although it is often used as such. If used accurately, the term caseous applies only to the gross pathologic cheeselike appearance of several necrotic lesions, including granulomas or neoplasms. There is no defined microscopic appearance that corresponds to the gross appearance of caseation; however, it usually has an eosinophilic granular quality and tends to destroy the underlying parenchymal architecture. Most necrotizing granulomas are caused by infection. Cultures should be sent at the time of surgery (either by the surgeon or by the pathologist after identification of a gross lesion). When confronted by necrotizing granulomas, staining for fungus and staining for acid-fast bacilli should be performed. Grocott methenamine silver stain is preferred for fungi because the periodic acid-Schiff stain tends not to stain 2 common lung pathogens: *Pneumocystis jiroveci* and *Histoplasma capsulatum*. In a study of solitary necrotizing granulomas, El-Zammar and Katzenstein[23] noted that in cases of tuberculosis (as well as histoplasmosis) the organisms were only identified in the central

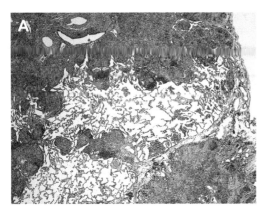
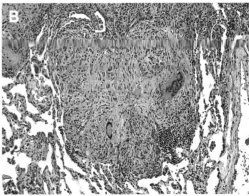

Fig. 12. (*A*) Sarcoidosis. In this low power view, the lymphangitic distribution of coalescent rounded granulomas is observed with aggregation around bronchovascular bundle (*upper left*) and interlobular septum lower right. The pleura shows mild involvement in this section. (*B*) Sarcoidosis. This high power view shows a rounded single granuloma composed of epithelioid histiocytes with occasional curved nuclei and occasional multinucleate giant cells.

necrotic portions of the granuloma. In other fungal diseases, the organisms were more randomly distributed throughout the granuloma. This information is helpful, as the biggest deterrent to identification of microorganisms on special stains is time. If the lesions look suspicious for infection, two or more blocks should be stained for microorganisms; however, pathologists should not perform stains on more blocks than they have time to carefully examine. The absence of identifiable organisms is not equivalent to the absence of infectious disease, and all cases should be correlated with clinical data and microbiologic cultures.

A small number of necrotizing granulomas are secondary to aspiration. The easiest method of recognizing such a process is when there are food particles within the granuloma. One of the more characteristic particles is leguminous pulse (**Fig. 13**). The cellulose shells and cotyledons form a rounded structure with internal smaller rounded starch granules. A vigorous giant cell reaction may be present in cases of aspiration. Acutely, one sees numerous neutrophils adjacent to the foreign material.

Interstitial Lung Disease with Associated Small Granulomas

Several diseases are characterized by the pattern of a diffuse or bronchiolocentric alveolar septal inflammatory infiltrate (NSIP or bronchiolocentric pattern) with scattered granulomas within the interstitium. The 2 most common diagnoses in this scenario are hypersensitivity pneumonia and atypical mycobacterial infection in an immunocompetent host (ie, hot tub lung).

Hypersensitivity pneumonia is an immunologically mediated pulmonary disease that results from a reaction to inhaled organic dusts.[11,25,26] The most common causes are molds, animal dander (bird antigens such as bloom), bacteria, and chemicals. The histologic findings in hypersensitivity pneumonia consist of what is sometimes referred to as a triad of 4 findings: (1a) a diffuse lymphoplasmacytic interstitial infiltrate, (1b) with bronchiolocentric accentuation, (2) poorly formed granulomas, and (3) foci of organizing pneumonia. The poorly formed granulomas of hypersensitivity pneumonia consist of loose aggregates of epithelioid histiocytes with or without multinucleate giant cells (**Fig. 14**). Their edges are poorly defined, and they tend to blend into the adjacent interstitium. Cholesterol clefts within giant cells are a common, but nonspecific, finding in hypersensitivity pneumonia, within

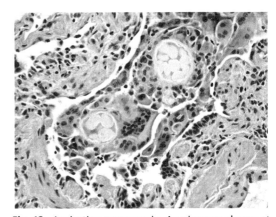

Fig. 13. Aspiration pneumonia. An airspace, shown at high magnification, contains several macrophages and multinucleated giant cells aggregating around aspirated foreign material with the characteristic appearance of leguminous pulse (bits of bean). Alveolar septa show mild chronic inflammation and type 2 pneumocyte hyperplasia.

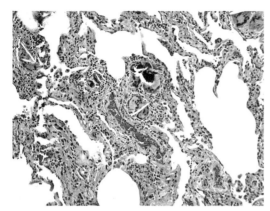

Fig. 14. Hypersensitivity pneumonia. The poorly formed granuloma of hypersensitivity pneumonia consists of a loose interstitial aggregate of multinucleate histiocytes with mild associated lymphocytic inflammation. One giant cell contains a chunky Schaumann body (cytoplasmic calcium carbonate), whereas another shows an acicular cleft consistent with cholesterol crystal.

granulomas or singly. Giant cells with cholesterol clefts are common in the airspaces in patients with physiologic obstruction. However, when present in the interstitium, they are more specific for hypersensitivity pneumonia.

Hot tub lung is a combination immunologic reaction and infection resulting from inhalation of aerosolized Mycobacterium avium-intracellulare complex (MAC), usually from indoor spas with Jacuzzi-like jets but also from contaminated showerheads in poorly ventilated rooms.[27,28] The biopsy in hot tub lung overlaps histologically with sarcoidosis and hypersensitivity pneumonia. The granulomas tend to be randomly distributed throughout the lung parenchyma, are usually well formed, and often occur as solitary granulomas rather than coalescent nodules. The granulomas of hot tub lung also commonly show a mild to moderate cuff of lymphocytes, unlike the usually naked granulomas of sarcoidosis. The results of special staining techniques for mycobacteria are almost always negative, but the techniques should be performed. Cultures of lung tissue or bronchial washings frequently reveal the organism; however, they may take weeks to grow out.

There are several other scenarios in which one sees MAC in immunocompetent patients: in patients with chronic obstructive pulmonary disease or bronchiectasis and in those with middle lobe syndrome (Lady Windermere syndrome).[29] In both settings, there is probable colonization and infection secondary to abnormal clearance of secretions.

Other Causes of Cellular Interstitial Pneumonia with Granulomas

Several drugs may result in a histologic picture indistinguishable from hypersensitivity pneumonitis. Some of the more common culprits are methotrexate,[30] nitrofurantoin,[31] and mesalazine.[32] A useful resource when investigating whether a particular drug may result in lung injury is the Web site of the Groupe d'Etudes de la Pathologie Pulmonaire Iatrogène (www.pneumotox.com).[33] Necrosis within the granulomas essentially eliminates drug reaction from the differential and makes infection the likely cause. Granulomas in cases of collagen vascular disease are relatively unusual; however, in cases in which there is an extensive lymphocytic infiltrate, one can find small scattered granulomas.[34] This is most common in cases of Sjögren syndrome. Necrotic nodules with peripheral palisading histiocytes may be observed in rheumatoid nodules as part of rheumatoid arthritis. Patients with inflammatory bowel disease may have small airway involvement with or without granulomatous inflammation.[35] Lung involvement is described in both patients with ulcerative colitis and those with Crohn disease, but granulomatous inflammation is more common in the latter. It is important to rule out a drug reaction in these patients because mesalazine (aka mesalamine or 5-aminosalicylic acid) may also cause this histologic picture. Patients with common variable immunodeficiency often show lymphocytic interstitial pneumonia. Occasional cases will show small poorly formed granulomas. This pattern of lung disease has been recently termed granulomatous lymphocytic interstitial lung disease.[36,37] Finding a rare nonnecrotizing granuloma in specimens resected for malignancy is relatively common. They may be a result of antigen stimulation by the tumor or may be related to prior infection or immune reaction. In these cases, obtaining stains on a single block is sufficient.

THIS LOOKS NORMAL, WHAT AM I MISSING

It is well known that when a person is concentrating on a specific problem, other obvious changes can occur without notice. This inattentional blindness[38] can occur in the interpretation of lung biopsies when the pathologist is focused on alveolar spaces and interstitium and the other compartments of the lung, particularly small airways and blood vessels, are ignored.

Obliterative Bronchiolitis

Obliterative bronchiolitis, also called constrictive bronchiolitis or cicatricial bronchiolitis, is a small airway disease characterized by concentric subepithelial scarring with narrowing of the bronchiolar lumens (Fig. 15),[17–19] In these cases, there are 2 primary difficulties in recognition. First, the bronchioles do not show extended long segments of fibrosis but rather show focal stenotic scarring. This leads to underrecognition due to the paucity of identifiable lesions. Second, the fibrotic lesions may completely obscure the normal appearance of the bronchiole, replacing it with a small nodular scar. To overcome these difficulties, 2 strategies may be used. First, multiple step sections may be obtained to increase the likelihood of observing pathologic changes, and, second, elastic tissue stains may be obtained to help identify the epithelial elastica within the scar. It is also helpful to remember that pulmonary arteries run alongside bronchioles in the centrilobular bronchovascular bundle. The identification of a scar adjacent to an artery is a clue to the diagnosis of obliterative bronchiolitis. Other histologic changes of obstruction may also be observed, including peribronchiolar foam cell accumulation and airspace cholesterol granuloma formation. Obliterative bronchiolitis is observed in chronic pulmonary transplant rejection, graft-versus-host disease, connective tissue disease, drug reactions, and postinfectious scarring.

Pulmonary Hypertension

Pulmonary hypertension may result from arterial or venous abnormalities. Pulmonary arterial disease is more common and is more readily identified histologically than its venous counterpart. The pulmonary arteries show luminal narrowing

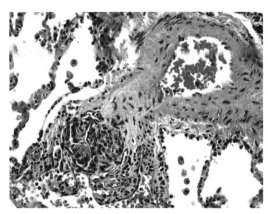

Fig. 16. Plexiform arteriopathy. A pulmonary artery shows mural disruption and emergence of a plexiform lesion characterized by a tangle collection of thin-walled vessels.

characterized by several histologic patterns. Plexiform arteriopathy is recognized by bulgelike tangled small vascular channels within or adjacent to small pulmonary arteries (Fig. 16). Thrombotic arteriopathy shows intimal thickening and luminal occlusion with histologic changes of recanalization. Other cases show only medial and intimal thickening. Elastic tissue stains may be helpful in identifying these lesions.

Pulmonary venous hypertension tends to be a more histologically subtle finding. Although pulmonary venoocclusive disease or occlusive venopathy may rarely be seen within the large veins in the interlobular septa, it is most often present in the smaller postcapillary venules within the lung parenchyma.[39] These small veins show intimal thickening by fibrosis. Elastic tissue stains are useful in these cases both to demonstrate the degree of fibrosis and to differentiate pulmonary veins (which have a single elastic layer) from pulmonary arteries (which have a dual elastic

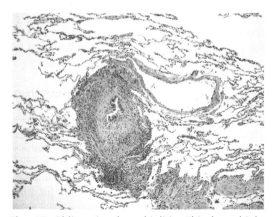

Fig. 15. Obliterative bronchiolitis. This bronchiole, present adjacent to its partnering pulmonary artery, shows luminal narrowing due to subepithelial scarring. The original diameter of the airway is approximated by the ring of surrounding submucosal smooth muscle.

Box 5
Clues for vascular disease

Pulmonary arterial hypertension

   Pulmonary atherosclerosis

   Plexiform lesions

Pulmonary venous disease

   Increased airspace siderophages

   Encrustation of vascular elastica

   Mild increase in alveolar septal cellularity

   Pulmonary capillary hemangiomatosislike changes

   Pulmonary venous intimal sclerosis

layer). As in other causes of increased pulmonary venous pressures (eg, sclerosing mediastinitis, congestive heart failure, mitral valve disease), there are additional histologic clues to prompt the pathologist to consider occlusive venopathy (**Box 5**).[40]

IS THERE A DIAGNOSIS THAT I AM FORGETTING

Absolutely. We cannot emphasize enough the value of putting together a strong team of clinicians, radiologists, and pathologists to minimize the chance of missing a diagnosis. A good clinician and radiologist can perform as the pathologist's alchemists; their data can turn a leaden descriptive diagnosis into a golden specific diagnosis.

REFERENCES

1. Tomashefski JF Jr. Pulmonary pathology of acute respiratory distress syndrome. Clin Chest Med 2000;21:435–66.
2. Beasley MB. The pathologist's approach to acute lung injury. Arch Pathol Lab Med 2010;134:719–27.
3. Ware LB, Matthay MA. The acute respiratory distress syndrome. N Engl J Med 2000;342:1334–49.
4. Epler GR. Bronchiolitis obliterans organizing pneumonia: definition and clinical features. Chest 1992; 102(Suppl 1):2S–6S.
5. Epler GR, Colby TV, McLoud TC, et al. Bronchiolitis obliterans organizing pneumonia. N Engl J Med 1985;312:152–8.
6. American Thoracic Society/European Respiratory Society International Multidisciplinary Consensus Classification of the Idiopathic Interstitial Pneumonias. This joint statement of the American Thoracic Society (ATS), and the European Respiratory Society (ERS) was adopted by the ATS board of directors, June 2001 and by the ERS Executive Committee, June 2001. Am J Respir Crit Care Med 2002;165:277–304.
7. Nicholson AG. Classification of idiopathic interstitial pneumonias: making sense of the alphabet soup. Histopathology 2002;41:381–91.
8. Beasley MB, Franks TJ, Galvin JR, et al. Acute fibrinous and organizing pneumonia: a histological pattern of lung injury and possible variant of diffuse alveolar damage. Arch Pathol Lab Med 2002;126: 1064–70.
9. Katzenstein AL, Myers JL. Idiopathic pulmonary fibrosis: clinical relevance of pathologic classification. Am J Respir Crit Care Med 1998,157.1301–15.
10. Travis WD, Matsui K, Moss J, et al. Idiopathic nonspecific interstitial pneumonia: prognostic significance of cellular and fibrosing patterns: survival comparison with usual interstitial pneumonia and desquamative interstitial pneumonia. Am J Surg Pathol 2000;24:19–33.
11. Trahan S, Hanak V, Ryu JH, et al. Role of surgical lung biopsy in separating chronic hypersensitivity pneumonia from usual interstitial pneumonia/idiopathic pulmonary fibrosis: analysis of 31 biopsies from 15 patients. Chest 2008;134:126–32.
12. Nicholson AG, Colby TV, Wells AU. Histopathological approach to patterns of interstitial pneumonia in patient with connective tissue disorders. Sarcoidosis Vasc Diffuse Lung Dis 2002;19:10–7.
13. Nakamura Y, Chida K, Suda T, et al. Nonspecific interstitial pneumonia in collagen vascular diseases: comparison of the clinical characteristics and prognostic significance with usual interstitial pneumonia. Sarcoidosis Vasc Diffuse Lung Dis 2003; 20(3):235–41.
14. Katzenstein AL, Fiorelli RF. Nonspecific interstitial pneumonia/fibrosis. Histologic features and clinical significance. Am J Surg Pathol 1994;18:136–47.
15. Katzenstein AL, Mukhopadhyay S, Zanardi C, et al. Clinically occult interstitial fibrosis in smokers: classification and significance of a surprisingly common finding in lobectomy specimens. Hum Pathol 2010; 41:316–25.
16. Utz JP, Swensen SJ, Gertz MA. Pulmonary amyloidosis. The Mayo Clinic experience from 1980 to 1993. Ann Intern Med 1996;124:407–13.
17. Couture C, Colby TV. Histopathology of bronchiolar disorders. Semin Respir Crit Care Med 2003;24: 489–98.
18. Cordier JF. Challenges in pulmonary fibrosis. 2: bronchiolocentric fibrosis. Thorax 2007;62:638–49.
19. Visscher DW, Myers JL. Bronchiolitis: the pathologist's perspective. Proc Am Thorac Soc 2006;3: 41–7.
20. Swigris JJ, Berry GJ, Raffin TA, et al. Lymphoid interstitial pneumonia: a narrative review. Chest 2002; 122.2150–04.
21. Hutton Klein JR, Tazelaar HD, Leslie KO, et al. One hundred consecutive granulomas in a pulmonary pathology consultation practice. Am J Surg Pathol 2010;34:1456–64.
22. Cheung OY, Muhm JR, Helmers RA, et al. Surgical pathology of granulomatous interstitial pneumonia. Ann Diagn Pathol 2003;7:127–38.
23. El-Zammar OA, Katzenstein AL. Pathological diagnosis of granulomatous lung disease: a review. Histopathology 2007;50:289–310.
24. Mukhopadhyay S, Gal AA. Granulomatous lung disease: an approach to the differential diagnosis. Arch Pathol Lab Med 2010;134:667–90.
25. Patel AM, Ryu JH, Reed CE. Hypersensitivity pneumonitis: current concepts and future questions. J Allergy Clin Immunol 2001;108:661–70.
26. Coleman A, Colby TV. Histologic diagnosis of extrinsic allergic alveolitis. Am J Surg Pathol 1988;12:514–8.

27. Agarwal R, Nath A. Hot-tub lung: hypersensitivity to Mycobacterium avium but not hypersensitivity pneumonitis. Respir Med 2006;100:1478.

28. Hanak V, Kalra S, Aksamit TR, et al. Hot tub lung: presenting features and clinical course of 21 patients. Respir Med 2006;100:610–5.

29. Kwon KY, Myers JL, Swensen SJ, et al. Middle lobe syndrome: a clinicopathological study of 21 patients. Hum Pathol 1995;26:302–7.

30. Imokawa S, Colby TV, Leslie KO, et al. Methotrexate pneumonitis: review of the literature and histopathological findings in nine patients. Eur Respir J 2000; 15:373–81.

31. Taskinen E, Tukiainen P, Sovijarvi AR. Nitrofurantoin-induced alterations in pulmonary tissue. A report on five patients with acute or subacute reactions. Acta Pathol Microbiol Scand A 1977;85(5):713–20.

32. Foster RA, Zander DS, Mergo PJ, et al. Mesalamine-related lung disease: clinical, radiographic, and pathologic manifestations. Inflamm Bowel Dis 2003;9(5):308–15.

33. Camus P, Fanton A, Bonniaud P, et al. Interstitial lung disease induced by drugs and radiation. Respiration 2004;71:301–26.

34. Colby TV. Pulmonary pathology in patients with systemic autoimmune diseases. Clin Chest Med 1998;19:587–612, vii.

35. Camus P, Colby TV. The lung in inflammatory bowel disease. Eur Respir J 2000;15:5–10.

36. Bates CA, Ellison MC, Lynch DA, et al. Granulomatous-lymphocytic lung disease shortens survival in common variable immunodeficiency. J Allergy Clin Immunol 2004;114(2):415–21.

37. Park JH, Levinson AI. Granulomatous-lymphocytic interstitial lung disease (GLILD) in common variable immunodeficiency (CVID). Clin Immunol 2010;134: 97–103.

38. Simons DJ, Chabris CF. Gorillas in our midst: sustained inattentional blindness for dynamic events. Perception 1999;28:1059–74.

39. Montani D, O'Callaghan DS, Savale L, et al. Pulmonary veno-occlusive disease: recent progress and current challenges. Respir Med 2010;104(Suppl 1): S23–32.

40. Lantuejoul S, Sheppard MN, Corrin B, et al. Pulmonary veno-occlusive disease and pulmonary capillary hemangiomatosis: a clinicopathologic study of 35 cases. Am J Surg Pathol 2006;30:850–7.

Idiopathic Pulmonary Fibrosis: Diagnosis and Epidemiology

Amy L. Olson, MD, MSPH*, Jeffrey J. Swigris, DO, MS

KEYWORDS

- Idiopathic pulmonary fibrosis • Diagnosis
- Epidemiology • Treatment

Idiopathic pulmonary fibrosis (IPF) is defined as a chronic fibrosing interstitial pneumonia of unknown cause with a histologic pattern of usual interstitial pneumonia (UIP) on surgical lung biopsy. IPF is a lung-limited process that tends to occur in older adults. It is the most common of the idiopathic interstitial pneumonias (IIPs), among which it has the worst prognosis, with median survival estimates ranging from 3 to 5 years after diagnosis.[1–3]

In 2000, the American Thoracic Society (ATS) and European Respiratory Society (ERS) published the first consensus statement providing guidelines on the diagnosis and treatment of IPF.[1] This statement presented, for the first time, diagnostic criteria for IPF and recommendations for treatment. Over the past decade, results from several studies have reshaped the thinking on IPF, and as a result, the guidelines have been recently revised using an evidence-based approach.[2] Meanwhile, several epidemiologic studies have yielded data that identify potential risk factors and that better define the societal burden of IPF. This article summarizes the approach to diagnosing IPF and reviews epidemiologic data on IPF.

THE DIAGNOSIS OF IPF

Over the past decade, emerging data have helped to refine the diagnostic criteria for IPF. In 2000, a collaborative effort among the ATS, ERS, and American College of Chest Physicians resulted in an international consensus statement for the diagnosis of IPF.[1] That statement, formulated on expert opinion and interpretation of available research at the time, held that a definitive diagnosis of IPF required a surgical lung biopsy showing a UIP pattern of lung injury and the following 3 criteria: (1) exclusion of other known causes of interstitial lung disease (ILD), including drug toxicities, environmental exposures, and collagen vascular diseases; (2) abnormal pulmonary function tests or impaired gas exchange; and (3) imaging consistent with this diagnosis. In the absence of a surgical lung biopsy, a diagnosis of probable IPF required all of the following 4 major criteria: (1) exclusion of other causes of ILD; (2) abnormal pulmonary function tests or impaired gas exchange; (3) bibasilar reticular abnormalities with minimal ground-glass opacities on high-resolution computed tomography (HRCT); and (4) transbronchial lung biopsy or bronchoalveolar lavage specimens without features to support an alternative diagnosis along with at least 3 of 4 minor criteria (age >50 years, the insidious onset of dyspnea, a duration of symptoms greater than 3 months, and bibasilar, inspiratory crackles).

Since that time, additional evidence has shown the value of HRCT in diagnosing IPF: when an experienced radiologist can say with high confidence that the pattern on HRCT is consistent with a histologic UIP pattern, UIP is the histologic pattern identified in more than 90% of cases.[4–7] Based on these and other data supporting the accuracy of HRCT, a surgical lung biopsy is no longer required for a definitive diagnosis of IPF in

Interstitial Lung Disease Program, Division of Pulmonary and Critical Care Medicine, Autoimmune Lung Center, National Jewish Health, 1400 Jackson Street, Denver, CO 80206, USA
* Corresponding author. Interstitial Lung Disease Program, Autoimmune Lung Center, National Jewish Health, 1400 Jackson Street, F-107, Denver, CO 80206.
E-mail address: olsona@njhealth.org

Clin Chest Med 33 (2012) 41–50
doi:10.1016/j.ccm.2011.12.001

cases with a radiologic UIP pattern and a compatible clinical presentation,[3] and the characteristic HRCT pattern of a UIP pattern of lung injury has been defined (**Box 1**). Given a characteristic HRCT pattern, the diagnosis of IPF still requires exclusion of other known causes of ILD, including domestic, occupational, or environmental exposures, connective tissue diseases, and drug toxicities.

For diagnosing IPF, the sensitivity of HRCT is significantly lower than its positive predictive value[4–9]; thus, when the characteristic HRCT pattern is absent, a surgical lung biopsy showing a UIP pattern is still required to make a definitive diagnosis of IPF.[3] Histologic criteria have been devised to allow pathologists to categorize findings in surgical lung biopsy specimens as definite, possible, probable,

---

Box 1
Criteria for a definite, possible, and inconsistent UIP pattern on HRCT scan

Definite UIP Pattern (requires all 4 of the following features)

Subpleural, basal predominance

Reticular abnormality

Honeycombing without traction bronchiectasis

Absence of features that are inconsistent with a UIP pattern (see "Possible UIP Pattern")

Possible UIP Pattern

Same as the criteria for a definite UIP pattern, although honeycombing is not present

Inconsistent with UIP Pattern (any of the following 7 features)

Upper-lung or midlung predominance

Peribronchovascular predominance

Extensive ground-glass abnormality (defined as the extent of the ground-glass abnormality is greater than the extent of the reticular abnormality)

Profuse micronodules

Discrete cysts

Diffuse mosaic attenuation or air-trapping (bilateral, in 3 of more lobes)

Consolidation in bronchopulmonary segments or lobes

Data from American Thoracic Society; European Respiratory Society. American Thoracic Society/European Respiratory Society International Multidisciplinary Consensus Classification of the Idiopathic Interstitial Pneumonias. This joint statement of the American Thoracic Society (ATS), and the European Respiratory Society (ERS) was adopted by the ATS board of directors, June 2001 and by the ERS Executive Committee, June 2001. Am J Respir Crit Care Med 2001;165:277–304.

---

or not UIP (**Box 2**). In addition, the recently published evidence-based guidelines provide a framework for interpreting permutations of HRCT and histologic data (**Table 1**).

Challenges in Diagnosing IPF

A threat to making a confident diagnosis of IPF arises when, as is the case in 12.5% to 26% of patients who have a multilobe surgical lung biopsy, a UIP pattern is found in samples from 1 lobe, but a different pattern is found in samples from another lobe (a scenario termed discordant UIP).[10,11] However, survival in patients with discordant UIP is similar to patients with concordant UIP (ie, surgical lung biopsy samples from all lobes having UIP patterns).[10,12] Thus, if a surgical lung biopsy is performed, multiple lobes should be sampled, and a diagnosis of definite IPF can be made when a UIP pattern is identified in any lobe (regardless of what is found in any other sample).

Making a diagnosis of IPF can be difficult, but the accuracy and confidence of an IPF diagnosis increases with multidisciplinary discussions among clinicians, radiologists, and pathologists. In a study of 58 consecutive cases of suspected IIP, Flaherty and colleagues[13] sequentially gave expert clinicians, radiologists, and pathologists more and more information about a case of ILD, and then allowed them to discuss their impressions as a group. As more information was divulged and cross-disciplinary discussions took place, the level of agreement about the diagnosis (and the degree of certainty in that diagnosis) improved. Not surprisingly, centers with expertise in IPF are more accurate at diagnosing IPF than community-based, referral practices.[5] For unclear reasons, early referral to such a center seems to improve survival in patients with IPF.[14]

THE EPIDEMIOLOGY OF IPF
Background

Epidemiology is defined as "the study of the distribution and determinants of health-related states or events (including disease)," and the goal of epidemiologists is to apply findings to control diseases or health issues.[15–17] Specific objectives include determining the extent and effects of disease: by defining its prevalence, incidence, and mortality; by identifying its risk factors or causes; and by examining its natural history and prognosis. This information then allows for the evaluation of preventative and therapeutic interventions, and builds a foundation for policies and regulatory decisions to be made that alleviate the burden of disease.[17]

The relative rarity of IPF has challenged investigators with an interest in its epidemiology, and

Box 2
Criteria for a definite, probable, possible, and inconsistent UIP pattern based on surgical lung biopsy

Definite UIP Pattern (requires all 4 of the following features)

Evidence of fibrosis/architectural distortion with or without honeycombing in a predominantly subpleural/paraseptal location

Fibrosis in a patchy distribution

Fibroblast foci

Absence of features suggesting a not UIP pattern (see "Not UIP Pattern")

Probable UIP Pattern (requires either the first 3 criteria of the fourth criteria)

Evidence of fibrosis/architectural distortion with or without honeycombing in a predominantly subpleural/paraseptal location

Either fibrosis in a patchy distribution or fibroblast foci

Absence of features suggesting a not UIP pattern (see "Not UIP Pattern")

Honeycomb changes alone

Possible UIP Pattern

Patchy or diffuse involvement with fibrosis with or without interstitial inflammation

Absence of features suggesting a not UIP pattern (see "Not UIP Pattern")

Not UIP Pattern

Hyaline membranes or organizing pneumonia (unless associated with an acute exacerbation of IPF)

Organizing pneumonia or granulomas (unless mild or occasional, respectively, but may otherwise suggest hypersensitivity pneumonitis)

Marked interstitial inflammation away from honeycombing

Predominant airway-centered disease

Other features suggesting an alternative diagnosis

Data from American Thoracic Society; European Respiratory Society. American Thoracic Society/European Respiratory Society International Multidisciplinary Consensus Classification of the Idiopathic Interstitial Pneumonias. This joint statement of the American Thoracic Society (ATS), and the European Respiratory Society (ERS) was adopted by the ATS board of directors, June 2001 and by the ERS Executive Committee, June 2001. Am J Respir Crit Care Med 2001;165:277–304.

Table 1
Criteria for a definite, probable, and possible diagnosis of IPF based on both HRCT pattern and surgical lung biopsy findings

HRCT Pattern	Surgical Lung Biopsy Pattern	Diagnosis of IPF
UIP	UIP	IPF
	Probable UIP	IPF
	Possible UIP	IPF
	Nonclassifiable fibrosis	IPF
	Not UIP	Not IPF
Possible UIP	UIP	IPF
	Probable UIP	IPF
	Possible UIP	Probable IPF
	Nonclassifiable fibrosis	Probable IPF
	Not UIP	Not IPF
Inconsistent with UIP	UIP	Possible IPF
	Probable UIP	Not IPF
	Possible UIP	Not IPF
	Nonclassifiable fibrosis	Not IPF
	Not UIP	Not IPF

Data from American Thoracic Society; European Respiratory Society. American Thoracic Society/European Respiratory Society International Multidisciplinary Consensus Classification of the Idiopathic Interstitial Pneumonias. This joint statement of the American Thoracic Society (ATS), and the European Respiratory Society (ERS) was adopted by the ATS board of directors, June 2001 and by the ERS Executive Committee, June 2001. Am J Respir Crit Care Med 2001;165:277–304.

in 1969,[19] IPF was not given a diagnostic code in the International Classification of Diseases (ICD) until the ninth revision (ICD-9) at the end of the 1970s.[20] This coding system gave investigators an opportunity to use ICD-coded mortality data to study the burden of IPF at the population level. Johnston and colleagues[21] did so, and published their results of mortality (discussed later) in 1990.

Mortality and Mortality Trends Over Time

Disease-specific mortality is calculated by determining the number of deaths per year resulting from a specific cause, divided by the number of persons alive in the midyear population. In a disease that is lethal, and when survival is short, as occurs in IPF, mortality serves as a surrogate for the incidence of disease.[17]

Death certificate and census data are vital statistics recorded in several countries, and these data have provided investigators with the means to study mortality and mortality trends over time. Little

before 1990, discouraged large-scale epidemiologic studies from being performed.[18] Although Leibow and Carrington first defined a UIP pattern is known about the validity of death certificate ICD coding in IPF, so results from studies using death certificate data should be interpreted with some caution. Investigators in the United Kingdom found that in 23 decedents with a diagnosis of IPF (ICD 9 code 516.3) recorded on a death certificate, 19 (83%) had premortem clinical information confirming either definite or possible IPF.[21] Conversely, among 45 patients with a premortem diagnosis of IPF (ICD-9 code 516.3), IPF was recorded on the death certificate only about 50% of the time. Before the ICD-10 coding system (which combines IPF and postinflammatory pulmonary fibrosis [PIPF]),[22] diagnostic transfer (or coding IPF as PIPF on the death certificate) was also reported to occur commonly. Of 20 decedents coded with PIPF (ICD-9 code 515) on the death certificate, nearly 50% had IPF (ICD-9 code 516.3) diagnosed before death. These data suggest IPF is likely underrecorded as the cause of death, and a significant proportion of decedents coded as dying from PIPF died of IPF. Although these findings are based on a small number of decedents from the United Kingdom, Coultas and Hughes[23] identified similar issues in mortality data from New Mexico.

Because the ICD-10 coding system combined PIPF and IPF into 1 diagnostic code (J84.1),[22] researchers calculating mortality with data after 1998 are likely including some decedents with progressive, fibrosing ILD that is not IPF. Investigators who have used this diagnostic code (J84.1) and who have systematically excluded cases with known-cause pulmonary fibrosis (PF) have termed this entity general PF.[24,25] Other investigators have not excluded concurrent conditions that may result in PF, and have termed this entity IPF clinical syndrome (IPF-CS).[26] Regardless of the precise diagnosis (ie, IPF vs other progressive, fibrotic ILD) for decedents in such studies, trends in mortality reveal that PF is a daunting and growing public health problem.[24–26]

Johnston and colleagues[21] were the first to calculate IPF (previously termed cryptogenic fibrosing alveolitis in the United Kingdom) mortality in a large-scale epidemiologic study. They found that in England and Wales, from 1979 to 1988, deaths from IPF (ICD-9 code, 516.3) more than doubled. IPF-associated mortality was more common in men (odds ratio [OR] = 2.24; 95% confidence interval [CI] = 2.11–2.38) and increased progressively with age: the risk of IPF in those 75 years old or older was 8 times the risk for those 45 to 54 years old. Greater mortality was found in the central, industrialized areas of England and Wales, suggesting environmental/occupational exposures could be a risk factor for IPF.

Hubbard and colleagues[27] extended on the work of Johnston and colleagues by investigating available mortality data for both IPF (ICD-9 code 516.3) and PIPF (ICD-9 code 515) from England, Wales, Scotland, Germany, Australia, New Zealand, Canada, and the United States from 1979 to 1992. They found that mortality from IPF was the highest in England and Wales and rates were increasing not only in these countries but also in Scotland, Australia, and Canada. Mortality from IPF was stable in New Zealand and Germany and had decreased over time in the United States. Mortality from PIPF was the highest in the United States, and increased over the study period in the United States, the United Kingdom, Canada, and Australia, with stable mortality again noted in New Zealand and Germany. The increase in mortality from PF could not be explained by diagnostic transfer (eg, a change in coding practices from PIPF to IPF, or PIPF to IPF over time), although systematic diagnostic transfer (always coding IPF as PIPF, because of different terminology and coding rules)[24] may have explained the higher mortality of PIPF in the United States.

Mannino and colleagues[24] examined PF mortality data in the United States from 1979 to 1991. To capture all decedents with IPF, given the coding issues noted earlier, these investigators defined PF by combing ICD-9 diagnostic codes 515 (PIPF) and 516.3 (IPF) and eliminated cases with concurrent diagnostic codes for conditions with known associations with PF, including radiation fibrosis, collagen vascular diseases, or asbestosis. Over that 13-year period, age-adjusted mortality from PF increased 4.7% in men (from 48.6 per million to 50.9 per million) and increased 27.1% in women (from 21.4 per million to 27.2 per million). PF-associated mortality increased with increasing age. States with the highest PF-associated mortality were in the west and southeast, and those with the lowest rates were in the midwest and northeast.

Data from the 1990s to early 2000 show a further increase, and acceleration, in PF-associated mortality. Using US mortality data from 1992 to 2003 and applying methods similar to Mannino and colleagues, Olson and colleagues[25] analyzed more than 28 million death records and found that the age-adjusted and standardized (to the year 2000) mortality increased 29.4% in men (from 49.7 deaths per million to 64.3 deaths per million) and 38.1% in women (from 42.3 deaths per million to 58.4 deaths per million) (Fig. 1). Rates increased with increasing age. Compared with the previous decade, mortality over this period increased at a significantly faster pace in both men and women. From 1992 to 2003, rates

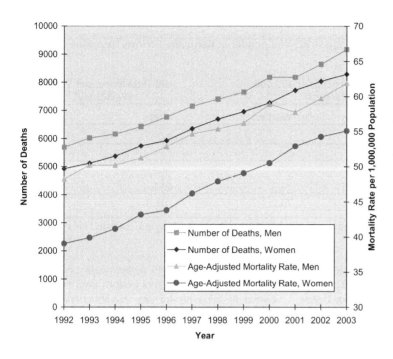

Fig. 1. Number of deaths per year and age-adjusted mortality in decedents with PF per 1,000,000 population from 1992 to 2003 in the United States. Mortality is standardized to the 2000 US census population. (*Reproduced from* Olson AL, Swigris JJ, Lezotte DC, et al. Mortality from pulmonary fibrosis increased in the United States from 1992 to 2003. Am J Respir Crit Care Med 2007;176:278; with permission.)

rose more steeply in women than men. Mortality was greater among white non-Hispanics than black non-Hispanics or Hispanics, suggesting that race and ethnicity may also play a role in the susceptibility to IPF.

Similar trends were recently reported in the United Kingdom: age-adjusted and sex-adjusted mortality from IPF-CS (ICD-9 code 515 or 516.3, or ICD-10 code J84.1) have reached 51 per million person-years (an increase of 5% per year since the late 1960s).[26] These studies suggest that, although once considered an orphan disease, PF (and PF-associated mortality) is more common than several common malignancies and is an important public health concern, particularly in elderly people.[25,26]

Prevalence and Incidence, and Trends Over Time

The prevalence of disease is defined as the number of persons with disease at a specific point in time divided by the total population at that time, and incidence is defined as the number of persons with newly diagnosed disease divided by the number of persons at risk for developing that disease over that period of time. Prevalence is a proportion; incidence is a rate. In disease processes in which the incidence and the duration of the disease are stable, the prevalence should reflect the incidence multiplied by the duration of the disease.[28]

Before 1994, little was known about the incidence or prevalence of ILD in general or IPF in particular.[29–31] Coultas and colleagues[32] performed one of the first large-scale epidemiologic investigations to determine the prevalence and incidence of IPF. Using several, broad case-finding methods, they established a population-based registry of ILD in Bernalillo County, New Mexico. From 1988 to 1993, they found that IPF was the most common ILD in this region, accounting for 22.5% of prevalent cases and 31.2% of incident cases. The prevalence and incidence of IPF was higher in men (20.2 cases per 100,000 persons and 13.2 cases per 100,000/y, respectively) than women (10.7 per 100,000 persons and 7.4 per 100,000/y, respectively). Both the prevalence and incidence of IPF increased dramatically with age (**Table 2**). Limitations to this study included that these data came from only 1 county in New Mexico, so it was not known whether these were applicable to the United States as a whole.

More than a decade later, Raghu and colleagues[33] determined the prevalence and incidence of IPF using a large health care claims database from a US health plan that covered approximately 3 million persons in 20 states. Using data from 1996 to 2000, they determined the prevalence and incidence of IPF using both a narrow and broad definition of IPF. The broad definition of IPF included any person 18 years of age or older, with 1 or more medical claims with a diagnosis of IPF (ICD-9 of 516.3), and without any other medical claims for a diagnosis of another ILD on or after the date of the last medical claim with

Table 2
The prevalence and incidence of IPF by age strata and gender in Bernalillo County, New Mexico from 1988 to 1993

Age Strata (y)	IPF (Prevalence, per 100,000 Persons)		IPF (Incidence, per 100,000 Persons/y)	
	Men	Women	Men	Women
35–44	2.7	–	4.0	–
45–54	8.7	8.1	2.2	4.0
55–64	28.4	5.0	14.2	10.0
65–74	104.6	72.3	48.6	21.1
≥75	174.7	73.2	101.9	57.0

Data from Coultas DB, Zumwalt RE, Black WC, et al. The epidemiology of interstitial lung diseases. Am J Respir Crit Care Med 1994;150:967–72.

this diagnostic code for IPF. The narrow definition of IPF included those criteria plus at least 1 claim for either a procedure code for surgical or transbronchial lung biopsy or a computed tomography scan of the thorax. They found that the overall prevalence of IPF was 14.0 or 42.7 per 100,000 persons, depending on whether the narrow or broad case definitions were used. These investigators found that the incidence of IPF was 6.8 or 16.3 per 100,000 persons per year, depending on whether the narrow or broad case definitions were used. Similar to Coultas and colleagues, they also found that both the prevalence and incidence increased with age (**Table 3**). Compared with Coultas and colleagues, Raghu and colleagues calculated prevalence and incidence estimates that were greater, suggesting the burden of disease had increased over time (see **Tables 2** and 3).

Studies performed outside the United States also suggest that the incidence of IPF has increased over time. Using a general practice database in the United Kingdom, Gribbin and colleagues[34]

examined persons with a diagnosis of IPF from 1991 to 2003. During this period, the overall incidence of IPF was 4.6 per 100,000 person-years (numbers slightly lower than reported by either Coultas and colleagues or Raghu and colleagues). However, this study suggested that the burden of IPF had increased over time: the incidence had more than doubled, a finding not explained by an aging population.

Similar to the case with mortality, it is unclear if these reported increases in incidence represent a true increase in disease occurrence or simply improved recognition of the disease. Case ascertainment may have increased over this period because of a growing use of HRCT in the evaluation of ILD. Increased public and community practice awareness of IPF may also account for these trends: during the 1990s, the first large, multicenter, therapeutic trial for IPF was conceptualized and began enrolling patients.[35]

Navaratnam and colleagues[26] reexamined the trends in incidence of PF in the United Kingdom through 2008. Using computerized primary care

Table 3
The prevalence and incidence of IPF by age strata and gender from a health care claims processing system of a large US health plan from 1996 to 2000 using the broad case definition (please see text)

Age Strata (y)	IPF (Prevalence, per 100,000 Persons)		IPF (Incidence, per 100,000 Persons/y)	
	Men	Women	Men	Women
35–44	4.9	12.7	1.1	5.4
45–54	22.3	22.6	11.4	10.9
55–64	62.8	50.9	35.1	22.6
65–74	148.5	106.7	49.1	36.0
≥75	276.9	192.1	97.6	62.2

Data from Raghu G, Weycker D, Edelsberg J, et al. Incidence and prevalence of idiopathic pulmonary fibrosis. Am J Respir Crit Care Med 2006;174:810–16.

records in the United Kingdom, they found that the incidence of IPF-CS (defined from 1965 to 1978 as ICD, eighth edition code 517, from 1979 to 1999 as ICD-9 code 516.3 and 515, and from 2000 onward as ICD-10 code J84.1) increased at a rate of approximately 5% per year.

Data from the United States, published within the past year, suggested a different trend. Fernandez-Perez and colleagues[36] analyzed data from Olmsted County, Minnesota to determine incidence and prevalence of IPF from 1997 to 2005. They screened 596 patients in a population-based registry for PF. Overall, the age-adjusted and sex-adjusted incidence was 8.8/100,000 person-years based on a narrow-case definition of IPF (UIP pattern on surgical lung biopsy or characteristic HRCT), and 17.4/100,000 person-years based on a broad case definition (UIP pattern on surgical lung biopsy or either definite or possible characteristic HRCT). The incidence was higher in men than in women, and the incidence increased with advancing age in men, and until the age of 80 years in women. Unlike any of the other investigators whose studies were described earlier, Fernandez-Perez and colleagues observed that the incidence significantly (P<.001) decreased over the study period (although peaks in incidence were noted in 1998 and 2001). In 2005, the age-adjusted and sex-adjusted prevalence of IPF was 27.9/100,000 and 63/100,000 (using the narrow and broad definition, respectively). However, given the aging population, these investigators project that the annual number of newly diagnosed cases of IPF in the US population by 2050 may reach 21,000. It is impossible to speculate whether these trends, observed in this 1 county, reflect the most current trends at a national or international level.

Risk Factors

Although IPF is defined as an idiopathic disease, epidemiologic studies have identified several risk factors (including environmental and occupational exposures) associated with the diagnosis. These studies tend to be case-control studies and are subject to bias: recall bias occurs when persons with disease recall exposures differently from those without the disease, and diagnosis misclassification bias occurs when the number of individuals incorrectly diagnosed with IPF is not equally distributed between those with and those without the risk factor.[07] Also, in case-control studies, the accurate assessment of dose and duration of exposure is challenging; thus, identifying a dose-response effect of the risk factor is frequently impossible.[38] Although case reports also suggest associations between IPF and several different exposures, the following discussion of exposures is limited to those in which the exposure was identified in 2 or more independent studies or via a meta-analysis. Clinical factors, including gastroesophageal reflux disease, diabetes, and infectious agents have been implicated as risk factors for IPF, but are beyond the scope of this review.[3]

Cigarette smoking

Several case-control studies have yielded data on the association between IPF and smoking. Baumgartner and colleagues[39] identified 248 IPF cases from 16 referral centers in the United States and matched these cases to 491 control individuals on sex, age, and geography. A smoking history was more common in those with IPF (72%) than controls (63%) (OR = 1.6; 95% CI = 1.1–2.4). Three other case-control studies from the United Kingdom and Japan found a similar association.[40–42] Scott and colleagues[30] found no association between IPF and smoking in a case-control study of 40 patients with IPF from Nottingham, United Kingdom and 106 matched controls. Of all the studies on the topic, this one included the fewest cases. In a meta-analysis of these 5 studies, patients with IPF were significantly more likely than controls to report a smoking history (OR = 1.58; 95% CI = 1.27–1.97).[38]

In an attempt to identify a dose-response relationship between smoking and IPF, Baumgartner and colleagues[39] observed that, when compared with individuals who had a 20–pack-year or fewer smoking history, those with a 21–pack-year to 40–pack-year history had a greater odds of developing IPF (OR = 2.26; 95% CI = 1.3–3.8); however, for those with a history greater than 40 pack-years, there was no further increase in the risk of developing IPF (OR = 1.12; 95% CI = 0.7 1.0). After adjusting for age, sex, and region of residency, Miyake and colleagues[42] found an association between IPF and smoking in those with a 20–pack-year to 39.9–pack-year history (OR = 3.23; 95% CI = 1.01–10.84), but not for those with either a fewer or greater pack-year history.

Environmental and Occupational Exposures

Because other environmental exposures (including asbestosis, silicosis, and coal workers' pneumoconiosis) are known to cause fibrotic lung disease,[43–45] IPF is more likely to occur in men than women (and men are more likely than women to work in jobs in which such exposures occur),[2] and IPF-associated mortality is higher in highly industrialized regions of some countries,[21] it has been hypothesized that environmental or occupational exposures may also be associated with IPF.

Metal dust

In several case-control studies and a meta-analysis, investigators have examined the association between a variety of environmental or occupational exposures and the risk of IPF. Each of the initial 5 studies yielded data that suggested an association between metal dust exposure and IPF (OR from the meta-analysis = 2.44, 95% CI = 1.74–3.40).[30,38,40–42,46] In 2 of these studies, a dose-response relationship was found.[40,46] In further support of this association, elemental microanalyses of hilar and mediastinal lymph nodes in patients with IPF have shown increased nickel,[47] silicon,[48] and aluminum[48] levels compared with controls.

In contrast, Gustafson and colleagues[49] recently found no association between metal dust exposure and IPF (OR = 0.9; 95% CI = 0.51–1.59) among 140 patients IPF and 757 matched controls in Sweden; they did not assess for a dose-response relationship.

Hubbard and colleagues[50] assembled a historical cohort from the pension-fund archives of employees who had worked for Rolls-Royce plc in the United Kingdom to determine the risk of IPF in those exposed to metal dust. Among members of this cohort, there were 20,526 total deaths, and 55 were IPF associated. The number of IPF-associated deaths in this cohort was significantly greater than expected based on national mortality (proportional mortality ratio = 1.39; 95% CI = 1.07–1.82). Among the 22 decedents with available archive data, a dose-response relationship between metal exposure and IPF was identified (OR per 10 years of exposure = 1.71; 95% CI = 1.09–2.68).

Using US death certificate data from 1999 to 2003 and available industry/occupation codes for a proportion of decedents with PF (ICD-10 code J84.1), Pinheiro and colleagues[51] found an increase in the proportionate mortality (PM) for those decedents whose industry was recorded as metal mining (PM = 2.4; 95% CI = 1.3–4.0) and those whose industry was recorded as fabricated structural metal products (PM = 1.9; 95% CI = 1.1–3.1).

Wood dust

In the studies mentioned earlier, and other case-controlled studies, researchers have examined the association between wood dust exposure and IPF.[30,38,40,42,46,52] Of the initial 5 studies, in only one did investigators observe a significantly increased risk of IPF in patients exposed to wood dust (OR = 1.71; 95% CI = 1.01–1.92).[40] However, when all of these studies were included in a meta-analysis, an increased risk of IPF was found in patients with exposure to wood dusts (OR = 1.94; 95% CI = 1.34–2.81).[38] In another study from Sweden, not included in the meta-analysis, there was no association between any wood dust and IPF among the entire study sample (OR = 1.2; 95% CI = 0.65–2.23); however, there was an increased risk of IPF in men exposed to birch dust (OR = 2.7, 95% CI = 1.30–5.65) or hardwood dust (OR = 2.7; 95% CI =1.14–6.52). No association between IPF and fur or fir dust was identified. This finding suggests that in addition to gender, specific types of dust may play a role in the pathogenesis of IPF.[49]

Sand, stone, and silica

Three of 4 case-control studies have found an increased risk of IPF in patients with exposures to sand, stone, or silica, with a summary OR of 1.97 (95% CI = 1.09–3.55).[30,38,40,46,52]

Farming and livestock

Agriculture/farming-related and livestock-related exposures have been found to be associated with IPF. In 2 case-control studies, 1 from the United States and 1 from Japan, workers in the agriculture or farming sectors were found to have an increased risk of IPF (meta-analysis OR = 1.65, 95% CI = 1.20–2.26).[38,41,46] The 1 study noted earlier from the United States and another study from the United Kingdom both found that exposure to livestock was associated with an increased risk of IPF (meta-analysis OR = 2.17, 95% CI = 1.28–3.68).[30,38,46] Further, Baumgartner and colleagues[46] identified a dose-response relationship between livestock exposure and IPF. After adjusting for age and smoking history, they found no increased risk for IPF among patients exposed for less than 5 years (OR = 2.1; 95% CI = 0.7–6.1), but a significantly increased risk for IPF among those with 5 or more years of exposure (OR = 3.3; 95% CI = 1.3–8.3).

SUMMARY

Over the last decade or two, results from several studies have advanced understanding of IPF: how it is diagnosed, its basic epidemiologic profile, and occupational or environmental exposures that may increase the risk for developing the disease. These results have reshaped how IPF is diagnosed, especially by highlighting the accuracy with which a characteristic HRCT identifies a UIP pattern of lung injury: patients with such an HRCT need not have a surgical lung biopsy for IPF to be diagnosed confidently. However, making a diagnosis of IPF is complex, and whether a surgical lung biopsy is indicated or not, diagnostic accuracy is improved with multidisciplinary discussions in centers that specialize in the care of patients with this disease. Over the same period, the burden of IPF seems to have increased, with some incidence and mortality estimates placing IPF on par with certain relatively common malignancies. Although through case-control and cohort studies investigators have identified risk factors for IPF, these studies do not prove causality, and further research is needed not only to better understand the underlying pathobiology of this complex disease but also to find effective therapies for it.

REFERENCES

1. American Thoracic Society. Idiopathic pulmonary fibrosis: diagnosis and treatment. International consensus statement. American Thoracic Society (ATS), and the European Respiratory Society (ERS). Am J Respir Crit Care Med 2000;161:646–64.

2. American Thoracic Society; European Respiratory Society. American Thoracic Society/European Respiratory Society International Multidisciplinary Consensus Classification of the Idiopathic Interstitial Pneumonias. This joint statement of the American Thoracic Society (ATS), and the European Respiratory Society (ERS) was adopted by the ATS board of directors, June 2001 and by the ERS Executive Committee, June 2001. Am J Respir Crit Care Med 2001;165:277–304.

3. Raghu G, Collard HR, Egan JJ, et al. An official ATS/ERS/JRS/ALAT statement: idiopathic pulmonary fibrosis: evidence-based guidelines for diagnosis and management. Am J Respir Crit Care Med 2011;183:788–824.

4. Raghu G, Mageto YN, Lockhart D, et al. The accuracy of the clinical diagnosis of new-onset idiopathic pulmonary fibrosis and other interstitial lung disease: a prospective study. Chest 1999;116: 1168–74.

5. Hunninghake GW, Zimmerman MB, Schwartz DA, et al. Utility of a lung biopsy for the diagnosis of idiopathic pulmonary fibrosis. Am J Respir Crit Care Med 2001;164:193–6.

6. Swensen SJ, Aughenbaugh GL, Meyers JL. Diffuse lung disease: diagnostic accuracy of CT in patients undergoing surgical biopsy of the lung. Radiology 1997;205:229–34.

7. Hunninghake GW, Lynch DA, Galvin JR, et al. Radiologic findings are strongly associated with a pathologic diagnosis of usual interstitial pneumonia. Chest 2003;124:1215–23.

8. MacDonald SL, Rubens MB, Hansell DM, et al. Nonspecific interstitial pneumonia and usual interstitial pneumonia: comparative appearances at and diagnostic accuracy of thin-section CT. Radiology 2001;221:600–5.

9. Johkoh T, Muller NL, Cartier Y, et al. Idiopathic interstitial pneumonias: diagnostic accuracy of thin-section CT in 129 patients. Radiology 1999;211: 555–60.

10. Monaghan H, Wells AU, Colby TV, et al. Prognostic implications of histologic patterns in multiple surgical lung biopsies from patients with idiopathic interstitial pneumonias. Chest 2004;125:522–6.

11. Flaherty KR, Travis WD, Colby TV, et al. Histopathologic variability in usual and nonspecific interstitial pneumonias. Am J Respir Crit Care Med 2001;164: 1722–7.

12. Flaherty KR, Thwaite EL, Kazerooni EA, et al. Radiological versus histological diagnosis in UIP and NSIP: survival implications. Thorax 2003;58: 143–8.

13. Flaherty KR, King TE, Raghu G, et al. Idiopathic interstitial pneumonia: what is the effect of a multidisciplinary approach to diagnosis? Am J Respir Crit Care Med 2004;170:904–10.

14. Lamas DJ, Kawut SM, Bagiella E, et al. Delayed access and survival in idiopathic pulmonary fibrosis: a cohort study. Am J Respir Crit Care Med 2011; 184(7):842–7.

15. World Health Organization. Epidemiology. Available at: http://www.who.int/topics/epidemiology/en/. Accessed June 15, 2011.

16. Last JM. A dictionary of epidemiology. 2nd edition. New York: Oxford University Press; 1998.

17. Gordis L. The epidemiologic approach to disease and intervention. In: Gordis L, editor. Epidemiology. 3rd edition. Philadelphia: Elsevier Saunders; 2004. p. 1–14.

18. Coultas DB, Hubbard R. Epidemiology of idiopathic pulmonary fibrosis. In: Lynch JP, editor. Idiopathic pulmonary fibrosis. New York: Marcel Dekker; 2004. p. 1–30.

19. Leibow AA, Carrington DB. The interstitial pneumonias. In: Simon M, Potchen EJ, LeMay M, editors. Frontiers of pulmonary radiology. New York: Grune & Stratton; 1969. p. 102–41.

20. World Health Organization. International classification of diseases 1975. 9th revision. Geneva (Switzerland): WHO; 1977.

21. Johnston I, Britton J, Kinnear W, et al. Rising mortality from cryptogenic fibrosing alveolitis. BMJ 1990;301:1017–21.

22. World Health Organization. ICD-10: international classification of diseases and related health problems, 10th revision. Geneva (Switzerland): WHO; 2003.

23. Coultas DB, Hughes MP. Accuracy or mortality data for interstitial lung disease in New Mexico, USA. Thorax 1996;51:717–20.

24. Mannino DM, Etzel RA, Parrish RG. Pulmonary fibrosis deaths in the United States, 1979-1991. Am J Respir Crit Care Med 1996;153:1548–52.

25. Olson AL, Swigris JJ, Lezotte DC, et al. Mortality from pulmonary fibrosis increased in the United States from 1992 to 2003. Am J Respir Crit Care Med 2007;176:277–84.

26. Navaratnam V, Fleming KM, West J, et al. The rising incidence of idiopathic pulmonary fibrosis in the UK. Thorax 2011;66:462–7.

27. Hubbard R, Johnston I, Coultas DB, et al. Mortality rates from cryptogenic fibrosing alveolitis in seven countries. Thorax 1996;51:711–6.

28. Gordis L. Measuring the occurrence of disease: I. Morbidity. In: Gordis L, editor. Epidemiology. 3rd edition. Philadelphia: Elsevier Saunders; 2004. p. 32–47.

29. Crystal RG, Bitterman PB, Rennard SI, et al. Interstitial lung diseases of unknown causes. Disorders characterized by chronic inflammation of the lower respiratory tract. N Engl J Med 1984;310:154–66, 235–44.

30. Scott J, Johnston I, Britton J. What causes cryptogenic fibrosing alveolitis? A case-control study of environmental exposure to dust. BMJ 1990;301: 1015–7.

31. U.S. Department of Health and Human Services. Vital and health statistics. National hospital discharge survey: annual summary, 1988. Hyattsville (MD): DHHS; 1991. No (PHS). p. 91–1101.

32. Coultas DB, Zumwalt RE, Black WC, et al. The epidemiology of interstitial lung diseases. Am J Respir Crit Care Med 1994;150:967–72.

33. Raghu G, Weycker D, Edelsberg J, et al. Incidence and prevalence of idiopathic pulmonary fibrosis. Am J Respir Crit Care Med 2006;174:810–6.

34. Gribbin J, Hubbard RB, Le Jeune I, et al. Incidence and mortality of idiopathic pulmonary fibrosis and sarcoidosis in the UK. Thorax 2006;61:980–5.

35. Raghu G, Brown KK, Bradford WZ, et al. A placebo controlled trial of interferon gamma-1b in patients with idiopathic pulmonary fibrosis. N Engl J Med 2004;350:125–33.

36. Fernández-Pérez ER, Daniels CE, Schroeder DR, et al. Incidence, prevalence, and clinical course of idiopathic pulmonary fibrosis. Chest 2010;137:129–37.

37. Gordis L. Case-control and cross-sectional studies. In: Gordis L, editor. Epidemiology. 3rd edition. Philadelphia: Elsevier Saunders; 2004. p. 159–76.

38. Taskar VS, Coultas DB. Is idiopathic pulmonary fibrosis an environmental disease? Proc Am Thorac Soc 2006;3:293–8.

39. Baumgartner KB, Samet JM, Stidley CA, et al. Cigarette smoking: a risk factor for idiopathic pulmonary fibrosis. Am J Respir Crit Care Med 1997;155:242–8.

40. Hubbard R, Lewis S, Richards K, et al. Occupational exposure to metal or wood dust and aetiology of cryptogenic fibrosing alveolitis. Lancet 1996;347: 284–9.

41. Iwai K, Mori T, Yamada N, et al. Idiopathic pulmonary fibrosis epidemiologic approaches to occupational exposure. Am J Respir Crit Care Med 1994;150: 670–5.

42. Miyaka Y, Sasaki S, Yokoyama T, et al. Occupational and environmental factors and idiopathic pulmonary fibrosis in Japan. Ann Occup Hyg 2005;49:259–65.

43. Weissman DN, Banks DE. Silicosis. In: Schwarz MI, King TE, editors. Interstitial lung disease. 4th edition. Ontario (Canada): BC Decker; 2003. p. 387–401.

44. Banks DE. Coal workers' pneumoconiosis. In: Schwarz MI, King TE, editors. Interstitial lung disease. 4th edition. Ontario (Canada): BC Decker; 2003. p. 402–17.

45. Steele M, Peterson MW, Schwarz DA. Asbestosis and asbestos-induced pleural fibrosis. In: Schwarz MI, King TE, editors. Interstitial lung disease. 4th edition. Ontario (Canada): BC Decker; 2003. p. 418–34.

46. Baumgarter KB, Samet JM, Coutas DB, et al. Occupational and environmental risk factors for idiopathic pulmonary fibrosis: a multicenter case-control study. Am J Epidemiol 2000;152:307–15.

47. Hashimoto H, Tajima H, Mizoguchi I, et al. Elemental analysis of hilar and mediastinal lymph nodes in idiopathic pulmonary fibrosis. Nihon Kyobu Shikkan Gakkai Zasshi 1992;30:2061–8 [in Japanese].

48. Kitamura H, Ichinose S, Hosoya T, et al. Inhalation of inorganic particles as a risk factor for idiopathic pulmonary fibrosis–elemental microanalysis of pulmonary lymph nodes obtained at autopsy cases. Pathol Res Pract 2007;203:575–85.

49. Gustafson T, Dahlman-Höglund A, Nilsson K, et al. Occupational exposure and severe pulmonary fibrosis. Respir Med 2007;110:2207–12.

50. Hubbard R, Cooper M, Antaoniak M, et al. Risk of cryptogenic fibrosing alveolitis in metal workers. Lancet 2000;355:466–7.

51. Pinheiro GA, Antao VC, Wood JM, et al. Occupational risks for idiopathic pulmonary fibrosis mortality in the United States. Int J Occup Environ Health 2008;14:117–23.

52. Mullen J, Hodgson MJ, DeGraff CA, et al. Case-control study of idiopathic pulmonary fibrosis and environmental exposures. J Occup Environ Med 1998;40: 363–7.

Idiopathic Pulmonary Fibrosis: Phenotypes and Comorbidities

Charlene D. Fell, MD, MSc, FRCPC

KEYWORDS

- Idiopathic pulmonary fibrosis • Phenotypes • Comorbidities
- Pulmonary hypertension • Emphysema

Idiopathic pulmonary fibrosis (IPF) is a progressive fatal disease of the lung with unknown etiology and limited treatment options. Once thought to be slowly progressive disease, more recent evidence suggests that there may be different phenotypes of IPF with different rates of disease progression. Furthermore, patients with comorbid disease, such as emphysema or pulmonary hypertension, do more poorly than those with IPF alone. Rapidly progressive IPF, combined emphysema and pulmonary fibrosis, and IPF with pulmonary hypertension may represent distinct disease phenotypes.[1]

Patients are often very discouraged to receive a diagnosis of IPF, given its poor prognosis and lack of readily available treatment options; however, much can be done to identify and alleviate symptoms from comorbidities, potentially improving the overall quality of life of these patients. This article describes emerging evidence to support the hypothesis that there is more than one phenotype for IPF and describes the common comorbidities seen in this disease.

ARE THERE DISTINCT PHENOTYPES IN IPF?

A phenotype is the outward manifestation of a gene or genes, may involve more than one organ system, and is dynamic, changing over time or in response to the environment.[2] In contrast, genotypes are stable over the life span of an individual. Defining a phenotype concisely and accurately is crucial, as phenotypes are used to predict prognosis, select patients for enrollment into clinical trials, and provide the foundation for studies exploring the pathobiology of disease. Some investigators have suggested that the lack of significant and reproducible results in recent therapeutic trials may be because of the inclusion of several different and yet to be characterized phenotypes in IPF.[3] Three distinct phenotypes of IPF have been proposed: combined emphysema and pulmonary fibrosis,[4] disproportionate pulmonary hypertension and IPF,[5] and IPF that is rapidly progressive.[3]

Combined Pulmonary Fibrosis and Emphysema

Smoking increases the risk of developing IPF,[6] and many patients exhibit features of IPF and emphysema. The prevalence of emphysema in patients with IPF was 30% in a retrospective study from Mexico[7] and 47% at the time of diagnosis and 55% during follow-up in a European cohort.[8] Early reports describe patients with a clinical presentation of severe dyspnea, pulmonary fibrosis, preserved lung volumes, and a markedly reduced transfer factor of the lung for carbon monoxide (T_{LCO}).[9,10] These patients had characteristic radiographic features including upper lobe predominant centrilobular or periseptal emphysema and lower lobe predominant pulmonary fibrosis (**Fig. 1**).[8,10] The syndrome of combined pulmonary fibrosis and emphysema (CPFE) was coined by Cottin and colleagues[8] in 2005 to describe this subgroup of patients with IPF.

Disclosure: Dr Fell has participated in scientific advisory boards for Actelion and InterMune.
Division of Respirology, University of Calgary, and Peter Lougheed Hospital, 3500 26th Avenue NE, Calgary, Alberta T1Y 6J4, Canada
E-mail address: cfell@ucalgary.ca

Clin Chest Med 33 (2012) 51–57
doi:10.1016/j.ccm.2011.12.005

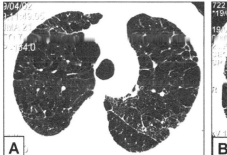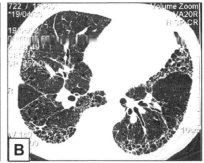

Fig. 1. High-resolution computed tomography images from a patient with combined pulmonary fibrosis and emphysema illustrating upper lobe emphysema (*A*) and lower lobe fibrosis with honeycomb change (*B*). (*From* Mejia M, Carrillo G, Rojas-Serrano J, et al. Idiopathic pulmonary fibrosis and emphysema: decreased survival associated with severe pulmonary arterial hypertension. Chest 2009;136:10–5; with permission.)

Patients with CPFE have worse survival than those with IPF alone (**Fig. 2**).[7] Prognosis of patients with concurrent pulmonary fibrosis and emphysema is even poorer if they develop pulmonary hypertension.[8] Indeed, pulmonary hypertension is the main determinant of mortality in these patients with relatively preserved lung volumes. Following changes in lung volume over time for this group will not be as informative as it is for patients with IPF alone. When patients develop restriction (forced vital capacity <50% predicted) in the setting of CPFE with pulmonary hypertension, the prognosis is grim.[7]

The pathobiology of CPFE has not been established. Cigarette smoke is the most important trigger, but other environmental exposures, such as agrochemical compounds, may also contribute.[11] It is not known whether CPFE develops in individuals who inherit susceptibility to both chronic obstructive pulmonary disease (COPD) and IPF or if there is a distinct genetic basis for the syndrome.

Management of patients with CPFE has not been established. Smoking cessation is of paramount importance. Oral corticosteroids and immunosuppressive therapy are ineffective.[8,9] Supplemental oxygen should be provided for hypoxemic patients. Antipulmonary hypertension therapy has not been specifically evaluated in this population.

Pulmonary Hypertension and IPF

Multiple studies have examined pulmonary hypertension in patients with IPF. Pulmonary hypertension is defined as a mean pulmonary arterial pressure (mPAP) of 25 mm Hg or higher at rest or 30 mm Hg or higher with exercise.[12] Echocardiography is recommended as a screening test for identifying patients with pulmonary hypertension[12]; however, in a study comparing echocardiographic and right heart catheterization data for patients with advanced lung disease waiting for lung transplantation, 48% of patients were misclassified with pulmonary hypertension.[13] Thus, echocardiographic data must be interpreted with caution and right heart catheterization is required to accurately confirm the presence and severity of pulmonary hypertension in the population with IPF.

Estimates of the prevalence of pulmonary hypertension in IPF range between 31% and 85%,[14–17] and are derived from data from patients awaiting lung transplantation. The incidence and severity of pulmonary hypertension increases with time[18] and thus the prevalence of pulmonary hypertension in the general IPF population may be lower.

Pulmonary hypertension in IPF is associated with a higher mortality,[16] especially in patients with combined emphysema and pulmonary fibrosis.[12,13] Although mPAP of 25 mm Hg or higher is an

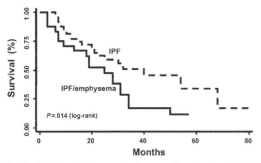

Fig. 2. Kaplan-Meier survival curve of patients with IPF and CPFE illustrating worse survival in the CPFE group. (*From* Mejia M, Carrillo G, Rojas-Serrano J, et al. Idiopathic pulmonary fibrosis and emphysema: decreased survival associated with severe pulmonary arterial hypertension. Chest 2009;136:10–5; with permission.)

accepted definition for pulmonary hypertension, a recent analysis demonstrated that mPAP higher than 17 mm Hg is the best discriminator of increased 5-year mortality for patients with IPF.[19]

Pulmonary hypertension in IPF is the result of several proposed pathophysiological mechanisms, including distortion and destruction of the vascular bed from fibrosis and chronic vasoconstriction attributable to hypoxemia.[5] Pulmonary hypertension usually develops in patients with severe IPF and is analogous to the development of pulmonary hypertension in other chronic lung diseases, such as COPD; however, there exists a subset of patients with IPF who develop pulmonary hypertension at earlier stages of the disease.[16,20,21] These patients are hypothesized to represent a distinct phenotype of disproportionate pulmonary hypertension in IPF.[5] Patients may have disproportionate pulmonary hypertension in IPF owing to episodic hypoxemia during sleep or exercise or may have an imbalance of angiogenesis and angiostasis in the lung.[5] Whether this represents a true novel phenotype remains to be explored, as do the underlying potential mechanisms of disproportional pulmonary hypertension in IPF.

Recent advances in the understanding of the pathobiology of pulmonary hypertension have resulted in the development of therapies that have greatly improved functional status and survival of select groups of patients with the disease.[22] Early trials of therapies for pulmonary hypertension in IPF provided promising results[23,24]; subsequent larger trials have failed to show a statistically significant benefit (**Table 1**). Whether this is because of a failure of individual drugs, limitations of clinical trial design, or a lack of effect of this class of drugs remains to be determined. Based on a lack of evidence, treatment of pulmonary hypertension in IPF is not recommended for most patients.[25]

Rapidly Progressive IPF

Patients with IPF may exhibit varying courses of their disease. some have slowly progressive disease, some experience acute exacerbations of IPF, and some experience a very rapid deterioration from the time of symptom onset (**Fig. 3**). Patients with rapid disease progression are hypothesized to represent a distinct phenotype of IPF. A recent study investigated this hypothesis by exploring gene expression and other biologic features of 26 patients with rapidly progressive disease (<6 months of symptoms) and 88 patients with slowly progressive disease (>24 months of symptoms).[3] There was a differential expression

Table 1
Outcomes of recent large clinical trials examining the therapeutic effect of pulmonary hypertension therapies for patients with IPF

Intervention TRIAL NAME	N	Primary Outcome	Status
Bosentan[61]			
BUILD 3	616	Death or disease progression	Negative
Sildenafil[62]			
STEP-IPF	180	Change in 6MWD	Negative
Ambrisentan[63]			
ARTEMIS-IPF	600	Death or disease progression	Negative
ARTEMIS-PH	225	Change in 6MWD	Terminated
Macitetan[64]			
MUSIC	156	Change in FVC	Negative

Abbreviations: ARTEMIS-IPF, Randomized Placebo-Controlled Study to Evaluate Safety and Effectiveness of Ambrisentan in IPF; ARTEMIS-PH, Study of Ambrisentan in Subjects with Pulmonary Hypertension Associated with Idiopathic Pulmonary Fibrosis; BUILD, Bosentan Use in Interstitial Lung Disease; FVC, forced vital capacity; MUSIC, Macitentan Use in an Idiopathic Pulmonary Fibrosis Clinical Study; STEP-IPF, Sildenafil Trial of Exercise Performance in Idiopathic Pulmonary Fibrosis; 6MWD, 6-minute walk distance.
Data from Refs.[61–64]

of genes between the groups, with the rapid progressors exhibiting upregulation of the several genes involved in cell motility, myofibroblast differentiation, coagulation, oxidative stress, and development, including the gene for the adenosine A_{2B} receptor. Immunohistochemical studies of lung biopsies from rapid progressors showed strong epithelial staining for the adenosine A_{2B} receptor, whereas biopsies from slow progressors and healthy controls did not.[3] The adenosine A_{2B} receptor is part of the pathway involved in the differentiation of lung fibroblasts into myofibroblasts, a step that is important in the pathogenesis of IPF.[26] These results suggest a biologically plausible mechanism underlying the difference between the proposed slow and rapid progressor phenotypes in IPF.

OTHER COMORBIDITIES IN IPF
Gastroeosophageal Reflux Disease

Evidence that gastroeosophageal reflux disease (GERD) is associated with IPF and recurrent silent

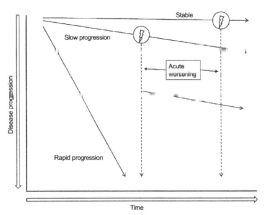

Fig. 3. Natural history of IPF. Most patients experience slow progression of the disease (Slow progression), whereas some have more stable disease (Stable). Patients with slow progression or stable disease may experience episodes of acute deterioration (lightening bolt; Acute worsening). A subset of patients have rapidly progressive disease (Rapid progression) and may encompass a distinct phenotype. (*Reprinted with* permission of the American Thoracic Society. Copyright © 2012 American Thoracic Society. Raghu G, Collard HR, Egan JJ, et al. An official ATS/ERS/JRS/ALAT statement: idiopathic pulmonary fibrosis: evidence-based guidelines for diagnosis and management. Am J Respir Crit Care Med 2011;183:788–824. Official Journal of the American Thoracic Society.)

aspiration of gastric acid is associated with acute exacerbations of IPF makes GERD an attractive hypothesis for the etiology of IPF.[27,28] Instillation of acid into the tracheobronchial tree produces pulmonary fibrosis in animal models[29,30] and aspiration of gastric contents can cause pulmonary fibrosis in humans.[31]

The prevalence of GERD in IPF is estimated to be between 66% and 87%.[28,32,33] Importantly, 33% to 53% of patients with documented acid reflux are asymptomatic.[28,32] In a study of patients with IPF being worked up for lung transplantation, symptoms of reflux were a poor predictor of acid reflux measured with esophageal pH monitoring with a sensitivity of 65% and specificity of 71%.[32] A small case series comparing bronchoalveolar lavage (BAL) pepsin levels found that patients with acute exacerbations of IPF had higher levels of BAL pepsin than patients with stable IPF.[34] In a recent study, patients with asymmetric IPF were more likely to have GERD and have experienced acute exacerbations of IPF than patients with symmetric IPF.[27] The investigators speculate that asymmetric IPF is caused by silent nocturnal aspiration and that acute exacerbations of IPF are also caused by silent aspiration.

There are limited data describing treatment outcomes for patients with IPF with silent GERD. A small series of 4 patients with IPF with silent GERD as documented by 24-hour pH measurements and treated with proton pump inhibitors and gastric fundoplication if required showed stabilization in lung function.[35] A retrospective study of patients with IPF waiting for lung transplantation found that those who underwent Nissan fundoplication for severe symptomatic acid reflux had an improved posttransplant course compared with patients who did not undergo the procedure.[36] Follow-up of these patients showed stabilization of oxygen requirements when compared with controls who had not had surgery. Recently, Lee and colleagues[37] examined the impact of GER-related variables, including GER symptoms, a diagnosis of GERD, and the use of medical and/or surgical therapies for GER, on survival time in patients with IPF. They found that the use of GER medications was associated with decreased radiologic fibrosis and was an independent predictor of longer survival time in patients with IPF.[37] Based on these data, the most recent guidelines on the diagnosis and management of IPF recommend treatment for silent GERD.[25] Treatment of nonacid reflux and treatment with fundoplication are not recommended.

Cardiovascular Disease and Venous Thromboembolic Disease

Several studies have demonstrated that patients with IPF have a higher risk of developing acute vascular disease (cardiovascular disease and venous thromboembolic disease) than those with other lung diseases or the general population. In an uncontrolled autopsy study of patients with IPF, 9 patients (21%) died of cardiovascular events.[38] A cross-sectional study of 630 patients referred for lung transplantation at a tertiary hospital demonstrated that patients with IPF have an increased risk of coronary artery disease identified at angiography than patients referred with other chronic lung disease (odds ratio [OR], 2.31; 95% confidence interval [CI], 1.11–4.82).[39] More recently, a large case-controlled study showed that patients with IPF are more likely to have a history of cardiovascular disease at the time of IPF diagnosis (OR, 1.53; 95% CI, 1.15–2.03) than controls and are more likely to have an acute coronary event during follow-up (relative risk 3.14; 95% CI, 2.02–4.87).[40] Patients with IPF were also shown to have an increased risk of angina, atrial fibrillation, deep venous thrombosis, and stroke in this study.

A large study of the Danish population examined whether thromboembolic disease is a risk factor for idiopathic interstitial pneumonia.[41] This study demonstrated that patients with deep venous thrombosis and pulmonary embolism have an increased risk of idiopathic interstitial pneumonia compared with controls (hazard ratio [HR] 1.3; 95% CI, 1.2–1.4; and HR 2.4; 95% CI, 2.3–2.6, respectively) with multivariate-adjusted analyses. In a study of all decedents in the United States between 1988 and 2007, the risk of death from venous thromboembolic disease was greater for patients with pulmonary fibrosis compared with the general population (OR 1.35, 95% CI 1.29–1.38, $P<.0001$), patients with lung cancer (OR 1.45, 95% CI 1.39–1.48, $P<.0001$), or patients with COPD (OR 1.55, 95% CI 1.49–1.59, $P<.0001$).[42]

Current guidelines on the management of IPF do not discuss the identification and management of comorbid vascular disease in patients with IPF; however, it is reasonable to screen patients for vascular disease on an annual basis or if they clinically deteriorate. In particular, when assessing a patient with a possible acute exacerbation of IPF, one must rule out cardiovascular disease and pulmonary embolism as causes of the deterioration.[43]

Lung Cancer

The risk of lung cancer for patients with IPF is high. When compared with that of the general population, the relative risk is 7.31 (95% CI, 4.47–11.93).[44] The prevalence of lung cancer among patients with IPF followed in national registries ranges between 4.4% and 9.8%.[44–46] In a retrospective cohort study, the cumulative incidence of lung cancer among patients with IPF was 3.3% at 1 year, 15.4% at 5 years, and 54.7% at 10 years.[47] The risk of developing lung cancer is greater for patients with IPF who are male ever-smokers.[44,46,47] There are 3 hypotheses to explain this relationship: pulmonary fibrosis causes lung cancer, lung cancer and/or its treatment causes pulmonary fibrosis, and/or common mediators cause lung cancer and pulmonary fibrosis.[48]

Treatment of lung cancer in idiopathic pulmonary fibrosis is fraught with difficulties, including acute exacerbations of pulmonary fibrosis/acute lung injury associated with surgical resection of cancers,[49,50] radiation therapy,[51] and chemotherapy.[52] Existing guidelines do not specifically address this issue and the decision to proceed with treatment of cancer in patients with IPF should be a carefully considered one.

Depression

Quality of life in patients with pulmonary fibrosis is poor[53,54] and associated with dyspnea and impaired pulmonary function.[55–58] Dyspnea in IPF affects health-related quality of life differently in men and women: in men, dyspnea worsens physical quality-of-life domains, and in women, it worsens emotional domains.[59] Twenty-three percent of patients with pulmonary fibrosis were found to have clinically significant depression in a recent study.[60] There is a strong correlation between depression and dyspnea in these patients; multivariate analysis suggests that depression is a major contributing factor in patients' perception of dyspnea and thus their quality of life.[60] Treating depression may improve patients' dyspnea and quality of life; this hypothesis needs testing in clinical trials.

SUMMARY

Patients with IPF face progressive dyspnea and disability, poor prognosis, and limited treatment options. Once thought to be a slowly progressive disease, IPF may have an accelerated variant phenotype. Combined pulmonary fibrosis and emphysema and disproportionate pulmonary hypertension in IPF may also be distinct phenotypes; further investigation is needed to characterize these phenotypes and determine if there is a plausible biologic explanation for these entities. Identification and management of comorbidities may improve the overall quality of life and well-being of these patients.

REFERENCES

1. King TE Jr, Pardo A, Selman M. Idiopathic pulmonary fibrosis. Lancet 2011;378:1949–61.
2. Schulze TG, McMahon FJ. Defining the phenotype in human genetic studies: forward genetics and reverse phenotyping. Hum Hered 2004;58:131–8.
3. Selman M, Carrillo G, Estrada A, et al. Accelerated variant of idiopathic pulmonary fibrosis: clinical behavior and gene expression pattern. PLoS One 2007;2:e482.
4. Cottin V, Cordier JF. The syndrome of combined pulmonary fibrosis and emphysema. Chest 2009;136:1–2.
5. Corte TJ, Wort SJ, Wells AU. Pulmonary hypertension in idiopathic pulmonary fibrosis: a review. Sarcoidosis Vasc Diffuse Lung Dis 2009;26:7–19.
6. Baumgartner KB, Samet JM, Stidley CA, et al. Cigarette smoking: a risk factor for idiopathic pulmonary fibrosis. Am J Respir Crit Care Med 1997;155:242–8.
7. Mejia M, Carrillo G, Rojas-Serrano J, et al. Idiopathic pulmonary fibrosis and emphysema: decreased survival associated with severe pulmonary arterial hypertension. Chest 2009;136:10–5.

8. Cottin V, Nunes H, Brillet P, et al. Combined pulmonary fibrosis and emphysema: a distinct underrecognised entity. Eur Respir J 2005;26:586–93.

9. Doherty MJ, Pearson MG, O'Grady EA, et al. Cryptogenic fibrosing alveolitis with preserved lung volumes. Thorax 1997;52:998–1002.

10. Wiggins J, Strickland B, Turner-Warwick M. Combined cryptogenic fibrosing alveolitis and emphysema: the value of high resolution computed tomography in assessment. Respir Med 1990;84:365–9.

11. Daniil Z, Koutsokera A, Gourgoulianis K. Combined pulmonary fibrosis and emphysema in patients exposed to agrochemical compounds. Eur Respir J 2006;27:434.

12. Barst RJ, McGoon M, Torbicki A, et al. Diagnosis and differential assessment of pulmonary arterial hypertension. J Am Coll Cardiol 2004;43:40S–7S.

13. Arcasoy SM, Christie JD, Ferrari VA, et al. Echocardiographic assessment of pulmonary hypertension in patients with advanced lung disease. Am J Respir Crit Care Med 2003;167:735–40.

14. Shorr AF, Wainright JL, Cors CS, et al. Pulmonary hypertension in patients with pulmonary fibrosis awaiting lung transplant. Eur Respir J 2007;30:715–21.

15. Agarwal R, Gupta D, Verma JS, et al. Noninvasive estimation of clinically asymptomatic pulmonary hypertension in idiopathic pulmonary fibrosis. Indian J Chest Dis Allied Sci 2005;47:267–71.

16. Lettieri CJ, Nathan SD, Barnett SD, et al. Prevalence and outcomes of pulmonary arterial hypertension in advanced idiopathic pulmonary fibrosis. Chest 2006;129:746–52.

17. Nadrous HF, Pellikka PA, Krowka MJ, et al. The impact of pulmonary hypertension on survival in patients with idiopathic pulmonary fibrosis. Chest 2005;128:616S–7S.

18. Nathan SD, Shlobin OA, Ahmad S, et al. Serial development of pulmonary hypertension in patients with idiopathic pulmonary fibrosis. Respiration 2008;76:288–94.

19. Hamada K, Nagai S, Tanaka S, et al. Significance of pulmonary arterial pressure and diffusion capacity of the lung as prognosticator in patients with idiopathic pulmonary fibrosis. Chest 2007;131:650–6.

20. Lederer DJ, Caplan-Shaw CE, O'Shea MK, et al. Racial and ethnic disparities in survival in lung transplant candidates with idiopathic pulmonary fibrosis. Am J Transplant 2006;6:398–403.

21. Nathan SD, Shlobin OA, Ahmad S, et al. Pulmonary hypertension and pulmonary function testing in idiopathic pulmonary fibrosis. Chest 2007;131:657–63.

22. Badesch DB, Abman SH, Simonneau G, et al. Medical therapy for pulmonary arterial hypertension: updated ACCP evidence-based clinical practice guidelines. Chest 2007;131:1917–28.

23. Collard HR, Anstrom KJ, Schwarz MI, et al. Sildenafil improves walk distance in idiopathic pulmonary fibrosis*. Chest 2007;131:897–9.

24. King TE Jr, Behr J, Brown KK, et al. BUILD-1: a randomized placebo-controlled trial of bosentan in idiopathic pulmonary fibrosis. Am J Respir Crit Care Med 2008;177:75–81.

25. Raghu G, Collard HR, Egan JJ, et al. An official ATS/ERS/JRS/ALAT statement: idiopathic pulmonary fibrosis: evidence-based guidelines for diagnosis and management. Am J Respir Crit Care Med 2011; 183:788–824.

26. Thannickal VJ, Loyd JE. Idiopathic pulmonary fibrosis: a disorder of lung regeneration? Am J Respir Crit Care Med 2008;178:663–5.

27. Tcherakian C, Cottin V, Brillet PY, et al. Progression of idiopathic pulmonary fibrosis: lessons from asymmetrical disease. Thorax 2011;66:226–31.

28. Raghu G, Freudenberger TD, Yang S, et al. High prevalence of abnormal acid gastro-oesophageal reflux in idiopathic pulmonary fibrosis. Eur Respir J 2006;27: 136–42.

29. Downs JB, Chapman RL Jr, Modell JH, et al. An evaluation of steroid therapy in aspiration pneumonitis. Anesthesiology 1974;40:129–35.

30. Moran TJ. Experimental aspiration pneumonia. IV. Inflammatory and reparative changes produced by intratracheal injections of autologous gastric juice and hydrochloric acid. AMA Arch Pathol 1955;60: 122–9.

31. Sladen A, Zanca P, Hadnott WH. Aspiration pneumonitis—the sequelae. Chest 1971;59:448–50.

32. Sweet MP, Patti MG, Leard LE, et al. Gastroesophageal reflux in patients with idiopathic pulmonary fibrosis referred for lung transplantation. J Thorac Cardiovasc Surg 2007;133:1078–84.

33. Han MK. High prevalence of abnormal acid gastro-oesophageal reflux in idiopathic pulmonary fibrosis. Eur Respir J 2006;28:884–5 [author reply: 5].

34. Lee J, Song J, Wolters P, et al. Bronchoalveolar lavage pepsin levels in acute exacerbations of idiopathic pulmonary fibrosis. Am J Respir Crit Care Med 2011;183:A3804.

35. Raghu G, Yang ST, Spada C, et al. Sole treatment of acid gastroesophageal reflux in idiopathic pulmonary fibrosis: a case series. Chest 2006;129:794–800.

36. Linden PA, Gilbert RJ, Yeap BY, et al. Laparoscopic fundoplication in patients with end-stage lung disease awaiting transplantation. J Thorac Cardiovasc Surg 2006;131:438–46.

37. Lee JS, Ryu JH, Elicker BM, et al. Gastroesophageal reflux therapy is associated with longer survival in patients with idiopathic pulmonary fibrosis. Am J Respir Crit Care Med 2011;184:1390–4.

38. Daniels CE, Yi ES, Ryu JH. Autopsy findings in 42 consecutive patients with idiopathic pulmonary fibrosis. Eur Respir J 2008;32:170–4.

39. Kizer JR, Zisman DA, Blumenthal NP, et al. Association between pulmonary fibrosis and coronary artery disease. Arch Intern Med 2004;164:551–6.

40. Hubbard RB, Smith C, Le Jeune I, et al. The association between idiopathic pulmonary fibrosis and vascular disease: a population-based study. Am J Respir Crit Care Med 2008;178:1257–61.

41. Sode BF, Dahl M, Nielsen SF, et al. Venous thromboembolism and risk of idiopathic interstitial pneumonia: a nationwide study. Am J Respir Crit Care Med 2010;181:1085–92.

42. Olson A, Sprunger D, Huie T, et al. The prevalence of venous thromboembolism (VTE) in pulmonary fibrosis (PF). Am J Respir Crit Care Med 2011;183: A5305.

43. Collard HR, Moore BB, Flaherty KR, et al. Acute exacerbations of idiopathic pulmonary fibrosis. Am J Respir Crit Care Med 2007;176:636–43.

44. Hubbard R, Venn A, Lewis S, et al. Lung cancer and cryptogenic fibrosing alveolitis. A population-based cohort study. Am J Respir Crit Care Med 2000;161:5–8.

45. Turner-Warwick M, Burrows B, Johnson A. Cryptogenic fibrosing alveolitis: clinical features and their influence on survival. Thorax 1980;35:171–80.

46. Harris JM, Johnston ID, Rudd R, et al. Cryptogenic fibrosing alveolitis and lung cancer: the BTS study. Thorax 2009;65:70–6.

47. Ozawa Y, Suda T, Naito T, et al. Cumulative incidence of and predictive factors for lung cancer in IPF. Respirology 2009;14:723–8.

48. Daniels CE, Jett JR. Does interstitial lung disease predispose to lung cancer? Curr Opin Pulm Med 2005;11:431–7.

49. Kushibe K, Kawaguchi T, Takahama M, et al. Operative indications for lung cancer with idiopathic pulmonary fibrosis. Thorac Cardiovasc Surg 2007;55:505–8.

50. Shintani Y, Ohta M, Iwasaki T, et al. Predictive factors for postoperative acute exacerbation of interstitial pneumonia combined with lung cancer. Gen Thorac Cardiovasc Surg 2010;58:182–5.

51. Takeda A, Enomoto T, Sanuki N, et al. Acute exacerbation of subclinical idiopathic pulmonary fibrosis triggered by hypofractionated stereotactic body radiotherapy in a patient with primary lung cancer and slightly focal honeycombing. Radiat Med 2008;26:504–7.

52. Isobe K, Hata Y, Sakamoto S, et al. Clinical characteristics of acute respiratory deterioration in pulmonary fibrosis associated with lung cancer following anti-cancer therapy. Respirology 2010; 15:88–92.

53. De Vries J, Kessels BL, Drent M. Quality of life of idiopathic pulmonary fibrosis patients. Eur Respir J 2001;17:954–61.

54. Swigris JJ, Kuschner WG, Jacobs SS, et al. Health-related quality of life in patients with idiopathic pulmonary fibrosis: a systematic review. Thorax 2005;60:588–94.

55. Martinez T, Pereira C, dos Santos M, et al. Evaluation of the short-form 36-item questionnaire to measure health-related quality of life in patients with idiopathic pulmonary fibrosis. Chest 2000;117:1627–32.

56. Chang JA, Curtis JR, Patrick DL, et al. Assessment of health-related quality of life in patients with interstitial lung disease. Chest 1999;116:1175–82.

57. Baddini Martinez JA, Martinez TY, Lovetro Galhardo FP, et al. Dyspnea scales as a measure of health-related quality of life in patients with idiopathic pulmonary fibrosis. Med Sci Monit 2002;8:R405–10.

58. Tzanakis N, Samiou M, Lambiri I, et al. Evaluation of health-related quality-of-life and dyspnea scales in patients with idiopathic pulmonary fibrosis. Correlation with pulmonary function tests. Eur J Intern Med 2005;16:105–12.

59. Han MK, Swigris J, Liu L, et al. Gender influences health-related quality of life in IPF. Respir Med 2010;104:724–30.

60. Ryerson CJ, Berkeley J, Carrieri-Kohlman VL, et al. Depression and functional status are strongly associated with dyspnea in interstitial lung disease. Chest 2011;139:609–16.

61. King TE Jr, Brown KK, Raghu G, et al. The BUILD-3 trial: a prospective, randomized, double-blind, placebo-controlled study of bosentan in idiopathic pulmonary fibrosis. Am J Respir Crit Care Med 2010;181:A6838.

62. The Idiopathic Pulmonary Fibrosis Clinical Research Network. A controlled trial of sildenafil in advanced idiopathic pulmonary fibrosis. N Engl J Med 2010; 363.620–8.

63. Gilead terminates phase III trial of ambrisentan in patients with idiopathic pulmonary fibrosis [press release]. Gilead Sciences, Inc; December 22, 2010. In press.

64. Actelion reports results of exploratory study with macitentan in patients with idiopathic pulmonary fibrosis promising long term safety and tolerability profile—efficacy data not supportive of Phase III in IPF [press release]. Actelion Pharmaceuticals Ltd; August 29, 2011. In press.

Acute Exacerbation of Idiopathic Pulmonary Fibrosis

Dong Soon Kim, MD, PhD

KEYWORDS

- Idiopathic pulmonary fibrosis • Acute exacerbation
- Incidence • Risk factors

Although idiopathic pulmonary fibrosis (IPF) is a chronic progressive and ultimately fatal disease, it has become clear that the clinical course of individual patients is highly variable and that the sudden deterioration of a patient's respiratory condition during a relatively stable course is not uncommon.[1,2] This deterioration can result from well-known causes such as infection, pulmonary embolism, congestive heart failure, pneumothorax, or drugs. However, in many cases the etiology is not certain despite rigorous searches, and these cases have been called acute exacerbation (AEx) of IPF under the assumption of sudden acceleration of the underlying disease process.[3–5] This phenomenon was recognized many years ago among pathologists as a diffuse alveolar damage (DAD) pattern superimposed on usual interstitial pneumonia (UIP),[6,7] and was also recognized clinically in Japan.[8–10] In the English literature, Kondoh and colleagues[4] first reported 3 cases of AEx in 1993; however, in Western countries it was taken as an extremely rare phenomenon until, in 2005, Martinez and colleagues[11] found an apparently acute and rapid progression of lung disease in almost half of the patients who died of an IPF-related cause among the placebo group of the randomized clinical trial of interferon-γ. Since then, several studies have reported the clinical significance of AEx-IPF; however, most of these were retrospective case series and the results were discordant. Therefore, in 2007 Collard and international experts summarized the state of knowledge at that time, and proposed consensus definition and diagnostic criteria to standardize the criteria for future research (**Box 1**).[5]

This review primarily discusses studies performed after this Consensus Perspective by Collard and colleagues.[5]

INCIDENCE

The true incidence of AEx is still not known. The results of the previous retrospective studies were highly variable, from 4.4% to 19% per year, probably because of the difference in case definition, method, and population. According to 2 recent retrospective studies, 1-year and 3-year incidence of AEx were 14.2% and 20.7% among 461 patients with IPF studied by Song and colleagues,[12] and 8.6% and 23.9% among 74 patients studied by Kondoh and colleagues.[13] However, the incidence rates in recent clinical trials were different (**Tables 1** and **2**). In most of the clinical trials, the AEx was infrequent (<4%) with few exceptions.[14,17] The reason for the difference in incidence is not clear.

AEx was the most common immediate cause of death (29%) in 42 autopsy cases with IPF.[23] In addition, composite data on IPF-related deaths prospectively recorded in recently published clinical studies[11,19,22,24,25] revealed that 30% of total deaths occurred as an acute worsening (less than 4 weeks) and 47% of the patients experienced subacute deterioration (over a period of 4 weeks to months) before their death.[2] In one other prospective clinical trial, patients with lower forced vital capacity (FVC) (<62% predicted) had more total and respiratory hospitalizations during subsequent follow-up.[11] A recent review of 461 patients with IPF by Song and colleagues[12]

Department of Pulmonary and Critical Care Medicine, Asan Medical Center, University of Ulsan, Seoul, Korea
E-mail address: dskim@amc.seoul.kr

Clin Chest Med 33 (2012) 59–68
doi:10.1016/j.ccm.2012.01.001
0272-5231/12/$ – see front matter © 2012 Elsevier Inc. All rights reserved.

Box 1
Proposed consensus criteria of acute exacerbation of IPF

1. Previous or concurrent diagnosis of idiopathic pulmonary fibrosis[a]
2. Unexplained worsening or development of dyspnea within 30 days
3. High-resolution computed tomography with new bilateral ground-glass abnormality[b] and/or consolidation superimposed on a background reticular or honeycomb pattern consistent with usual interstitial pneumonia (UIP) pattern[c]
4. No evidence of pulmonary infection by endotracheal aspirate or bronchoalveolar lavage[c]
5. Exclusion of alternative causes including: left heart failure, pulmonary embolism, and identifiable cause of acute lung injury[d]

Patients with idiopathic clinical worsening who fail to meet all 5 criteria due to missing data should be termed suspected acute exacerbations.

[a] If the diagnosis of idiopathic pulmonary fibrosis is not previously established according to American Thoracic Society/European Respiratory Society consensus criteria (2), this criterion can be met by the presence of radiologic and/or histopathologic changes consistent with usual interstitial pneumonia pattern on the current evaluation.
[b] If no previous high-resolution computed tomography is available, the qualifier "new" can be dropped.
[c] Evaluation of samples should include studies for routine bacterial organisms, opportunistic pathogens, and common viral pathogens.
[d] Causes of acute lung injury include sepsis, aspiration, trauma, reperfusion pulmonary edema, pulmonary contusion, fat embolization, inhalational injury, cardiopulmonary bypass, drug toxicity, acute pancreatitis, transfusion of blood products, and stem cell transplantation.
From Collard HR, Moore BB, Flaherty KR, et al. Acute exacerbations of idiopathic pulmonary fibrosis. Am J Respir Crit Care Med 2007;176(7):636–43; with permission.

---

revealed that low FVC was a significant risk factor for AEx, and Kondoh and colleagues[13] reported that decline in FVC at 6 months was an independent risk factor along with an initially high modified Medical Research Council scale. These data suggested that many AExs may be terminal events occurring during the relatively later course of the disease. Therefore, the overall incidence of AEx

Table 1
Incidence of acute exacerbation of IPF reported in randomized controlled clinical trials

Name	Pirfenidone Azuma[14]		Pirfenidone Taniguchi[15]			CAPACITY1[16]			CAPACITY2[16]	
AEx Criteria	JRS†		JRS†			Collard + Pao$_2$			Collard + Pao$_2$	
Duration	9 mo		52 wk			77 wk			77 wk	
	PR	Control	PR-High	PR-Low	Control	PR-High	PR-Low	Control	PR-High	Control
No.	72	35	108	55	104	174	87	174	171	(173)
AEx (%)	0	13.9	5.6	5.5	4.8	1.1	1.1	1.7	1.2	0.6
Age (y)	64.0	64.3	65.4	63.9	64.7	65.7	68	66.3	66.8	67.0
Nonsmoker	11	6	20.4	21.8	20.2	32	31	29	35	37.0
FVC	81.6	78.4	77.3	76.2	79.1	74.5	76.4	76.2	74.9	73.1
DLco	57.6	57.7	52	54	55	46.4	47.2	46.1	47.8	47.4

Abbreviations: AEx, acute exacerbation; DLco, carbon monoxide diffusing capacity; FVC, forced vital capacity; Ima, imatinib; PR, pirfenidone.
CAPACITY: Clinical studies assessing pirfenidone in idiopathic pulmonary fibrosis: research of efficacy and safety outcomes: 2 randomized trials.[16]
Diagnostic criteria of acute exacerbation:
JRS†: Japanese Respiratory Society criteria: (1) manifestation of all of the following: worsening, otherwise unexplained clinical features within 1 month, progression of dyspnea over a few days to less than 5 weeks, + (2) new radiographic/high-resolution computed tomography (HRCT) parenchymal abnormalities without pneumothorax or pleural effusion (eg, new, superimposed round-glass opacities), + (3) a decrease in the Pao$_2$ by 10 mm Hg or more, and (4) exclusion of apparent infection based on absence of *Aspergillus* and *Pneumococcus* antibodies in blood, urine for *Legionella pneumophila*, and sputum cultures.
Collard & Pao$_2$: Collard's criteria + reduction of Pao$_2$ more than 10 mm Hg.

Table 2
Incidence of acute exacerbation of IPF reported in randomized controlled clinical trials

Name	Kubo[17]		IFIGENIA[18]		INSPIRE[19]		BUILD-1[20]		BUILD-3[21]		Imatinib[22]	
AEx Criteria[a]	[b]		Respiratory failure		Acute respiratory failure		Acute decompensation of IPF		Acute exacerbation of IPF		Acute worsening of IPF	
Duration	3 y		1 y		537 d		12 mo		20 mo		96 wk	
	AC	Control	NAC	Control	IF-g	Control	Bos	Control	Bos	Control	Ima	Control
No.	23	33	80	75	551	275	71	83	407	209	59	60
AEx (%)	16	21	6	1	2	—	1.4	3.6	4.7	2.9	8.5	1.7
Age (y)	71	68	62	64	66	659	65	65	64	63	66	68
Nonsmoker	100	100	38.8	30.7	28	31	—	—	38	32	28	36
FVC	69	71	80	75	72	73	66	70	75	73	64	66
DLco	59	63	79	74	47	47	42	41	48	48	40	39

Abbreviations: AC, anticoagulation; Bos, bosentan; NAC, N-acetylcysteine.

IFIGENIA: Idiopathic Pulmonary Fibrosis International Group Exploring N-Acetylcysteine I Annual.[18]

INSPIRE: Effect of interferon gamma-1b on survival in patients with idiopathic pulmonary fibrosis (INSPIRE): a multicentre, randomized, placebo-controlled trial.[19]

BUILD-1 (Bosentan Use in Interstitial Lung Disease-1): a randomized placebo-controlled trial of bosentan in idiopathic pulmonary fibrosis.[20]

BUILD-3 (Bosentan Use in Interstitial Lung Disease-3): a randomized, controlled trial of bosentan in idiopathic pulmonary fibrosis.[21]

Imatinib: treatment for idiopathic pulmonary fibrosis: Randomized placebo-controlled trial results.[22]

Diagnostic criteria of acute exacerbation:

Kubo: (1) exacerbation of dyspnea within a few weeks; (2) newly developing diffuse pulmonary infiltrates on chest radiographs or HRCT; (3) deterioration of hypoxemia (Pao_2/fraction of inspired oxygen <300); and (4) absence of infectious pneumonia, heart failure, and sepsis.

BUILD-1: acute decompensation (unexplained rapid deterioration over 4 weeks with increased dyspnea requiring hospitalization and oxygen supplementation $\geq$5 L/min to maintain a resting oxygen saturation (arterial blood gas; Sao_2) $\geq$90% or Pao_2 $\geq$55 mm Hg (sea level) or 50 mm Hg (above 1400 m)).

[a] Not specified but the data are mentioned as.

[b] Kubo: (1) exacerbation of dyspnea within a few weeks; (2) newly developing diffuse pulmonary infiltrates on chest radiographs or HRCT; (3) deterioration of hypoxemia (Pao_2/fraction of inspired oxygen <300); and (4) absence of infectious pneumonia, heart failure, and sepsis.

likely varies depending on the patient population, and this may explain the low incidence of AEx in those clinical trials where most of the enrolled patients were stable and mild to moderate in severity.

RISK FACTORS
Ethnic or Genetic Factors

Epidemiologic data suggest that Japanese persons suffer more frequently from DAD, due to various causes such as drugs[26]; for example, 5.8% of Japanese patients on gefitinib therapy developed interstitial lung disease, a frequency 10- to 100-fold higher than for patients of other genetic backgrounds.[27] The incidence of AEx in clinical trials conducted in Japan seems to be higher than that in other countries. However, this observation should be interpreted cautiously, because the study design and criteria for AEx were different in these studies. This point should

be pursued further in the global multinational clinical trials. Of interest is that genetic and ethnic disparities exist in acute lung injury, a condition clinically and histopathologically similar to AEx-IPF, and may be worthy of investigation as well.[28]

Other Factors

As stated earlier, low lung function as indicated by low FVC, higher dyspnea score, and more decline in FVC at 6 months were reported as significant risk factors for AEx.[12,13] In the study by Song and colleagues,[12] never-smokers had higher risk, whereas higher body mass index was reported by Kondoh and colleagues[13] as another independent risk factor.

ETIOLOGY

The etiology and pathobiology of AEx-IPF is still unknown, but several potential causes have been proposed.

Infection

Because of the similarity in clinical features between infection and AEx-IPF and also the potentially increased susceptibility to infection in these patients secondary to therapy or underlying disease, it is difficult to exclude the possibility of infection for the diagnosis of AEx-IPF. In a murine model, infection with gammaherpesvirus caused exacerbation of established fluorescein isothiocyanate–induced fibrosis manifested by increased total lung collagen, histologic changes of acute lung injury, and diminished lung function.[29] Some or many patients with clinically diagnosed AEx-IPF may have hidden infection despite vigorous clinical workup. In one prospective study conducted to investigate the possible role of *Chlamydophila pneumoniae* infection in triggering AEx, 2 of 27 AEx-IPF cases showed a significant increase in antibody response.[30] Huie and colleagues[31] reported that a detailed diagnostic evaluation including viral culture, antigen-based testing, or molecular testing for respiratory viruses and atypical pathogens revealed a potential infectious etiology in up to one-third of cases in their 27 patients with fibrotic lung disease hospitalized for an acute respiratory decline (including 10 definite AEx and 9 suspected AEx), although the causative role of these infections was not certain. However, recently Wootton and colleagues[32] confirmed the absence of viral infection in the majority of the bronchoalveolar lavage (BAL) fluid prospectively collected in the early phase of 43 AEx-IPF cases using the most current genomics-based technologies (multiplex polymerase chain reaction, pan-viral microarray, and high-throughput cDNA sequencing), also using the patients with stable IPF and acute lung injury as control group. The investigators found torque teno virus in 12 BAL fluids; however, it was present in a similar percentage of acute respiratory distress syndrome (ARDS) control patients, suggesting that its presence is not specific for AEx-IPF, but rather may be associated with acute lung injury in general. These data suggest that infection may not be the cause of most cases of AEx-IPF, although there is still a possibility of viral triggering of acute lung injury and disappearance at the time of clinical presentation.

Gastroesophageal Reflux

There is a growing interest in the role of gastroesophageal reflux disease (GERD) and occult aspiration in patients with IPF.[33] The symptoms of GERD are frequent in patients with IPF, and stabilization of lung function and reduced oxygen requirements after the medical therapy or a fundoplication[34] suggest a possible association of this condition with disease progression in IPF. Aspiration of gastric contents can cause acute lung injury manifested by DAD on lung biopsy,[35] and this has been proposed as one possible cause of AEx-IPF.[5,33] A recent study on BAL pepsin level of 24 AEx-IPF cases and 30 stable IPF controls showed measurable BAL pepsin in most patients with stable IPF, suggesting that occult aspiration is common in IPF. Eight (33%) of the AEx-IPF cases had high BAL pepsin levels (above the 95th percentile of the stable control population, 70 ng/mL).[36] Although the relationship is modest, this finding provides evidence that occult aspiration may be one important cause of AEx-IPF.

Other Possibilities

Another possible but not yet studied determinant of AEx is air pollution. Because the respiratory system is directly exposed to inhaled environmental substances and the relationship between ambient air pollution exposure and exacerbation of airway disease (eg, asthma, chronic obstructive pulmonary disease) is well established, it could possibly exacerbate the underlying parenchymal lung disease in IPF.

PATHOGENESIS AND PATHOBIOLOGY

It is not yet certain whether AEx-IPF represents an acceleration of the pathobiologic process of the primary disease or represents a clinically occult and unrecognized extrinsic trigger such as a viral infection or silent aspiration. In this paradigm, AEx-IPF may be the sequela of an acute direct stress or injury superimposed on already fibrotic lung, with an acceleration of the underlying fibroproliferative process of IPF. Indeed, the finding of subpleural fibrosis with fibroblastic foci, a typical feature of UIP in half of the autopsies of acute interstitial pneumonia (AIP) reported by Araya and colleagues,[37] suggests that some or many of the cases of AIP, especially in old age, may be actually the AEx of subclinical IPF.

A recent biomarker study comparing AEx-IPF and ARDS may shed some light on this question.[38] Although the histology of AEx-IPF is similar to fibroproliferative ARDS, the plasma biomarker profile is different. In early ARDS, the levels of the receptor for advanced glycation end products (RAGE), a marker of type I alveolar epithelial cell injury/proliferation, proinflammatory cytokines, markers of endothelial dysfunction, activated coagulation, and inhibited fibrinolysis were all elevated, whereas AEx-IPF group had lower levels of RAGE and higher levels of KL-6 and SP-D (markers of type II alveolar epithelial cell proliferation and/or injury).[38] The absence of a type I cell injury signature combined with an exuberant elevation of type II cell markers provides support for the hypothesis that AEx-IPF is predominantly a manifestation of the underlying disease process accelerating, rather than the result of a second injury. In such a context, all the pathogenetic processes of IPF itself may be responsible for AEx-IPF. Konish and colleagues[39] showed that the global gene expression patterns of IPF-AEx were almost identical to those of stable IPF, although a set of different gene (epithelial injury and proliferation and apoptosis of epithelium) expression was enhanced in patients with AEx-IPF compared with stable IPF.

PRECIPITATING FACTORS
Lung Resection

There are many reports about the occurrence of AEx after lung resection. Sakamoto and colleagues[40] reported that 3 of 39 patients with IPF developed AEx after the operation (2 lobectomy, 1 biopsy). Shintani and colleagues[41] reported similar results; 15% (6 of 40 patients) of the patients with UIP and lung cancer developed postoperative AEx. Regarding other aspects, Saito and colleagues[42] found that the incidence of ARDS was 2% among 487 lung cancer surgery procedures, but 86% of these ARDS cases occurred in patients with histologically proved interstitial pneumonia. A histopathologic finding of interstitial pneumonia was the only predictor of ARDS (31.8% in interstitial pneumonia–positive group vs 1.5% in interstitial pneumonia–negative group), suggesting a high frequency of AEx of IPF after the surgery for lung cancer.[42] The underlying mechanism of this is not clear. Sakamoto and colleagues[40] suggested oxygen supplementation at a high concentration and/or prolonged mechanical ventilation as possible etiologic factors. In animal experiments, pneumonectomy alone can cause noncritical lung injury and amplify the inflammatory response and fibrosis to bleomycin.[43]

Surgical Lung Biopsy

Not only lung resection but also surgical lung biopsy can precipitate AEx.[44,45] According to Kondoh and colleagues,[44] among the 236 consecutive patients with interstitial pneumonia who underwent a surgical lung biopsy, 5 (2.1%) (IPF, 3; nonspecific interstitial pneumonia, 1; cryptogenic organizing pneumonia, 1) developed AEx, and the extent of the parenchymal involvement was significantly greater on the nonbiopsied (ie, the mechanically ventilated) side.

Lung Cancer Chemotherapy

Many chemotherapeutic agents, especially newly developed drugs, can provoke interstitial pneumonia and may mimic AEx in the patients with preexisting IPF. Minegishi and colleagues[46] reported that the incidence of acute respiratory deterioration related to anticancer treatment was 22.7% among 120 patients with lung cancer accompanied by idiopathic interstitial pneumonia.

Bronchoalveolar Lavage

There have been several case reports of AEx developing after BAL procedures, although the possibility of infection was not completely excluded.[3,8,47]

BIOMARKERS

In addition to serum KL-6, neutrophil elastase, and lactate dehydrogenase (LDH) levels, which have been suggested as markers of AEx-IPF,[48] there are several new possible biomarkers.

α-Defensins

α-Defensins, a family of mammalian neutrophil peptides, can stimulate collagen synthesis from lung fibroblasts via β-catenin signaling,[49] and their plasma level was reported to be higher in patients with IPF compared with healthy subjects.[50] Plasma levels of α-defensins also correlated with the clinical course of AEx-IPF, and BAL fluid levels had an inverse correlation with the arterial oxygen tension (Pao_2) and pulmonary function. Using gene expression microarrays of lung tissues, Konishi and colleagues[39] demonstrated that α-defensins and CCNA2 were among the most upregulated genes in AEx-IPF and that α-defensin levels were elevated in the peripheral blood of patients with AEx-IPF, although there was no evidence of an infectious or overwhelming inflammatory etiology.

ST2 Protein

The human ST2 gene can be induced by growth stimulation in fibroblastic cells, and soluble ST2 protein is expressed preferentially in T-helper type 2 (Th2) cells by proinflammatory stimuli such as tumor necrosis factor–α and interleukin-1β. Tajima and colleagues[51] reported that serum ST2 levels in AEx-IPF were significantly higher than those in the stable IPF group or the healthy controls, correlated statistically with LDH and C-reactive protein, and inversely correlated with Pao_2.

Circulating Fibrocytes

Moeller and colleagues[52] reported that circulating fibrocytes were significantly elevated in patients with stable IPF (n = 51), with a further increase during AEx (n = 7), and that they were an independent predictor of early mortality. The level in the ARDS control group (n = 10) were not different, suggesting that fibrocytes may be more indicative of fibrotic tissue injury or repair and not a reflection of acute lung injury per se.

Annexin-1

Using serologic identification of antigens by recombinant expression cloning (SEREX) analysis, Kurosu and colleagues[53] identified 5 antibodies as novel biomarker candidates for AEx-IPF. Among them, antibody to annexin-1 was detected in 47% of the sera and 53% of the BAL fluid from patients with AEx. The N-terminal portion of annexin-1 induced marked proliferative responses of CD4-positive T cells, suggesting that annexin-1 is an autoantigen that raises both antibody production and T-cell response in AEx.[53]

PATHOLOGY

The histologic pattern of AEx is acute lung injury superimposed on underlying UIP. In the published literature, acute injury consists of diffuse alveolar damage in the vast majority of cases, and much more rarely profuse organizing pneumonia or extensive fibroblastic foci. Patients with organizing pneumonia or extensive fibroblast foci may do better than those with DAD.[54] An interesting observation on the relationship between histopathologic features and the course of IPF by Titto and colleagues[55] in 76 patients with UIP (64 IPF, 12 connective tissue disease [CTD]-UIP) was that there was no correlation between the clinical severity of an AEx and the extent of DAD. Six of 11 patients had widespread DAD in their necroscopic samples, but without clinical signs of an AEx before death. Furthermore, only 2 of 6 patients with clinical signs of pneumonia revealed typical histopathologic features of pneumonia, whereas 2 other patients with typical pneumonia in necropsy lung samples did not have any changes of pneumonia before death. The investigators also found that the number of fibroblastic foci in lung samples before death is associated with poor survival but not with DAD, which is a common feature in necropsy specimens of patients with UIP. Fibroblastic foci did not predict AEx-IPF.

RADIOLOGY

The radiologic findings of AEx-IPF are newly developed ground-glass opacities superimposed on peripheral basal reticulation and/or honeycombing on high-resolution computed tomography (HRCT). By reviewing the HRCT of 64 AEX episodes of 58 patients with IPF, Akira and colleagues[56] found that peripheral pattern was most common (n = 34), followed by diffuse pattern (n = 16) and multifocal pattern, and strong correlations were observed between CT patterns (diffuse versus multifocal and peripheral) and survival.

DIAGNOSIS

To standardize future research investigation on AEx, international experts proposed perspective diagnostic criteria, stated in **Box 1**. Although most of the previous criteria included increasing hypoxemia (a decline in Pao_2 more than 10 mm Hg compared with preexacerbation status), in this perspective criteria, the abnormal gas exchange criterion was deliberately omitted because it was thought to add little specificity. It was recommended that endotracheal aspiration or BAL be used to exclude possible infection, recognizing that the most difficult step in the diagnosis of AEx-IPF is the exclusion of infection. If these data are unavailable (BAL or endotracheal aspirate are often difficult to obtain clinically), but the case is otherwise consistent, the diagnosis is suspected AEx.[5] By contrast, the exclusion of other alternative causes, such as heart failure or pulmonary embolism, is left intentionally vague. Later, Wuyts and colleagues[57] proposed a complementary diagnostic algorithm using D-dimers, echocardiography, pulmonary embolism CT, and BAL; however, this algorithm needs validation in more prospective studies.

TREATMENT

High-dose corticosteroid, sometimes as pulse therapy with or without immunosuppressive agents in combination with a broad spectrum of antimicrobial coverage, was used in most of the AEx patients reported in the literature, and is recommended for use by the recent international evidence-based treatment guideline document for IPF.[58] However, the efficacy of these therapies is uncertain and survival is still very poor.[5,12] Therefore, many innovative procedures have been tried.

- A few articles have reported a better outcome for patients treated with cyclosporine A. In a study by Inase and colleagues',[59] long-term survival was possible in 4 of 7 patients on cyclosporine A. Sakamoto and colleagues[60] reported an improved mean survival in 11 patients treated with cyclosporine A (286 days) in comparison with 11 patients in the non–cyclosporine A group (mean: 60 days). However, these are all noncontrolled retrospective studies with very small cohorts.

- There are several case reports from Japan on the effect of direct hemoperfusion with a polymyxin B–immobilized fiber column, which adsorbs neutrophils on AEx-IPF.[61,62]
- Another small study in Japan reported improved survival in AEx-IPF patients treated with sivelestat (a neutrophil elastase inhibitor)[63] or tacrolimus.[64]
- One prospective study showed improved survival with anticoagulation therapy, mostly attributable to improved mortality for AEx; however, the study was not blinded, had disproportionate dropout, and had an unusually high incidence of AEx in both groups.[17]
- A double-blind, randomized, placebo-controlled trial of pirfenidone on 107 patients showed fewer episodes of AEx-IPF in the pirfenidone group (0%) than in the placebo group (13.9%).[24] However, the results were not confirmed in another larger trial in the same country,[15] Japan.

ACUTE RESPIRATORY WORSENING OF OTHER CONDITIONS

Acute respiratory worsening may occur in other types of idiopathic interstitial pneumonia and CTD-related interstitial pneumonia. Park and colleagues[65] reported 6 cases among 74 idiopathic nonspecific interstitial pneumonia and 4 among 93 CTD-related interstitial pneumonia (mostly rheumatoid arthritis–related UIP). Later, Suda and colleagues[66] reported 6 patients among 83 CTD-related interstitial pneumonia (5 rheumatoid arthritis and one primary Sjögren syndrome), 5 (83.3%) of whom died of respiratory failure. This phenomenon was actually reported earlier, although the investigators did not use the same terminology. In 1999, study of follow-up CT on 29 patients with rheumatoid arthritis–related interstitial pneumonia by Akira and colleagues[67] showed that 6 patients among 19 with UIP-pattern disease developed rapidly progressing ground-glass opacity with fulminant clinical course. All died, and an autopsy in one patient showed both UIP and an organizing DAD pattern. Also, Dawson and colleagues[68] reported that 2 patients among 29 with rheumatoid arthritis–related interstitial pneumonia showed sudden deterioration with occurrence of a new ground-glass pattern disease. Whether these non-IPF cases of acute respiratory deterioration represent AEx as discussed above remains to be seen.

SUMMARY

Despite considerable remaining uncertainty, the weight of the evidence to date suggests AEx of IPF involves the sudden acceleration of the underlying fibroproliferative process of IPF. In some cases it may be triggered by infection, especially viral infection, aspiration of gastric contents, or mechanical stress by surgery, BAL, or hyperinflation. The reported incidence is highly variable, with lower incidence in many randomized clinical trials than in retrospective cohorts. Recent large clinical studies have suggested lower FVC (ie, more severe physiologic impairment) to be a risk factor. Unfortunately, there remains no proven effective treatment and high mortality.

ACKNOWLEDGMENTS

The author extends appreciation to H.R. Collard for the collaboration in the clinical research of AEx-IPF and also for reviewing the manuscript.

REFERENCES

1. Kim DS, Collard HR, King TE Jr. Classification and natural history of the idiopathic interstitial pneumonias. Proc Am Thorac Soc 2006;3(4):285–92.
2. Ley B, Collard HR, King TE Jr. Clinical course and prediction of survival in idiopathic pulmonary fibrosis. Am J Respir Crit Care Med 2011;183(4):431–40.
3. Kim DS, Park JH, Park BK, et al. Acute exacerbation of idiopathic pulmonary fibrosis: frequency and clinical features. Eur Respir J 2006;27(1):143–50.
4. Kondoh Y, Taniguchi H, Kawabata Y, et al. Acute exacerbation in idiopathic pulmonary fibrosis. Analysis of clinical and pathologic findings in three cases. Chest 1993;103(6):1808–12.
5. Collard HR, Moore BB, Flaherty KR, et al. Acute exacerbations of idiopathic pulmonary fibrosis. Am J Respir Crit Care Med 2007;176(7):636–43.
6. Colby TV. Interstitial disease. In: Colby TV, Lombard CM, Yousem SA, et al, editors. Atlas of pulmonary surgical pathology. Philadelphia: WB Saunders; 1991. p. 227–306.
7. Kitaichi M. Pathologic features and the classification of interstitial pneumonia of unknown etiology. Bull Chest Dis Res Inst Kyoto Univ 1990;23(1–2):1–18.
8. Suga T, Sugiyama Y, Ohno S, et al. Two cases of IIP which developed acute exacerbation after bronchoalveolar lavage. Nihon Kyobu Shikkan Gakkai Zasshi 1994;32(2):174–8 [in Japanese].

9. Horio H, Nomori H, Morinaga S, et al. Exacerbation of idiopathic interstitial pneumonia after lobectomy for lung cancer. Nihon Kyobu Shikkan Gakkai Zasshi 1996;34(4):439–43 [in Japanese].

10. Takahashi T, Munakata M, Ohtsuka Y, et al. Effects of corticosteroid pulse treatment on outcomes in acute exacerbations of idiopathic interstitial pneumonia. Nihon Kyobu Shikkan Gakkai Zasshi 1997;35(1):9–15 [in Japanese].

11. Martinez FJ, Safrin S, Weycker D, et al. The clinical course of patients with idiopathic pulmonary fibrosis. Ann Intern Med 2005;142(12 Pt 1):963–7.

12. Song JW, Hong SB, Lim CM, et al. Acute exacerbation of idiopathic pulmonary fibrosis: incidence, risk factors and outcome. Eur Respir J 2011;37(2):356–63.

13. Kondoh Y, Taniguchi H, Katsuta T, et al. Risk factors of acute exacerbation of idiopathic pulmonary fibrosis. Sarcoidosis Vasc Diffuse Lung Dis 2010;27(2):103–10.

14. Azuma A, Nukiwa T, Tsuboi E, et al. Double-blind, placebo-controlled trial of pirfenidone in patients with idiopathic pulmonary fibrosis. Am J Respir Crit Care Med 2005;171(9):1040–7.

15. Taniguchi H, Ebina M, Kondoh Y, et al. Pirfenidone in idiopathic pulmonary fibrosis. Eur Respir J 2010;35(4):821–9.

16. Noble PW, Albera C, Bradford WZ, et al. Pirfenidone in patients with idiopathic pulmonary fibrosis (CAPACITY): two randomised trials. Lancet 2011;377(9779):1760–9.

17. Kubo H, Nakayama K, Yanai M, et al. Anticoagulant therapy for idiopathic pulmonary fibrosis. Chest 2005;128(3):1475–82.

18. Demedts M, Behr J, Buhl R, et al. High-dose acetylcysteine in idiopathic pulmonary fibrosis. N Engl J Med 2005;353(21):2229–42.

19. Fernandez Perez ER, Daniels CE, Schroeder DR, et al. Incidence, prevalence, and clinical course of idiopathic pulmonary fibrosis: a population-based study. Chest 2010;137(1):129–37.

20. King TE Jr, Behr J, Brown KK, et al. BUILD-1: a randomized placebo-controlled trial of bosentan in idiopathic pulmonary fibrosis. Am J Respir Crit Care Med 2008;177(1):75–81.

21. King TE Jr, Brown KK, Raghu G, et al. BUILD-3: a randomized, controlled trial of bosentan in idiopathic pulmonary fibrosis. Am J Respir Crit Care Med 2011;184(1):92–9.

22. Raghu G, Brown KK, Costabel U, et al. Treatment of idiopathic pulmonary fibrosis with etanercept: an exploratory, placebo-controlled trial. Am J Respir Crit Care Med 2008;178(9):948–55.

23. Daniels CE, Yi ES, Ryu JH. Autopsy findings in 42 consecutive patients with idiopathic pulmonary fibrosis. Eur Respir J 2008;32(1):170–4.

24. Daniels CE, Lasky JA, Limper AH, et al. Imatinib treatment for idiopathic pulmonary fibrosis: randomized placebo-controlled trial results. Am J Respir Crit Care Med 2010;181(6):604–10.

25. King TE Jr, Albera C, Bradford WZ, et al. Effect of interferon gamma-1b on survival in patients with idiopathic pulmonary fibrosis (INSPIRE): a multicentre, randomised, placebo-controlled trial. Lancet 2009;374(9685):222–8.

26. Azuma A, Kudoh S. High prevalence of drug-induced pneumonia in Japan. Japan Med Assoc J 2007;50:405–11.

27. Azuma A, Hagiwara K, Kudoh S. Basis of acute exacerbation of idiopathic pulmonary fibrosis in Japanese patients. Am J Respir Crit Care Med 2008;177(12):1397–8 [author reply: 1398].

28. Barnes KC. Genetic determinants and ethnic disparities in sepsis-associated acute lung injury. Proc Am Thorac Soc 2005;2(3):195–201.

29. McMillan TR, Moore BB, Weinberg JB, et al. Exacerbation of established pulmonary fibrosis in a murine model by gammaherpesvirus. Am J Respir Crit Care Med 2008;177(7):771–80.

30. Tomioka H, Sakurai T, Hashimoto K, et al. Acute exacerbation of idiopathic pulmonary fibrosis: role of Chlamydophila pneumoniae infection. Respirology 2007;12(5):700–6.

31. Huie TJ, Olson AL, Cosgrove GP, et al. A detailed evaluation of acute respiratory decline in patients with fibrotic lung disease: aetiology and outcomes. Respirology 2010;15(6):909–17.

32. Wootton SC, Kim DS, Kondoh Y, et al. Viral infection in acute exacerbation of idiopathic pulmonary fibrosis. Am J Respir Crit Care Med 2011;183(12):1698–702.

33. Lee JS, Collard HR, Raghu G, et al. Does chronic microaspiration cause idiopathic pulmonary fibrosis? Am J Med 2010;123(4):304–11.

34. Linden PA, Gilbert RJ, Yeap BY, et al. Laparoscopic fundoplication in patients with end-stage lung disease awaiting transplantation. J Thorac Cardiovasc Surg 2006;131(2):438–46.

35. Travis WD, Colby TV, Koss MN, et al. Lipoid pneumonia and chronic fibrosis. In: King DW, editor. Non-neoplastic disorders of the lower respiratory tract. Washington, DC: American Registry of Pathology and the Armed Forces Institute of Pathology; 2002.

36. Lee JS, Song JW, Wolters PJ, et al. Bronchoalveolar lavage pepsin in acute exacerbation of idiopathic pulmonary fibrosis. ERJ Express 2011. DOI:10.1183/09031936.00050911.

37. Araya J, Kawabata Y, Jinho P, et al. Clinically occult subpleural fibrosis and acute interstitial pneumonia a precursor to idiopathic pulmonary fibrosis? Respirology 2008;13(3):408–12.

38. Collard HR, Calfee CS, Wolters PJ, et al. Plasma biomarker profiles in acute exacerbation of idiopathic pulmonary fibrosis. Am J Physiol Lung Cell Mol Physiol 2010;299(1):L3–7.

39. Konishi K, Gibson KF, Lindell KO, et al. Gene expression profiles of acute exacerbations of idiopathic pulmonary fibrosis. Am J Respir Crit Care Med 2009;180(2):167–75.

40. Sakamoto S, Homma S, Mun M, et al. Acute exacerbation of idiopathic interstitial pneumonia following lung surgery in 3 of 68 consecutive patients: a retrospective study. Intern Med 2011;50(2):77–85.

41. Shintani Y, Ohta M, Iwasaki T, et al. Predictive factors for postoperative acute exacerbation of interstitial pneumonia combined with lung cancer. Gen Thorac Cardiovasc Surg 2010;58(4):182–5.

42. Saito H, Minamiya Y, Nanjo H, et al. Pathological finding of subclinical interstitial pneumonia as a predictor of postoperative acute respiratory distress syndrome after pulmonary resection. Eur J Cardiothorac Surg 2011;39(2):190–4.

43. Kakizaki T, Kohno M, Watanabe M, et al. Exacerbation of bleomycin-induced injury and fibrosis by pneumonectomy in the residual lung of mice. J Surg Res 2009;154(2):336–44.

44. Kondoh Y, Taniguchi H, Kitaichi M, et al. Acute exacerbation of interstitial pneumonia following surgical lung biopsy. Respir Med 2006;100(10):1753–9.

45. Utz JP, Ryu JH, Douglas WW, et al. High short-term mortality following lung biopsy for usual interstitial pneumonia. Eur Respir J 2001;17(2):175–9.

46. Minegishi Y, Takenaka K, Mizutani H, et al. Exacerbation of idiopathic interstitial pneumonias associated with lung cancer therapy. Intern Med 2009; 48(9):665–72.

47. Hiwatari N, Shimura S, Takishima T, et al. Bronchoalveolar lavage as a possible cause of acute exacerbation in idiopathic pulmonary fibrosis patients. Tohoku J Exp Med 1994;174(4):379–86.

48. Yokoyama A, Kohno N, Fujino S, et al. Circulating interleukin-6 levels in patients with bronchial asthma. Am J Respir Crit Care Med 1995;151(5):1354–8.

49. Han W, Wang W, Mohammed KA, et al. Alpha-defensins increase lung fibroblast proliferation and collagen synthesis via the beta-catenin signaling pathway. FEBS J 2009;276(22):6603–14.

50. Mukae H, Iiboshi H, Nakazato M, et al. Raised plasma concentrations of alpha-defensins in patients with idiopathic pulmonary fibrosis. Thorax 2002;57(7):623–8.

51. Tajima S, Oshikawa K, Tominaga S, et al. The increase in serum soluble ST2 protein upon acute exacerbation of idiopathic pulmonary fibrosis. Chest 2003;124(4):1206–14.

52. Moeller A, Gilpin SE, Ask K, et al. Circulating fibrocytes are an indicator of poor prognosis in idiopathic pulmonary fibrosis. Am J Respir Crit Care Med 2009; 179(7):588–94.

53. Kurosu K, Takiguchi Y, Okada O, et al. Identification of annexin 1 as a novel autoantigen in acute exacerbation of idiopathic pulmonary fibrosis. J Immunol 2008;181(1):756–67.

54. Churg A, Muller NL, Silva CI, et al. Acute exacerbation (acute lung injury of unknown cause) in UIP and other forms of fibrotic interstitial pneumonias. Am J Surg Pathol 2007;31(2):277–84.

55. Tiitto L, Bloigu R, Heiskanen U, et al. Relationship between histopathological features and the course of idiopathic pulmonary fibrosis/usual interstitial pneumonia. Thorax 2006;61(12):1091–5.

56. Akira M, Kozuka T, Yamamoto S, et al. Computed tomography findings in acute exacerbation of idiopathic pulmonary fibrosis. Am J Respir Crit Care Med 2008;178(4):372–8.

57. Wuyts WA, Thomeer M, Dupont LJ, et al. An algorithm to tackle acute exacerbations in idiopathic pulmonary fibrosis. Am J Respir Crit Care Med 2008;177(12):1397 [author reply: 1398].

58. Raghu G, Collard HR, Egan JJ, et al, ATS/ERS/JRS/ALAT Committee on Idiopathic Pulmonary Fibrosis. An official ATS/ERS/JRS/ALAT statement: idiopathic pulmonary fibrosis: evidence-based guidelines for diagnosis and management. Am J Respir Crit Care Med 2011;183:788–824.

59. Inase N, Sawada M, Ohtani Y, et al. Cyclosporin A followed by the treatment of acute exacerbation of idiopathic pulmonary fibrosis with corticosteroid. Intern Med 2003;42(7):565–70.

60. Sakamoto S, Homma S, Miyamoto A, et al. Cyclosporin A in the treatment of acute exacerbation of idiopathic pulmonary fibrosis. Intern Med 2010; 49(2):109–15.

61. Seo Y, Abe S, Kurahara M, et al. Beneficial effect of polymyxin B-immobilized fiber column (PMX) hemoperfusion treatment on acute exacerbation of idiopathic pulmonary fibrosis. Intern Med 2006;45(18): 1033–8.

62. Miyamoto K, Tasaka S, Hasegawa N, et al. Effect of direct hemoperfusion with a polymyxin B immobilized fiber column in acute exacerbation of interstitial pneumonia and serum indicators. Nihon Kokyuki Gakkai Zasshi 2009;47(11):978–84 [in Japanese].

63. Nakamura M, Ogura T, Miyazawa N, et al. Outcome of patients with acute exacerbation of idiopathic interstitial fibrosis (IPF) treated with sivelestat and the prognostic value of serum KL-6 and surfactant protein D. Nihon Kokyuki Gakkai Zasshi 2007; 45(6):455–9 [in Japanese].

64. Horita N, Akahane M, Okada Y, et al. Tacrolimus and steroid treatment for acute exacerbation of idiopathic pulmonary fibrosis. Intern Med 2011;50(3): 189–95.

65. Park IN, Kim DS, Shim TS, et al. Acute exacerbation of interstitial pneumonia other than idiopathic pulmonary fibrosis. Chest 2007;132(1):214–20.

66. Suda T, Kaida Y, Nakamura Y, et al. Acute exacerbation of interstitial pneumonia associated with collagen vascular diseases. Respir Med 2009; 103(6):846–53.

67. Akira M, Sakatani M, Hara H. Thin-section CT findings in rheumatoid arthritis-associated lung disease: CT patterns and their courses. J Comput Assist Tomogr 1999;23(6):941–8.

68. Dawson JK, Fewins HE, Desmond J, et al. Predictors of progression of HRCT diagnosed fibrosing alveolitis in patients with rheumatoid arthritis. Ann Rheum Dis 2002;61(6):517–21.

Idiopathic Pulmonary Fibrosis: Pathobiology of Novel Approaches to Treatment

Toby M. Maher, MB, MSc, PhD, MRCP[a,b,c,*]

KEYWORDS

- Idiopathic pulmonary fibrosis • Wound healing
- Clinical trials • Extra-cellular matrix

Idiopathic pulmonary fibrosis is a nonmalignant disease, yet it carries a prognosis akin to, or even worse than, many cancers. Until recently, lung transplantation has been the only therapeutic intervention that has offered any prospect of improved survival for individuals with IPF. The past decade has, however, witnessed an explosion of interest in IPF. Triggered by improved clinical phenotyping, this interest has led to major developments in understanding of disease pathogenesis. The first true multicenter randomized trial of therapy for IPF began in 1999 and results were published in 2004.[1] Since then there has been an exponential increase in the recruitment of IPF patients to clinical trials and several novel drugs have been subjected to rigorous assessment. This has stimulated the development of several compounds designed specifically for the treatment of IPF, resulting in a pharmaceutical development pipeline that offers the genuine promise of future treatments of this devastating disease.

This article seeks to review the mechanisms of action of potential IPF therapies with reference to current disease understanding and to highlight areas of IPF disease biology that afford attractive targets for the development of the treatments of tomorrow.

THE PATHOGENESIS OF IPF: SHIFTING PARADIGMS

Understanding of the mechanisms involved in the pathogenesis of IPF has greatly evolved during the past 2 to 3 decades. The realization, as outlined in the first American Thoracic Society/European Respiratory Society (ATS/ERS) consensus statement, that IPF is an entity distinct from the other idiopathic interstitial pneumonias, has been an important contributor to this evolution.[2] Clearer case definition coupled with the advent of high-resolution CT—which has enabled accurate, noninvasive, differentiation of IPF from other diffuse parenchymal lung diseases—has greatly improved both clinical and scientific research into IPF. Hypotheses concerning the cause and pathogenesis of IPF have been important in shaping research priorities and treatment stratagems. Conversely, new insights into the molecular processes underlying the development of IPF have resulted in the advancement of new hypotheses concerning the pathogenesis of IPF.[3,4]

Historically, IPF was considered an inflammatory or autoimmune condition. This idea was based in part on the belief that desquamative interstitial pneumonia represented an early stage in the

Disclosures: I am in receipt of an unrestricted academic industry grant from GlaxoSmithKline (GSK). In the past 3 years I have received advisory board or consultancy fees from Actelion, Boheringer Ingleheim, GSK, Respironics, and Sanofi-Aventis.
[a] Interstitial Lung Disease Unit, Royal Brompton Hospital, Sydney Street, London SW3 6NP, UK
[b] National Heart and Lung Institute, Imperial College London, South Kensington, London SW& 2AZ, UK
[c] Centre for Respiratory Research, Rayne Institute, University College London, 5 University Street, London WC1E 6JF, UK
* Interstitial Lung Disease Unit, Royal Brompton Hospital, Sydney Street, London SW3 6NP, UK.
E-mail address: t.maher@rbht.nhs.uk

chestmed.theclinics.com

development of IPF.[2,5] As cogently argued by Katzenstein and Myers, the evidence underpinning this belief is untenable.[5] Instead, it is appreciated that at a molecular level IPF is characterized by the apparently unopposed activation of multiple pathways involved in wound healing. The purpose of the normal wound healing process is to restore tissue integrity, structure, and function after injury. In the early stages of wound healing there is tissue expansion with the laying down of granulation tissue; this is associated with migration to the site of injury of fibroblasts that then proliferate, transform into myofibroblasts, and rapidly synthesize extracellular matrix (ECM). Once structural integrity is restored to a tissue and re-epithelialization of the basement membrane has occurred, the profibrotic phase of tissue repair switches off and resorbtion of the ECM, with fibroblast apoptosis and architectural remodeling of tissue, occurs.[6–8]

In IPF, by contrast, there is an imbalance between the profibrotic mediators that promote ECM expansion, fibroblast recruitment, proliferation and differentiation, and antifibrotic mediators that drive the process of tissue remodelling.[9] Several strands of evidence point to repetitive alveolar epithelial injury as an important driver for the development of this imbalance. Damage and necrosis of alveolar epithelial cells with areas of basement membrane denudation are a consistent finding in IPF.[10,11] These areas of epithelial damage correspond to sites of microscopic alveolar injury and invariably overlie fibroblastic foci.[12] Areas of alveolar epithelial cell apoptotic activity in IPF are also found at sites adjacent to fibroblastic foci and to a lesser extent within histologically normal alveoli and in epithelium lining honeycom spaces.[13–15] In animal models, induction of widespread epithelial injury and apoptosis alone is sufficient to induce the development of fibrosis, whereas inhibition of epithelial cell death abrogates the development of bleomycin-induced fibrosis.[16,17]

A variety of factors may contribute to alveolar epithelial cell injury. The lung is continuously exposed to a multitude of noxious and potentially injurious stimuli. These range from cigarette smoke to pollutants, dusts, and infectious agents. These and many other factors have the potential to cause lung epithelial cell injury and death. Epidemiologic studies, across centers and countries, consistently show that cigarette smoking and exposure to wood dusts, metal dusts, and mineral dusts are associated with an increased odds ratio for the subsequent development of IPF.[18–20] Similarly, past viral infection with particular viral subtypes has been reported, in some cases, associated with the subsequent development of IPF.[21] The sum of these observations suggests that IPF arises, in genetically susceptible individuals, as the consequence of an aberrant wound healing response that develops after repetitive, multifactorial, epithelial injury (**Fig. 1**).[3] This shift in paradigm has led to a corresponding evolution in treatment development for IPF. Historical approaches to treatment of IPF have centered on anti-inflammatory and immunomodulatory agents. Current pharmaceutical developments in IPF

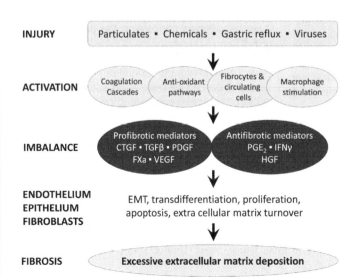

Fig. 1. A schematic outlining the proposed pathogenetic events involved in the development of IPF. Injury activates multiple inflammatory, cell signaling, and repair pathways. Activation of these cascades causes an imbalance in profibrotic and antifibrotic mediators. In turn these mediators activate multiple cell types, causing changes in cellular functioning and cell-cell interactions that ultimately result in progressive fibrosis. EMT, epithelial-mesenchymal transition; HGF, hepatocyte growth factor.

target modulation of wound healing cascades with the intent of blocking the mechanisms integral to fibrogenesis.

TREATMENT DEVELOPMENT CHALLENGES: AN EMBARRASSMENT OF RICHES BUT A LACK OF TOOLS

Even a cursory review of the IPF literature discloses that a vast number of mediators, growth factors, cytokines, and signalling pathways are differentially regulated in IPF lung compared with normal control lung. This should, however, come as no surprise given the complexity, pleiotropism, and biologic redundancy that characterize the normal wound healing response. One of the major challenges confronting IPF researchers is separating key initiating events and pathways integral to the development of fibrosis from downstream changes that occur in response to these initial triggers. Because of this, when attempting to identify potential therapeutic targets in IPF, it is possible to make a cogent argument for targeting any of tens, if not hundreds, of mediators or signaling pathways.

This embarrassment of riches when it comes to potential drug targets is compounded by a lack of effective tools for validating candidate therapeutic molecules. Although it is possible to imagine a series of key in vitro and in vivo experiments by which to judge putative IPF therapies, there remain many unknowns. For instance, which is the most important in vitro endpoint in fibroblast culture experiments? Is it inhibition of fibroblast proliferation, blocking of collagen and ECM synthesis, preventing transformation of fibroblasts to a myofibroblast phenotype, or induction of fibroblast apoptosis? Which, if any, of the several available animal models best recapitulates human disease and should, therefore, be used to facilitate drug discovery? Whilst these unknowns make drug development in IPF challenging it is reassuring to note the dramatic increase in early and late phase trials in IPF that has occurred over the last decade. Furthermore, it is noteworthy that these trials have now translated in to the first licensed therapy for IPF in Europe, Japan and India.[22] With this in mind what can we learn from previous IPF treatment strategies and completed clinical trials and how will this inform the development of novel treatments over the coming decade?

THE IPF TREATMENT LANDSCAPE: PAST AND PRESENT

The belief that the development and progression of IPF were driven by uncontrolled inflammation underpins what has, until only recently, been the standard therapeutic approach for IPF. Even now, prednisolone, either alone, or in combination with azathioprine, is widely used as first-line treatment of many patients with IPF. Yet there is a lack of robust trial evidence to support this approach and evidence that there is predates the current classification of IPF.[23] Clinical experience indicates that combined immunosuppression frequently fails to prevent inexorable progression of disease in individuals with IPF, an observation borne out by a systematic review of the small number of trials that have been conducted to assess the use of prednisolone and other immunosuppressants in the treatment of IPF.[24] Inflammation, however, does play a role in the normal wound healing process and although not the primary driver of IPF, it may be an important contributory factor in the evolution of progressive fibrosis. The on-going, National Institutes of Health–funded, triple-arm PANTHER-IPF study (NCT00650091) has been designed, in part, to assess the efficacy of prednisolone and azathioprine (together with N-acetylcysteine [NAC]) as a treatment of IPF. Although the study has yet to report, it has recently been announced, after an interim safety analysis, that the arm consisting of prednisolone, azathioprine, and NAC has been discontinued because of an excess of mortality and adverse events compared with the placebo arm. This announcement, even in lieu of the final published data, effectively signals the end of combination immunosuppression as a treatment of IPF.

In the past decade, the majority of compounds that have been trialed in IPF have been targeted at mechanisms involved in the wound healing cascade or have been administered with the aim of augmenting lung defense mechanisms against alveolar epithelial injury. Two new treatments have reached the clinic for IPF during the past 5 years. Although not universally accepted and receiving only lukewarm endorsement in the current ATS/ERS/Japanese Respiratory Society/Latin American Thoracic Association guidelines for IPF,[25] the progress of NAC and pirfenidone from trial compounds to viable therapies for IPF provides encouragement that treatments currently in development may ultimately prove beneficial.

NAC acts on the lung to increase intracellular and extracellular levels of glutathione and exerts an antioxidant effect.[26] The bronchial and alveolar epithelium, through exposure to ambient air and a wide range of pollutants, are constantly under high levels of oxidative stress. Evolution has equipped the lung with several protective mechanisms to counter the potentially deleterious consequences of reactive oxygen species (ROS) and free radical exposure. In IPF, there is evidence that these antioxidant mechanisms are impaired and that this in turn contributes to epithelial injury and apoptosis. Levels of the key endogenous antioxidant glutathione are 4 times lower in the BAL fluid of individuals with IPF compared with healthy controls.[27] This observation led to a pilot study in which 12 weeks of treatment with NAC was shown sufficient to increase BAL glutathione levels.[28] This in turn led to the development of the multicenter IFIGENIA trial and this study became the first prospective IPF trial to report a positive outcome. In total, 155 patients with IPF were enrolled, with 80 assigned to treatment with NAC. After 12 months of treatment, there was a slower rate of loss of vital capacity (VC) in the NAC-treated group with VC 0.18 L (9%) better than that observed in the placebo-treated arm. Similarly, there was a slowing in the deterioration of the diffusing capacity of lung for carbon monoxide by 24% in the NAC-treated IPF patients.[26] The study has attracted criticism for lack of a true placebo arm (all patients in the study, in addition to taking the study drug or placebo, were on prednisolone and azathioprine), a high dropout rate, and results that have yet to be replicated. These issues will be addressed by the ongoing PANTHER-IPF.

Pirfenidone has recently become the first therapy to be licensed in Europe, India, and Japan as a treatment of IPF. Preclinical data point to pirfenidone as a broad-spectrum but low-potency kinase inhibitor that exerts a combination of anti-inflammatory, antifibrotic, and antioxidant actions.[22] When administered in the fibrotic phase of the murine bleomycin-induced, pulmonary fibrosis model, pirfenidone causes a reduction in fibrosis with a corresponding reduction in levels of transforming growth factor (TGF)-β, basic fibroblast growth factor, and platelet-derived growth factor (PDGF).[29,30] Pirfenidone has also been shown, in rodents, to down-regulate transcription of procollagens 1 and 3 and the collagen-specific molecular chaperone HSP47.[31] Pirfenidone has been tested in 4 multicenter clinical trials.[32–34] In 3 of these 4 studies, pirfenidone has slowed disease progression compared with placebo. In the largest of the studies, CAPACITY 2, forced vital capacity (FVC) decline in the placebo group was 12.4% during 72 weeks. In the pirfenidone group (2403 mg per day), this decline was reduced to 8 (P = .001).[34,35] In the parallel and nearly identical CAPACITY 1 study, the rate of decline in the pirfenidone-treated subjects was similar (−9.0% for 72 weeks); however, the rate of decline in the placebo group was only −9.6%, resulting in a failure of the study to achieve its primary endpoint. This issue notwithstanding, in both CAPACITY studies,

changes in secondary measures were consistent in pointing to an effect of pirfenidone versus placebo. Taken together, the trial results for NAC and pirfenidone suggest that a strategy of preventing epithelial injury and down-regulating wound healing/profibrotic pathways has the potential to alter disease behavior in IPF.

WHAT CAN BE LEARNT FROM IPF TRAIL FAILURES?

During the past decade, several potential treatments of IPF have failed to show efficacy in phase III clinical trials. It is worth considering these agents for the insights they provide into the pathogenetic processes in IPF. Interferon gamma-1b was the first compound to be tested in a true randomized placebo controlled trial in IPF.[1] The rationale underlying the use of interferon gamma-1b in IPF was the observation that there exists an imbalance between profibrotic T_H2 cytokines and antifibrotic T_H1 cytokines, including interferon (IFN)-γ, in the lungs of patients with IPF. In vitro IFN-γ suppresses fibroblast proliferation and ECM production.[36] In in vivo animal studies, IFN-γ is effective in down-regulating TGF-β, PDGF, interleukin (IL)-4, IL-6, and IL-13.[37] In the first IFN-γ multicenter clinical trial, active treatment showed a trend toward decreased mortality with a post hoc subgroup analysis suggesting a survival advantage in subjects with mild disease.[1] In a parallel pharmacodynamic study, Streiter and colleagues[38] were able to show that treatment with IFN-γ led to detectable decreases in CXCL5, PDGF, and type 1 procollagen in bronchoalveolar lavage (BAL) fluid. Despite these findings, the INSPIRE study, the largest prospective clinical trial performed in IPF to date, failed to show any survival advantage associated with IFN-γ treatment.[39]

Endothelin (ET)-1 is a polypeptide cytokine that acts via ET receptors A and B and is secreted by endothelial cells and principally causes vasoconstriction. It has also been shown to stimulate fibroblast proliferation, chemotaxis, and ECM production.[40,41] ET receptor antagonists have revolutionized the treatment of pulmonary hypertension. The finding that ET is found in elevated concentrations in IPF BAL fluid and that ET-1 overexpression causes chronic progressive fibrosis in mice were key observations that drove the development of trials of ET receptor antagonism in IPF.[42,43] Yet clinical trials of the potent ET receptor antagonists, bosentan, ambrisentan, and macitentan, have all failed to demonstrate a significant treatment benefit in IPF compared with placebo.[44,45]

Imatinib mesylate, a tyrosine kinase inhibitor with activity against a variety of targets, including PDGF receptors and discoidin domain receptor (DDR)-1 and DDR-2, has been demonstrated in vitro to exert potent antiproliferative effects on fibroblasts.[46] Imatinib blocks fibroblast to myofibroblast transformation and ECM synthesis through inhibition of TGF-β and PDGF.[46] In animal models, imatinib blocks the development of fibrosis when dosed before lung injury but, importantly, lacks efficacy in murine bleomycin-induced fibrosis when dosed during the late fibrotic phase.[46] These observations, however, led to a phase II multicenter clinical trial in IPF that again failed to demonstrate any benefit of active treatment compared with placebo.[47]

So what do these trial failures reveal about IPF? They confirm that understanding of the intricate interaction of the different pathways involved in the development and progression of fibrosis remains rudimentary. It is possible that these interventions failed because they were simply targeting downstream consequences of more important upstream events. Equally, targeting of individual receptors, cytokines, or tyrosine kinases may be doomed to failure because of the considerable redundancy and pleiotropism that exist in the normal process of wound healing. These clinical studies confirm that current preclinical tools, including in vitro and in vivo disease models, are flawed as measures of potential therapeutic efficacy. Furthermore, not only preclinical tools but also clinical tools are limited. The growth in IPF clinical trials in the past few years has highlighted the challenge of identifying appropriate trial endpoints. The ideal endpoint of mortality requires unfeasibly long or large studies, so the majority of clinical trialists in IPF have accepted FVC as the most appropriate measure of IPF disease progression. There remains considerable debate, however, as to whether this should be handled as a categorical (eg, change greater than or less than 10%) or continuous variable and for what period of time change should be measured (for instance, the recent BIBF 1120 study was 48 weeks in duration but the pirfenidone CAPACITY studies were performed for 72 weeks[34,48]). These observations, coupled with the cost of undertaking of large-scale phase III studies in IPF, have also raised interest in finding biomarkers that correlate with future disease progression. The ability to identify individuals at greatest risk of disease progression during the succeeding 12 months would permit enrichment in study populations with a corresponding reduction in required sample sizes. Prior decline in lung function remains the only

clear predictor of poor short-term outcome.[49,50] Recent proteomic studies, however, suggest that serum biomarkers may permit identification of individuals with progressive disease.[51]

Notwithstanding the negative outcomes from many of these studies, experience gained from clinical trials coupled with a growing understanding of the pathogenetic mechanisms at play in IPF has seen an explosion in early-stage clinical trials in IPF.

EMERGING TREATMENT TARGETS IN IPF

Several novel therapies targeting a variety of pathways important in wound healing are in early-phase trials in patients with IPF. Many more compounds are in the preclinical development phase. The remainder of this article considers potential therapeutic targets in IPF with particular reference to those being explored in currently active clinical trials programs (overviewed in **Fig. 2**).

Protein and Receptor Kinases

Protein-tyrosine kinases are enzymes that modify other proteins through the process of phosphorylation; this results in functional changes in the target protein that include altered enzymatic activity, changes in cellular localization, or association with other proteins.[52] There are 518 protein kinases encoded for in the human genome and approximately 30% of proteins may be modified by kinase activity.[53] Some of these genes encode for receptor tyrosine kinases (RTKs), transmembrane receptors containing an extracellular ligand-binding domain, and an intracellular catalytic protein-tyrosine kinase domain. Key signaling pathways activated by RTKs include the extracellular signal–regulated kinase (ERK) and mitogen-activated protein kinase (MAPK) pathway, the phosphatidylinositol 3-kinase (Pi3K)-Akt pathway, and the Janus kinase–signal transducer of activator of transcription (JAK-STAT) pathway. The consequences of activation of these RTKs and downstream intracellular protein kinases are complex and depend on a variety of factors, including cell type and signaling pathway activated. Protein kinases, however, exert a huge range of important effects, including control of cell proliferation, mitogenesis, survival, motility, and metabolism.[52] As such, the protein kinases and the RTKs are integral to the processes involved in fibrogenesis and in many cases act as the downstream mediators of key growth factors, such as TGF-β.[54] Specific pathways, such as the Wnt signaling pathway, have been shown up-regulated in IPF lung tissue compared with control and in vitro in fibroblasts and in vivo

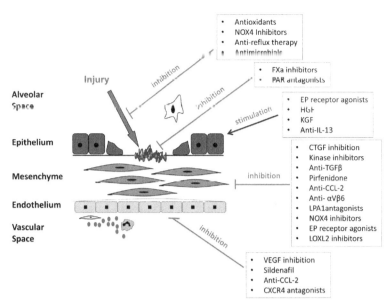

Fig. 2. Current understanding of the pathogenesis of IPF suggests that repetitive alveolar epithelial injury results in basement membrane denudation and activation of key pathways involved in the wound healing response. This in turn leads to fibroblast proliferation, transformation of fibroblasts to myofibroblasts, and expansion of the ECM. These effects are augmented by the influx of circulating inflammatory cells, including the putative bone marrow–derived fibroblast precursor, the fibrocyte. Various treatments are in development targeting different aspects of IPF disease pathogenesis, through inhibition of fibrogenesis, through promotion of antifibrotic pathways, or through reduction of alveolar injury. HGF, hepatocyte growth factor; KGF, keratinocyte growth factor.

in animal models have been shown to be important contributors to the development of fibrosis.[55,56]

As the downstream activators of multiple signaling pathways, the protein kinases represent an attractive and tractable target for novel treatment developments in IPF. In the cancer field, a range of protein kinase inhibitors has been developed with the aim of inhibiting proliferation and survival of malignant cells.[52] By analogy it might be expected that the same approach of protein kinase inhibition could be effective in preventing fibroblast proliferation and survival in IPF.[52] As described previously, imatinib mesylate, an inhibitor of the Abl protein-tyrosine kinase, failed to show effectiveness in a placebo-controlled trial in IPF.[47] BIBF 1120, a compound developed for the treatment of malignancy, acts as an inhibitor of 3 RTKs— vascular endothelial growth factor (VEGF) receptor, PDGF receptor, and fibroblast growth factor (FGF) receptor.[57] In a recently reported phase II trial of 432 subjects with IPF, BIBF 1120, at a dose of 150 mg twice daily, reduced FVC decline to 0.06 L for 1 year compared with 0.19 L in the placebo group. In addition to the reduction in FVC decline, acute exacerbations were reduced from 15.7 to 2.7 per 100 patient years in the 150-mg twice-daily group compared with placebo. Overall the drug was well tolerated with gastrointestinal upset the predominant dose-limiting side effect.[48] Parallel

phase III trials are currently ongoing to validate these findings (NCT01335477 and NCT01335464).

Interleukin 13 and Type 2 Helper T-Cell Cytokines

As discussed previously, IPF is characterized by an imbalance between type 1 helper T-cell (T_H1) and type 2 helper T-cell (T_H2) cytokines that favors fibroproliferation. There is a growing body of evidence to support key roles for the archetypal T_H2 cytokine IL-13 in the development of fibrosis.[9] IL-13 is found in increased levels in the BAL fluid of patients with pulmonary fibrosis compared with controls.[58] In mice, transgenic overexpression of IL-13 is, in itself, sufficient to trigger the development of subepithelial fibrosis.[59] In vitro, IL-13 triggers fibroblast proliferation, ECM synthesis, and fibroblast to myofibroblast transformation via TGF-β–dependant and TGF-β–independent pathways.[60,61] IL-13 also induces epithelial apoptosis.[62] IL-13 knockout mice are protected from developing fibrosis induced by a range of profibrotic stimuli, including fluorescein isothiocyanate.[63] Targeted inhibition of IL-13, with an IL-13 fusion protein combined to *Pseudomonas* exotoxin, from 21 to 28 days after bleomycin challenge in rodents is sufficient to attenuate the development of pulmonary fibrosis.[64] IL-13 has also been shown an important mediator of fibrosis in the liver.[9] Furthermore, there is an overlap of signaling pathways between IL-13 and both TGF-β and the chemokine CCL2.[65] In pulmonary fibroblasts, CCL2 seems to be a downstream effector of TGF-β and IL-13 with inhibition of CCL2 resulting in a reduction of the profibrotic effects of both IL-13 and TGF-β. These data provide a compelling argument for the role of IL-13 in the pathobiology of IPF. This is of particular interest because several pharmaceutical companies have produced monoclonal antibodies that target IL-13. From an IPF perspective the most advanced of these is QAX576 (Novartis, Basel, Switzerland); this antibody is currently being tested in a multicenter phase II study (NCT01266135). A human-specific anti-CCL2 monoclonal antibody (CNTO 888, Centocor, Horsham, PA, USA) is being studied in a phase II trial in IPF (NCT00786201).

Acute Exacerbations as a Therapeutic Target

Since the reclassification of IPF in 2001, it has become increasingly clear that for a significant minority of patients, periods of relative disease stability are punctuated by episodes of unheralded rapid decline (in clinical trials this number has consistently been between 15% and 20% of IPF patients per year[48,66]) which, on biopsy, are characterized by the finding of diffuse alveolar damage.[66] These episodes, termed *acute exacerbations*, have been defined as increasing symptoms occurring for 30 or fewer days that are associated with new parenchymal infiltrates on chest radiograph or CT in the absence of infection, pulmonary edema, or emboli.[67] Whether acute exacerbations arise due to a cryptogenic flare-up of the underlying disease process or alternatively represent the sequelae of episodes of occult infection remains unclear. In favor of the idea that infection may be an important initiator of acute exacerbations is the observation that disease course and prognosis are identical in patients with cryptogenic acute exacerbations and those who acutely deteriorate due to culture-proved respiratory tract infection.[68]

Collard and colleagues[69] recently demonstrated, by measuring a range of plasma biomarkers, that there is evidence of epithelial cell damage and activation of wound healing pathways, such as the coagulation cascade in individuals undergoing acute exacerbations. These pathways differ from those activated in individuals with acute lung injury. It has also been demonstrated that levels of fibrocytes, circulating immune active, bone marrow–derived cells believed to be fibroblast precursors, increase dramatically in acute exacerbations and reduce again during remission.[70] Viruses have been proposed as having the potential to trigger acute exacerbations of IPF and in animal models gammaherpesvirus infection has been shown to mimic acute exacerbations in mice with established fibrosis.[71] Wootton and colleagues,[72] however, have recently applied molecular microbiologic techniques to serum and BAL from 43 subjects undergoing acute exacerbation and found evidence of specific viruses in only 4 individuals. Similarly, Konishi and colleagues[73] compared gene expression profiles from 8 lung samples obtained during acute exacerbations with 23 samples obtained from patients with stable IPF. They did not identify up-regulation of any gene transcripts believed to associate with viral or bacterial infection. The investigators did, however, find an increase in transcripts of genes involved in epithelial apoptosis and epithelial response to injury. One interpretation of current data on acute exacerbations is that these episodes are probably triggered by any of several stimuli, all of which share the capacity to cause epithelial injury and death. Stimuli include viral and bacterial infection, drugs, microaspiration, and excessive alveolar stretch (which can occur during single lung ventilation at time of surgical biopsy).

Better understanding of the causes of acute exacerbations should provide novel targets for treatment. The significant contribution made to morbidity and mortality in IPF by acute exacerbations makes them an attractive target for intervention. In the systemic vasculitidies, such as Wegener granulomatosis, it has been demonstrated that bacterial infection and chronic carriage of *Staphylococcus aureus* are important triggers for exacerbations of the disease. Prophylactic treatment with the antibiotic co-trimoxazole has been shown to have an important effect in reducing disease relapses in individuals with Wegener granulomatosis.[74] In a small pilot study of 14 subjects with chronic fibrosing lung disease of varying causes, co-trimoxazole led to an improvement in FVC after 3 months and was associated with reductions in serum levels of VEGF.[75] These results led on to the development in the United Kingdom of a multicenter study of co-trimoxazole in patients with IPF and idiopathic fibrosing nonspecific interstitial pneumonia (Treating Interstitial Pneumonia with the Addition of Co-trimoxazole [TIPAC] study, ISRCTN 22201583). The study has completed recruitment and is due to report in the near future. A strategy of antibiotic prophylaxis that proves effective in preventing either acute exacerbations or disease progression in IPF may pave the way to trials of antibiotics, such as macrolides, that combine antibacterial, antiviral, and anti-inflammatory effects. This approach is particularly attractive because these agents have shown efficacious in preventing exacerbations of other respiratory disorders, such as asthma and COPD.[76,77]

The Coagulation Cascade

One of the earliest components activated in the wound healing process is the coagulation cascade. In normal wound healing this activation results in the deposition of fibrin, which enables hemostasis, and provides a provisional ECM, which maintains tissue structural integrity and provides a scaffold to which inflammatory cells and fibroblasts can migrate.[78] The coagulation cascade relies on the highly complex interaction of many molecules that ensure a balance between the activation and inhibition of clotting. In IPF there is evidence of activation of the coagulation cascade with fibrin deposition in alveolar spaces and activated tissue factor (TF) localizing to the alveolar epithelium.[79] Furthermore, thrombin and factor (F) Xa are elevated in the BAL fluid of patients with IPF.[80] FXa has recently been demonstrated to be locally produced by alveolar epithelium and acts as a potent inducer of fibroblast to myofibroblast differentiation through proteinase-activated receptor (PAR) 1 and integrin $\alpha V\beta 5$–mediated activation of TGF-β.[81] In animal models of fibrosis, underexpression or overexpression of various components of the coagulation cascade, including urokinase plasminogen activator, tissue plasminogen activator, and plasminogen activator inhibitor 1, all modulate the response to fibrogenic stimuli.[82]

As well as driving the development of a fibrin clot, molecules within the coagulation cascade are able to exert other profibrotic effects. The PARs are a family of 4 transmembrane G-coupled receptors, which, as their name suggests, are activated by the proteolytic unmasking of a tethered ligand.[78] Individual PARs are activated by different members of the coagulation cascade. FXa (or a complex of TF-FVIIa-FXa) activates PAR1 and PAR2. PAR1 is responsible for mediating a range of cellular responses to both thrombin and FXa. These responses include the release of proinflammatory cytokines (IL-1β, IL-6, monocyte chemoattractant protein-1, and TNF-α), activation of latent TGF-β, stimulation of fibroblast differentiation and ECM production, and alveolar epithelial apoptosis.[83,84] In support of a role for PAR1 in fibrosis, PAR1 knockout mice are protected from the development of bleomycin-induced fibrosis.[85] PAR1 may not, however, be the only PAR involved

in the development of fibrosis. Wygrecka and colleagues[86] recently demonstrated that local production of FVII by lung epithelial cells activates PAR2, which, in turn, stimulates fibroblast ECM production. This process is potentiated by TF but inhibited by TF antisense oligonucleotides.

These data support an important role for the coagulation cascade in both directly and indirectly driving the development of fibrosis in IPF. Further support for the importance of the coagulation cascade has been provided by a small Japanese study by Kubo and colleagues[87] assessing the role of anticoagulation (in the form of warfarin or low molecular weight heparin) in patients hospitalized due to worsening IPF. In this study anticoagulation conferred a survival benefit compared with standard care alone. The small size of the study as well as enrolment criteria that are not applicable to the majority of patients with IPF has meant that it has not been possible for anticoagulant therapy to be recommended for IPF.[25] This study has, however, provided the impetus for the IPFnet to develop the AntiCoagulant Effectiveness in Idiopathic Pulmonary Fibrosis (ACE-IPF) study (NCT00957242), a randomized, multicenter trial comparing warfarin to placebo. Although yet to be published, it has recently been reported that the ACE-IPF trial has been closed to further enrolment after an interim safety analysis. It may be that the well-recognized bleeding risks associated with warfarin outweigh any benefit in IPF and other, safer coagulation-targeted approaches may prove more effective as treatments of IPF. Potential coagulation pathway–specific therapies include the use of specific FXa inhibitors (these are currently used for thromboprophylaxis post–orthopedic surgery) or specific PAR antagonists, several of which are in early-stage development.

Eicosanoids

The eicosanoids are a family of potent, biologically active, lipid mediators, including prostaglandins, thromboxane, and leukotrienes (LTs).[88] All are synthesized from membrane phospholipid-derived arachiodonic acid. In general, LTs exert profibrotic effects on a range of structural cells in the lung whereas prostanoids are antifibrotic. Prostaglandin E2 (PGE^2) is the most abundant prostanoid found in the healthy lung. In IPF, however, PGE^2 levels are reduced and this occurs because of a failure of induction of the key synthetic enzyme cyclooxygenase (COX)-2.[89,90] This failure of induction of PGE^2 contributes to unopposed fibroblast proliferation and synthesis of collagen, fibroblast transition to a myofibroblast phenotype, and fibroblast resistance to apoptosis.[14,91–94] The reduction in PGE^2

also renders the alveolar epithelium more sensitive to apoptotic stimuli.[14] PGE[2] exerts its effects via 4 transmembrane G-protein–coupled receptors, E-prostanoid (EP) receptors 1–4. Nebulization of PGE[2], a strategy that could be considered a method for replenishing deficient levels in IPF, is limited by the side effect of cough.[89] The tussive effect of PGE[2] has recently been shown mediated via EP3[95–98] whereas the majority, if not all, of the antifibrotic effects of PGE[2] are mediated through either EP2 or EP4. These receptors, therefore, represent potentially attractive therapeutic targets in IPF.

In contrast to PGE[2], the cysteinyl LTs are found at increased concentrations in IPF lung.[99] This is postulated to occur because failure of COX-2 induction results in arachidonic acid preferentially metabolized by the 5-lipoxygenase pathway into LTs, especially LTB[4].[88] The LTs stimulate macrophages to produce a range of profibrotic cytokines and growth factors, including IL-6, IL-8, IL-13, TNF-α, and FGF.[100,101] the LTs stimulate the alveolar epithelium to produce TGF-β and the induce fibroblast proliferation and ECM production.[100,102] In rodents the LT antagonist monteleukast has been shown to attenuate the development of bleomycin-induced fibrosis when dosed prophylactically (ie, before the administration of bleomycin).[103] LT antagonists have been shown safe and well tolerated in the treatment of asthma and thus might be considered a potential therapeutic option in IPF.

NADPH Oxidase Proteins

As suggested by the results of the IFIGENIA study, oxidative stress is an important contributor to epithelial injury in IPF and seems to be a key contributor to the pathogenesis of IPF.[26] Oxidative stress may occur through exposure of the lung to exogenously and endogenously generated ROS. ROS are generated as a by-product of respiration and have also been shown to play a role in intracellular and extracellular signaling mechanisms and are utilized by neutrophils as a mechanism for killing microbes. NADPH oxidase (NOX) proteins are membrane associated enzymes that catalyze the reduction of oxygen through the use of NADPH as an electron donor.[104] The NOX proteins can be divided into 3 distinct groups with one of these consisting of the proteins NOX1–4.[105] These enzymes are ubiquitously expressed and play several important roles. NOX-derived ROS can react with specific proteins to alter their activity and localization. The interaction of ROS with tyrosine kinases inhibits the catalytic cysteine residue of the enzymes, thus inhibiting their effects. Of the specific enzymes, NOX2 is involved in neutrophil

oxygen burst killing of microbes whereas NOX4 acts to constitutively generate extracellular H[2]O[2].[106]

NOX4 has recently been shown up-regulated in pulmonary fibroblasts derived from IPF patients.[107,108] TGF-β stimulates NOX4 production by healthy and fibrotic lung fibroblasts.[108] In the murine model of bleomycin-induced pulmonary fibrosis, NOX4 is up-regulated, and pharmacologic and siRNA inhibition of NOX4 results in abrogation of fibrosis.[107] Similarly, in vitro in human lung fibroblasts NOX4 inhibition blocks TGF-β-induced fibroblast to myofibroblast transformation and ECM synthesis and also protects alveolar epithelial cells from apoptosis.[108] NOX4 may potentially also contribute to the development of hypoxia-induced pulmonary hypertension.[109] Although NOX4 inhibitors are yet to enter clinical trials, Laleu and colleagues[110] have recently reported on the development of a first-in-class, NOX4-selective, orally available compound that has shown promise in preclinical studies as a potential treatment of IPF.

Transforming Growth Factor β

TGF-β consists of a family of 3 structurally and functionally related protein isoforms—TGF-β[1], TGF-β[2], and TGF-β[3]. TGF-β[1] has been consistently shown elevated in IPF and exerts a series of potent profibrotic effects on a range of cell types, including induction of mononuclear cell and fibroblast chemotaxis, stimulation of fibroblast proliferation and differentiation into myofibroblasts, protection of myofibroblasts from apoptosis, promotion of ECM production, stimulation of cytokine (IL-1, TNF-α, PDGF, and TGF-β) release by phagocytes, down-regulation of matrix metalloproteinases, and upregulation of tissue inhibitor of metalloproteinase (TIMP) and plasminogen activator inhibitor.[99,111–115]

In rodents, transient, adenoviral vector-mediated, overexpression of the active form of TGF-β1 (but not the inactive latent form) results in a rapidly progressive and severe fibrosis with little inflammatory cell infiltration.[116] This TGF-β-induced fibrosis is typified by an increase in ECM content of the lungs and also by the presence of myofibroblasts. Blocking of the effect of TGF-β, by the administration of soluble TGF-β receptors, attenuates the development of bleomycin-induced pulmonary fibrosis in hamsters.[117] In vitro the selectively induced overexpression of TGF-β by rat airway epithelial cells results, after 14 days, in the development of lesions resembling the fibroblastic foci of IPF.[111]

Inactive, latency-activated peptide (LAP)-bound TGF-β is secreted by cells. TGF-β then undergoes activation either through proteolytic cleavage of

LAP or through the proteolytic-independent interaction of LAP with integrins or thrombospondin-1.[118,119] Once activated, TGF-β signals via several single-pass serine/threonine kinase receptors.[120] Stimulation of these receptors in turn leads to activation of either canonical (via Smad 2/3) or noncanonical pathways (including MAPK and Pi3K pathways) that ultimately control the downstream effects of TGF-β. Although TGF-β plays an integral role in the development of fibrosis in IPF, it also has a key function in maintaining cellular homeostatic mechanisms. There is, therefore, a well-founded concern that therapeutic targeting of TGF-β may have significant deleterious consequences.[121] This concern notwithstanding, several approaches for targeting TGF-β are in varying stages of pharmacologic development. Genzyme (Cambridge, MA, USA) has recently tested a TGF-β neutralizing antibody, GC1008, in a phase I clinical trial in IPF (NCT00125385). Inhibitors of the TGF-β receptor, ALK5, have been developed for several indications but their use has been limited by concerns regarding potential toxicity.[122] An alternative strategy to inhibit TGF-β signaling is to block activation. Recent studies have demonstrated that integrins, especially αVβ6, are up-regulated at sites of tissue injury.[83] Integrin-targeted therapy, therefore, potentially offers a mechanism by which TGF-β can be preferentially targeted at sites of fibrosis.[123] A humanized monoclonal antibody against the αVβ6 integrin (STX-100, Stromedix, Cambridge, MA, USA) is currently being assessed in a phase I trial in IPF (NCT01371305). Lysophosphatidic acid (LPA), a bioactive phospholipid derivative found in increased concentration in IPF lung compared with control, functions in part through αVβ6-mediated activation of TGF-β.[124] An orally active antagonist of the LPA1 receptor has recently been demonstrated to inhibit the development of murine bleomycin-induced fibrosis and is predicted to enter clinical trials in the near future.[125,126]

Connective Tissue Growth Factor

Connective tissue growth factor (CTGF) is a potent inducer of fibroblast proliferation, chemotaxis, and ECM deposition, which is found in elevated concentrations in BAL fluid from IPF patients.[127] CTGF is produced by epithelial, endothelial, and mesenchymal cells, with TGF-β the principle mediator of CTGF production by fibroblasts.[128] Overexpression of TGF-β in the mouse lung results in a severe fibrotic reaction.[116] By contrast Smad3 knockout mice are resistant to TGF-β–induced fibrosis and this resistance is associated with a failure to induce CTGF gene expression.[129] Overexpression, induced by adenoviral gene transfer, of CTGF in mice results,

at 14 days, in patchy fibrosis, fibroblast differentiation into myofibroblasts, and increased total lung collagen.[130,131] These changes, however, all resolve by day 28, suggesting that CTGF is capable of inducing but not sustaining a fibrotic response within the lungs.[130] Similarly, in mice, administration of both TGF-β and CTGF accentuates the extent of bleomycin-induced fibrosis compared with administration of either factor alone, suggesting a synergy between the 2 proteins.[132] An anti-CTGF antibody has been shown to inhibit murine bleomycin-induced pulmonary fibrosis.[133] A phase I trial of an anti-CTGF antibody (FG-3019, FibroGen, San Francisco, CA, USA) has recently been completed (NCT00074698) and a phase IIa trial is recruiting in the United States (NCT01262001).

SUMMARY

IPF is a complex disease characterized by abnormalities in multiple pathways involved in the normal wound healing response. Better understanding of the pathobiology of the disease has led to a dramatic increase in the past decade in the number of clinical trials of novel therapies for IPF. With the recent licensing of pirfenidone in Europe, India, and Japan, these trials are beginning to result in the availability of treatments proved to alter the progression of the disease. Even so, pirfenidone only slows, but does not halt, disease progression and there remains a huge gulf between the effectiveness of available treatment of IPF and the expectations of patients with the disease. It is hoped, therefore, that some of the targets described in this article will prove amenable to therapies that improve outcomes for individuals with IPF. Nonetheless, in a condition characterized by multiple overlapping pathways, many of which are pleiotropic and display considerable redundancy, truly effective treatment may require combinations of drugs, with each targeting individual disease mechanisms. The licensing of pirfenidone affords the opportunity for the development of randomized control trials assessing combination therapy for IPF akin to that used by oncologists in the management of malignancy. These challenges notwithstanding, the current pharmacologic development landscape in IPF offers genuine hope that the treatment options available for sufferers with this appalling disease should continue to improve in the coming few years.

REFERENCES

1. Raghu G, Brown KK, Bradford WZ, et al. A placebo-controlled trial of interferon gamma-1b in patients with idiopathic pulmonary fibrosis. N Engl J Med 2004;350(2):125–33.

2. American Thoracic Society, European Respiratory Society. American Thoracic Society/European Respiratory Society International Multidisciplinary Consensus Classification of the Idiopathic Interstitial Pneumonias. This joint statement of the American Thoracic Society (ATS), and the European Respiratory Society (ERS) was adopted by the ATS board of directors, June 2001 and by the ERS Executive Committee, June 2001. Am J Respir Crit Care Med 2002;165(2):277–304.

3. Maher TM, Wells AU, Laurent GJ. Idiopathic pulmonary fibrosis: multiple causes and multiple mechanisms? Eur Respir J 2007;30(5):835–9.

4. Selman M, King TE, Pardo A. Idiopathic pulmonary fibrosis: prevailing and evolving hypotheses about its pathogenesis and implications for therapy. Ann Intern Med 2001;134(2):136–51.

5. Katzenstein AL, Myers JL. Idiopathic pulmonary fibrosis: clinical relevance of pathologic classification. Am J Respir Crit Care Med 1998;157(4 Pt 1):1301–15.

6. Baum CL, Arpey CJ. Normal cutaneous wound healing: clinical correlation with cellular and molecular events. Dermatol Surg 2005;31(6):674–86.

7. Desmouliere A, Chaponnier C, Gabbiani G. Tissue repair, contraction, and the myofibroblast. Wound Repair Regen 2005;13(1):7–12.

8. Lorena D, Uchio K, Costa AM, et al. Normal scarring: importance of myofibroblasts. Wound Repair Regen 2002;10(2):86–92.

9. Wynn TA. Integrating mechanisms of pulmonary fibrosis. J Exp Med 2011;208(7):1339–50.

10. Myers JL, Katzenstein AL. Epithelial necrosis and alveolar collapse in the pathogenesis of usual interstitial pneumonia. Chest 1988;94(6):1309–11.

11. Kuhn C III, Boldt J, King TE Jr, et al. An immunohistochemical study of architectural remodeling and connective tissue synthesis in pulmonary fibrosis. Am Rev Respir Dis 1989;140(6):1693–703.

12. Kuhn C, McDonald JA. The roles of the myofibroblast in idiopathic pulmonary fibrosis. Ultrastructural and immunohistochemical features of sites of active extracellular matrix synthesis. Am J Pathol 1991;138(5):1257–65.

13. Lappi Blanco E, Soini Y, Paakko P. Apoptotic activity is increased in the newly formed fibromyxoid connective tissue in bronchiolitis obliterans organizing pneumonia. Lung 1999;177(6):367–76.

14. Maher TM, Evans IC, Bottoms SE, et al. Diminished prostaglandin E2 contributes to the apoptosis paradox in idiopathic pulmonary fibrosis. Am J Respir Crit Care Med 2010;182(1):73–82.

15. Uhal BD, Joshi I, Hughes WF, et al. Alveolar epithelial cell death adjacent to underlying myofibroblasts in advanced fibrotic human lung. Am J Physiol 1998;275(6 Pt 1):L1192–9.

16. Hagimoto N, Kuwano K, Miyazaki H, et al. Induction of apoptosis and pulmonary fibrosis in mice in response to ligation of Fas antigen. Am J Respir Cell Mol Biol 1997;17(3):272–8.

17. Wang R, Ibarra-Sunga O, Verlinski L, et al. Abrogation of bleomycin-induced epithelial apoptosis and lung fibrosis by captopril or by a caspase inhibitor. Am J Physiol Lung Cell Mol Physiol 2000;279(1):L143–51.

18. Antoniou KM, Hansell DM, Rubens MB, et al. Idiopathic pulmonary fibrosis: outcome in relation to smoking status. Am J Respir Crit Care Med 2008;177(2):190–4.

19. Hubbard R, Lewis S, Richards K, et al. Occupational exposure to metal or wood dust and aetiology of cryptogenic fibrosing alveolitis. Lancet 1996;347(8997):284–9.

20. Baumgartner KB, Samet JM, Coultas DB, et al. Occupational and environmental risk factors for idiopathic pulmonary fibrosis: a multicenter case-control study. Collaborating Centers. Am J Epidemiol 2000;152(4):307–15.

21. Egan JJ, Stewart JP, Hasleton PS, et al. Epstein-Barr virus replication within pulmonary epithelial cells in cryptogenic fibrosing alveolitis. Thorax 1995;50(12):1234–9.

22. Maher TM. Pirfenidone in idiopathic pulmonary fibrosis. Drugs Today (Barc) 2010;46(7):473–82.

23. Raghu G, Depaso WJ, Cain K, et al. Azathioprine combined with prednisone in the treatment of idiopathic pulmonary fibrosis: a prospective double-blind, randomized, placebo-controlled clinical trial. Am Rev Respir Dis 1991;144(2):291–6.

24. Richeldi L, Davies HR, Ferrara G, et al. Corticosteroids for idiopathic pulmonary fibrosis. Cochrane Database Syst Rev 2003;(3):CD002880.

25. Raghu G, Collard HR, Egan JJ, et al. An official ATS/ERS/JRS/ALAT statement: idiopathic pulmonary fibrosis: evidence-based guidelines for diagnosis and management. Am J Respir Crit Care Med 2011;183(6):788–824.

26. Demedts M, Behr J, Buhl R, et al. High-dose acetylcysteine in idiopathic pulmonary fibrosis. N Engl J Med 2005;353(21):2229–42.

27. Cantin AM, Hubbard RC, Crystal RG. Glutathione deficiency in the epithelial lining fluid of the lower respiratory tract in idiopathic pulmonary fibrosis. Am Rev Respir Dis 1989;139(2):370–2.

28. Behr J, Maier K, Degenkolb B, et al. Antioxidative and clinical effects of high-dose N-acetylcysteine in fibrosing alveolitis. Adjunctive therapy to maintenance immunosuppression. Am J Respir Crit Care Med 1997;156(6):1897–901.

29. Iyer SN, Gurujeyalakshmi G, Giri SN. Effects of pirfenidone on transforming growth factor-beta gene expression at the transcriptional level in bleomycin

hamster model of lung fibrosis. J Pharmacol Exp Ther 1999;291(1):367–73.

30. Oku H, Shimizu T, Kawabata T, et al. Antifibrotic action of pirfenidone and prednisolone: different effects on pulmonary cytokines and growth factors in bleomycin-induced murine pulmonary fibrosis. Eur J Pharmacol 2008;590(1–3):400–8.

31. Kakugawa T, Mukae H, Hayashi T, et al. Pirfenidone attenuates expression of HSP47 in murine bleomycin-induced pulmonary fibrosis. Eur Respir J 2004;24(1):57–65.

32. Azuma A, Nukiwa T, Tsuboi E, et al. Double-blind, placebo-controlled trial of pirfenidone in patients with idiopathic pulmonary fibrosis. Am J Respir Crit Care Med 2005;171(9):1040–7.

33. Taniguchi H, Ebina M, Kondoh Y, et al. Pirfenidone in idiopathic pulmonary fibrosis. Eur Respir J 2010; 35(4):821–9.

34. Noble PW, Albera C, Bradford WZ, et al. Pirfenidone in patients with idiopathic pulmonary fibrosis (CAPACITY): two randomised trials. Lancet 2011; 377(9779):1760–9.

35. Richeldi L, du Bois RM. Pirfenidone in idiopathic pulmonary fibrosis: the CAPACITY program. Expert Rev Respir Med 2011;5(4):473–81.

36. Narayanan AS, Whithey J, Souza A, et al. Effect of gamma-interferon on collagen synthesis by normal and fibrotic human lung fibroblasts. Chest 1992; 101(5):1326–31.

37. Wen FQ, Liu XD, Terasaki Y, et al. Interferon-gamma reduces interleukin-4- and interleukin-13-augmented transforming growth factor-beta2 production in human bronchial epithelial cells by targeting Smads. Chest 2003;123(Suppl 3): 372S–3S.

38. Strieter RM, Starko KM, Enelow RI, et al. Effects of interferon-gamma 1b on biomarker expression in patients with idiopathic pulmonary fibrosis. Am J Respir Crit Care Med 2004;170(2):133–40.

39. King TE Jr, Albera C, Bradford WZ, et al. Effect of interferon gamma-1b on survival in patients with idiopathic pulmonary fibrosis (INSPIRE): a multicentre, randomised, placebo-controlled trial. Lancet 2009;374(9685):222–8.

40. Shi-Wen X, Chen Y, Denton CP, et al. Endothelin-1 promotes myofibroblast induction through the ETA receptor via a rac/phosphoinositide 3-kinase/Akt-dependent pathway and is essential for the enhanced contractile phenotype of fibrotic fibroblasts. Mol Biol Cell 2004;15(6):2707–19.

41. Xu SW, Howat SL, Renzoni EA, et al. Endothelin-1 induces expression of matrix-associated genes in lung fibroblasts through MEK/ERK. J Biol Chem 2004;279(22):23098–103.

42. Giaid A, Michel RP, Stewart DJ, et al. Expression of endothelin-1 in lungs of patients with cryptogenic fibrosing alveolitis. Lancet 1993;341(8860):1550–4.

43. Park SH, Saleh D, Giaid A, et al. Increased endothelin-1 in bleomycin-induced pulmonary fibrosis and the effect of an endothelin receptor antagonist. Am J Respir Crit Care Med 1997; 156(2 Pt 1):600–0.

44. King TE Jr, Brown KK, Raghu G, et al. BUILD-3: a randomized, controlled trial of bosentan in idiopathic pulmonary fibrosis. Am J Respir Crit Care Med 2011;184(1):92–9.

45. King TE Jr, Behr J, Brown KK, et al. BUILD-1: a randomized placebo-controlled trial of bosentan in idiopathic pulmonary fibrosis. Am J Respir Crit Care Med 2008;177(1):75–81.

46. Daniels CE, Wilkes MC, Edens M, et al. Imatinib mesylate inhibits the profibrogenic activity of TGF-beta and prevents bleomycin-mediated lung fibrosis. J Clin Invest 2004;114(9):1308–16.

47. Daniels CE, Lasky JA, Limper AH, et al. Imatinib treatment for idiopathic pulmonary fibrosis: randomized placebo-controlled trial results. Am J Respir Crit Care Med 2010;181(6):604–10.

48. Richeldi L, Costabel U, Selman M, et al. Efficacy of a tyrosine kinase inhibitor in idiopathic pulmonary fibrosis. N Engl J Med 2011;365(12):1079–87.

49. Zappala CJ, Latsi PI, Nicholson AG, et al. Marginal decline in forced vital capacity is associated with a poor outcome in idiopathic pulmonary fibrosis. Eur Respir J 2010;35(4):830–6.

50. Latsi PI, du Bois RM, Nicholson AG, et al. Fibrotic idiopathic interstitial pneumonia: the prognostic value of longitudinal functional trends. Am J Respir Crit Care Med 2003;168(5):531–7.

51. Richards TJ, Kaminski N, Baribaud F, et al. Peripheral blood proteins predict mortality in idiopathic pulmonary fibrosis. Am J Respir Crit Care Med 2011. [Epub ahead of print].

52. Grimminger F, Schermuly RT, Ghofrani HA. Targeting non-malignant disorders with tyrosine kinase inhibitors. Nat Rev Drug Discov 2010;9(12):956–70.

53. Manning G, Whyte DB, Martinez R, et al. The protein kinase complement of the human genome. Science 2002;298(5600):1912–34.

54. Garneau-Tsodikova S, Thannickal VJ. Protein kinase inhibitors in the treatment of pulmonary fibrosis. Curr Med Chem 2008;15(25):2632–40.

55. Konigshoff M, Kramer M, Balsara N, et al. WNT1-inducible signaling protein-1 mediates pulmonary fibrosis in mice and is upregulated in humans with idiopathic pulmonary fibrosis. J Clin Invest 2009;119(4):772–87.

56. Konigshoff M, Balsara N, Pfaff EM, et al. Functional Wnt signaling is increased in idiopathic pulmonary fibrosis. PLoS One 2008;3(5):e2142.

57. Antoniu SA, Kolb MR. Intedanib, a triple kinase inhibitor of VEGFR, FGFR and PDGFR for the treatment of cancer and idiopathic pulmonary fibrosis. IDrugs 2010;13(5):332–45.

58. Hancock A, Armstrong L, Gama R, et al. Production of interleukin 13 by alveolar macrophages from normal and fibrotic lung. Am J Respir Cell Mol Biol 1998; 18(1):60–5.

59. Zhu Z, Homer RJ, Wang Z, et al. Pulmonary expression of interleukin-13 causes inflammation, mucus hypersecretion, subepithelial fibrosis, physiologic abnormalities, and eotaxin production. J Clin Invest 1999;103(6):779–88.

60. Ingram JL, Rice AB, Geisenhoffer K, et al. IL-13 and IL-1beta promote lung fibroblast growth through coordinated up-regulation of PDGF-AA and PDGF-Ralpha. FASEB J 2004;18(10):1132–4.

61. Kaviratne M, Hesse M, Leusink M, et al. IL-13 activates a mechanism of tissue fibrosis that is completely TGF-beta independent. J Immunol 2004;173(6):4020–9.

62. Lee CG, Kang HR, Homer RJ, et al. Transgenic modeling of transforming growth factor-beta(1): role of apoptosis in fibrosis and alveolar remodeling. Proc Am Thorac Soc 2006;3(5):418–23.

63. Kolodsick JE, Toews GB, Jakubzick C, et al. Protection from fluorescein isothiocyanate-induced fibrosis in IL-13-deficient, but not IL-4-deficient, mice results from impaired collagen synthesis by fibroblasts. J Immunol 2004;172(7):4068–76.

64. Jakubzick C, Choi ES, Joshi BH, et al. Therapeutic attenuation of pulmonary fibrosis via targeting of IL-4- and IL-13-responsive cells. J Immunol 2003; 171(5):2684–93.

65. Murray LA, Hackett TL, Warner SM, et al. BMP-7 does not protect against bleomycin-induced lung or skin fibrosis. PLoS One 2008;3(12):e4039.

66. Martinez FJ, Safrin S, Weycker D, et al. The clinical course of patients with idiopathic pulmonary fibrosis. Ann Intern Med 2005;142(12 Pt 1):963–7.

67. Collard HR, Moore BB, Flaherty KR, et al. Acute exacerbations of idiopathic pulmonary fibrosis. Am J Respir Crit Care Med 2007;176(7):636–43.

68. Huie TJ, Moss M, Frankel SK. What can biomarkers tell us about the pathogenesis of acute exacerbations of idiopathic pulmonary fibrosis? Am J Physiol Lung Cell Mol Physiol 2010;299(1):L1–2.

69. Collard HR, Calfee CS, Wolters PJ, et al. Plasma biomarker profiles in acute exacerbation of idiopathic pulmonary fibrosis. Am J Physiol Lung Cell Mol Physiol 2010;299(1):L3–7.

70. Moeller A, Gilpin SE, Ask K, et al. Circulating fibrocytes are an indicator of poor prognosis in idiopathic pulmonary fibrosis. Am J Respir Crit Care Med 2009;179(7):588–94.

71. McMillan TR, Moore BB, Weinberg JB, et al. Exacerbation of established pulmonary fibrosis in a murine model by gammaherpesvirus. Am J Respir Crit Care Med 2008;177(7):771–80.

72. Wootton SC, Kim DS, Kondoh Y, et al. Viral infection in acute exacerbation of idiopathic pulmonary fibrosis. Am J Respir Crit Care Med 2011;183(12): 1698–702.

73. Konishi K, Gibson KF, Lindell KO, et al. Gene expression profiles of acute exacerbations of idiopathic pulmonary fibrosis. Am J Respir Crit Care Med 2009;180(2):167–75.

74. Zycinska K, Wardyn KA, Zielonka TM, et al. Co-trimoxazole and prevention of relapses of PR3-ANCA positive vasculitis with pulmonary involvement. Eur J Med Res 2009;14(Suppl 4):265–7.

75. Varney VA, Parnell HM, Salisbury DT, et al. A double blind randomised placebo controlled pilot study of oral co-trimoxazole in advanced fibrotic lung disease. Pulm Pharmacol Ther 2008; 21(1):178–87.

76. Johnston SL, Blasi F, Black PN, et al. The effect of telithromycin in acute exacerbations of asthma. N Engl J Med 2006;354(15):1589–600.

77. Albert RK, Connett J, Bailey WC, et al. Azithromycin for prevention of exacerbations of COPD. N Engl J Med 2011;365(8):689–98.

78. Chambers RC. Procoagulant signalling mechanisms in lung inflammation and fibrosis: novel opportunities for pharmacological intervention? Br J Pharmacol 2008;153(S1):S367–78.

79. Imokawa S, Sato A, Hayakawa H, et al. Tissue factor expression and fibrin deposition in the lungs of patients with idiopathic pulmonary fibrosis and systemic sclerosis. Am J Respir Crit Care Med 1997;156(2 Pt 1):631–6.

80. Gunther A, Mosavi P, Ruppert C, et al. Enhanced tissue factor pathway activity and fibrin turnover in the alveolar compartment of patients with interstitial lung disease. Thromb Haemost 2000;83(6): 853–60.

81. Scotton CJ, Krupiczojc MA, Konigshoff M, et al. Increased local expression of coagulation factor X contributes to the fibrotic response in human and murine lung injury. J Clin Invest 2009;119(9): 2550–63.

82. Eitzman DT, McCoy RD, Zheng X, et al. Bleomycin-induced pulmonary fibrosis in transgenic mice that either lack or overexpress the murine plasminogen activator inhibitor-1 gene. J Clin Invest 1996;97(1): 232–7.

83. Jenkins RG, Su X, Su G, et al. Ligation of protease-activated receptor 1 enhances alpha(v)beta6 integrin-dependent TGF-beta activation and promotes acute lung injury. J Clin Invest 2006; 116(6):1606–14.

84. Naldini A, Pucci A, Carney DH, et al. Thrombin enhancement of interleukin-1 expression in mononuclear cells: involvement of proteinase-activated receptor-1. Cytokine 2002;20(5):191–9.

85. Howell DC, Johns RH, Lasky JA, et al. Absence of proteinase-activated receptor-1 signaling affords protection from bleomycin-induced lung

inflammation and fibrosis. Am J Pathol 2005; 166(5):1353–65.

86. Wygrecka M, Kwapiszewska G, Jablonska E, et al. Role of protease-activated receptor-2 in idiopathic pulmonary fibrosis. Am J Respir Crit Care Med 2011;183(12):1703–14.

87. Kubo H, Nakayama K, Yanai M, et al. Anticoagulant therapy for idiopathic pulmonary fibrosis. Chest 2005;128(3):1475–82.

88. Huang SK, Peters-Golden M. Eicosanoid lipid mediators in fibrotic lung diseases: ready for prime time? Chest 2008;133(6):1442–50.

89. Borok Z, Gillissen A, Buhl R, et al. Augmentation of functional prostaglandin E levels on the respiratory epithelial surface by aerosol administration of prostaglandin E. Am Rev Respir Dis 1991; 144(5):1080–4.

90. Wilborn J, Crofford LJ, Burdick MD, et al. Cultured lung fibroblasts isolated from patients with idiopathic pulmonary fibrosis have a diminished capacity to synthesize prostaglandin E2 and to express cyclooxygenase-2. J Clin Invest 1995; 95(4):1861–8.

91. Keerthisingam CB, Jenkins RG, Harrison NK, et al. Cyclooxygenase-2 deficiency results in a loss of the anti-proliferative response to transforming growth factor-beta in human fibrotic lung fibroblasts and promotes bleomycin-induced pulmonary fibrosis in mice. Am J Pathol 2001;158(4): 1411–22.

92. McAnulty RJ, Hernandez-Rodriguez NA, Mutsaers SE, et al. Indomethacin suppresses the anti-proliferative effects of transforming growth factor-beta isoforms on fibroblast cell cultures. Biochem J 1997;321(Pt 3):639–43.

93. Kolodsick JE, Peters-Golden M, Larios J, et al. Prostaglandin E2 inhibits fibroblast to myofibroblast transition via E. prostanoid receptor 2 signaling and cyclic adenosine monophosphate elevation. Am J Respir Cell Mol Biol 2003;29(5): 537–44.

94. Lama V, Moore BB, Christensen P, et al. Prostaglandin E2 synthesis and suppression of fibroblast proliferation by alveolar epithelial cells is cyclooxygenase-2-dependent. Am J Respir Cell Mol Biol 2002;27(6):752 8.

95. Maher SA, Birrell MA, Belvisi MG. Prostaglandin E2 mediates cough via the EP3 receptor: implications for future disease therapy. Am J Respir Crit Care Med 2009;180(10):923–8.

96. Huang SK, Wettlaufer SH, Chung J, et al. Prostaglandin E2 inhibits specific lung fibroblast functions via selective actions of PKA and Epac-1. Am J Respir Cell Mol Biol 2008;39(4):482–9.

97. Huang S, Wettlaufer SH, Hogaboam C, et al. Prostaglandin E(2) inhibits collagen expression and proliferation in patient-derived normal lung fibroblasts via E prostanoid 2 receptor and cAMP signaling. Am J Physiol Lung Cell Mol Physiol 2007;292(2):L405–13.

98. Moore BB, Ballinger MN, White ES, et al. Bleomycin induced E prostanoid receptor changes alter fibroblast responses to prostaglandin E2. J Immunol 2005;174(9):5644–9.

99. Wardlaw AJ, Hay H, Cromwell O, et al. Leukotrienes, LTC4 and LTB4, in bronchoalveolar lavage in bronchial asthma and other respiratory diseases. J Allergy Clin Immunol 1989;84(1):19–26.

100. Bosse Y, Thompson C, McMahon S, et al. Leukotriene D4-induced, epithelial cell-derived transforming growth factor beta1 in human bronchial smooth muscle cell proliferation. Clin Exp Allergy 2008;38(1):113–21.

101. Phan SH, McGarry BM, Loeffler KM, et al. Leukotriene C4 binds to rat lung fibroblasts and stimulates collagen synthesis. Adv Prostaglandin Thromboxane Leukot Res 1987;17B:997–9.

102. Peres CM, Aronoff DM, Serezani CH, et al. Specific leukotriene receptors couple to distinct G proteins to effect stimulation of alveolar macrophage host defense functions. J Immunol 2007;179(8): 5454–61.

103. Shimbori C, Shiota N, Okunishi H. Effects of montelukast, a cysteinyl-leukotriene type 1 receptor antagonist, on the pathogenesis of bleomycin-induced pulmonary fibrosis in mice. Eur J Pharmacol 2011;650(1):424–30.

104. Crestani B, Besnard V, Boczkowski J. Signalling pathways from NADPH oxidase-4 to idiopathic pulmonary fibrosis. Int J Biochem Cell Biol 2011; 43(8):1086–9.

105. Brown DI, Griendling KK. Nox proteins in signal transduction. Free Radic Biol Med 2009;47(9): 1239–53.

106. Chan EC, Jiang F, Peshavariya HM, et al. Regulation of cell proliferation by NADPH oxidase-mediated signaling: potential roles in tissue repair, regenerative medicine and tissue engineering. Pharmacol Ther 2009;122(2):97–108.

107. Hecker L, Vittal R, Jones T, et al. NADPH oxidase-4 mediates myofibroblast activation and fibrogenic responses to lung injury. Nat Med 2009;15(9): 1077–81.

108. Amara N, Goven D, Prost F, et al. NOX4/NADPH oxidase expression is increased in pulmonary fibroblasts from patients with idiopathic pulmonary fibrosis and mediates TGFbeta1-induced fibroblast differentiation into myofibroblasts. Thorax 2010; 65(8):733–8.

109. Lu X, Murphy TC, Nanes MS, et al. PPAR{gamma} regulates hypoxia-induced Nox4 expression in human pulmonary artery smooth muscle cells through NF-{kappa}B. Am J Physiol Lung Cell Mol Physiol 2010;299(4):L559–66.

110. Laleu B, Gaggini F, Orchard M, et al. First in class, potent, and orally bioavailable NADPH oxidase isoform 4 (Nox4) inhibitors for the treatment of idiopathic pulmonary fibrosis. J Med Chem 2010; 53(21):7715–30.

111. Xu YD, Hua J, Mui A, et al. Release of biologically active TGF-beta1 by alveolar epithelial cells results in pulmonary fibrosis. Am J Physiol Lung Cell Mol Physiol 2003;285(3):L527–39.

112. Hagimoto N, Kuwano K, Inoshima I, et al. TGF-beta 1 as an enhancer of Fas-mediated apoptosis of lung epithelial cells. J Immunol 2002;168(12):6470–8.

113. Coker RK, Laurent GJ, Jeffery PK, et al. Localisation of transforming growth factor beta1 and beta3 mRNA transcripts in normal and fibrotic human lung. Thorax 2001;56(7):549–56.

114. Zhang HY, Phan SH. Inhibition of myofibroblast apoptosis by transforming growth factor beta(1). Am J Respir Cell Mol Biol 1999;21(6):658–65.

115. Coker RK, Laurent GJ, Shahzeidi S, et al. Transforming growth factors-beta 1, -beta 2, and -beta 3 stimulate fibroblast procollagen production in vitro but are differentially expressed during bleomycin-induced lung fibrosis. Am J Pathol 1997;150(3):981–91.

116. Sime PJ, Xing Z, Graham FL, et al. Adenovector-mediated gene transfer of active transforming growth factor-beta1 induces prolonged severe fibrosis in rat lung. J Clin Invest 1997;100(4):768–76.

117. Wang Q, Wang Y, Hyde DM, et al. Reduction of bleomycin induced lung fibrosis by transforming growth factor beta soluble receptor in hamsters. Thorax 1999;54(9):805–12.

118. Munger JS, Huang X, Kawakatsu H, et al. The integrin alpha v beta 6 binds and activates latent TGF beta 1: a mechanism for regulating pulmonary inflammation and fibrosis. Cell 1999;96(3):319–28.

119. Ide M, Ishii H, Mukae H, et al. High serum levels of thrombospondin-1 in patients with idiopathic interstitial pneumonia. Respir Med 2008;102(11): 1625–30.

120. Weiss CH, Budinger GR, Mutlu GM, et al. Proteasomal regulation of pulmonary fibrosis. Proc Am Thorac Soc 2010;7(1):77–83.

121. Hawinkels LJ, Ten Dijke P. Exploring anti-TGF-beta therapies in cancer and fibrosis. Growth Factors 2011;29(4):140–52.

122. de Gouville AC, Huet S. Inhibition of ALK5 as a new approach to treat liver fibrotic diseases. Drug News Perspect 2006;19(2):85–90.

123. Horan GS, Wood S, Ona V, et al. Partial inhibition of integrin alpha(v)beta6 prevents pulmonary fibrosis without exacerbating inflammation. Am J Respir Crit Care Med 2008;177(1):56–65.

124. Xu MY, Porte J, Knox AJ, et al. Lysophosphatidic acid induces alphavbeta6 integrin-mediated TGF-beta activation via the LPA2 receptor and the small G protein G alpha(q). Am J Pathol 2009;174(4): 1264–79.

125. Swaney JS, Chapman C, Correa LD, et al. Pharmacokinetic and pharmacodynamic characterization of an oral lysophosphatidic acid type 1 receptor-selective antagonist. J Pharmacol Exp Ther 2011; 336(3):693–700.

126. Swaney JS, Chapman C, Correa LD, et al. A novel, orally active LPA(1) receptor antagonist inhibits lung fibrosis in the mouse bleomycin model. Br J Pharmacol 2010;160(7):1699–713.

127. Allen JT, Knight RA, Bloor CA, et al. Enhanced insulin-like growth factor binding protein-related protein 2 (Connective tissue growth factor) expression in patients with idiopathic pulmonary fibrosis and pulmonary sarcoidosis. Am J Respir Cell Mol Biol 1999;21(6):693–700.

128. Kelly M, Kolb M, Bonniaud P, et al. Re-evaluation of fibrogenic cytokines in lung fibrosis. Curr Pharm Des 2003;9(1):39–49.

129. Bonniaud P, Kolb M, Galt T, et al. Smad3 null mice develop airspace enlargement and are resistant to TGF-beta-mediated pulmonary fibrosis. J Immunol 2004;173(3):2099–108.

130. Bonniaud P, Martin G, Margetts PJ, et al. Connective tissue growth factor is crucial to inducing a profibrotic environment in "fibrosis-resistant" BALB/c mouse lungs. Am J Respir Cell Mol Biol 2004; 31(5):510–6.

131. Bonniaud P, Margetts PJ, Kolb M, et al. Adenoviral gene transfer of connective tissue growth factor in the lung induces transient fibrosis. Am J Respir Crit Care Med 2003;168(7):770–8.

132. Wang Q, Usinger W, Nichols B, et al. Cooperative interaction of CTGF and TGF-beta in animal models of fibrotic disease. Fibrogenesis Tissue Repair 2011;4(1):4.

133. Wang X, Wu G, Gou L, et al. A novel single-chain-Fv antibody against connective tissue growth factor attenuates bleomycin-induced pulmonary fibrosis in mice. Respirology 2011; 16(3):500–7.

Management of Idiopathic Pulmonary Fibrosis

Stefania Cerri, MD, PhD, Paolo Spagnolo, MD, PhD,
Fabrizio Luppi, MD, PhD, Luca Richeldi, MD, PhD*

KEYWORDS

- Idiopathic pulmonary fibrosis • Pirfenidone
- Corticosteroids • Randomized controlled trials
- Comorbidities

Idiopathic pulmonary fibrosis (IPF) represents one of the most challenging diseases for chest physicians. The diagnostic process is complex and requires close interaction with different specialists. The prognosis of IPF is invariably poor. Notwithstanding the many treatments used in clinical practice and evaluated in the context of controlled randomized trials, the modalities for the follow-up of patients with IPF are poorly defined. Given the lack of proof for most interventions, all decisions need to be extensively discussed and agreed upon with the patient and their families. As a consequence, few respiratory disorders require of chest physicians more interactive skills and more dedication than IPF.

PHARMACOLOGIC TREATMENTS

The pharmacologic approach to IPF management has changed as the understanding of the pathogenesis of the disease has evolved over the last decade. The initial thinking was in favor of a disease triggered by a persistent inflammatory process, resulting in the induction of fibrosis and scarring of the lungs. As such, several trials were performed evaluating the efficacy of drugs that primarily exert their functions by suppressing inflammatory or immune responses (such as corticosteroids and nonsteroid immunomodulatory agents). Current treatment approaches favor agents with antifibrotic properties. A systematic assessment of the evidence available for different therapeutic options in IPF has been recently published as an evidence-based guideline.[1] A summary of the therapeutic recommendations listed in this important document, formulated according to the Grades of Recommendation Assessment, Development and Evaluation methodology,[2] along with the reported voting results from the committee members, is provided in **Table 1**.

Anti-Inflammatory and Immunomodulatory Drugs

Patients with IPF have been (and most still continue to be) treated in many parts of the world with corticosteroids. A summary of the results available for the efficacy of corticosteroid in IPF was first published in 2003 as a Cochrane systematic review,[3] when no high-quality studies were identified and only nonrandomized, retrospective, studies were available. Hence, there was a major lack of evidence supporting the use of corticosteroids in the treatment of IPF. An update of that same systematic review, published in 2010,[4] did not identify any new additional randomized clinical trial on the use of steroids in IPF, thus confirming the persisting lack of evidence for their use in the management of IPF. This issue has been also reassessed in the current evidence-based guidelines,[1]

Financial disclosures: S.C., P.S. and F.L. have nothing to disclose; L.R. reports receiving consulting fees from Boehringer Ingelheim, Intermune, Celgene and Gilead and lecture fees from Intermune.
Center for Rare Lung Diseases, Department of Oncology, Hematology and Respiratory Diseases, University Hospital Policlinico of Modena, Via del Pozzo 71, 41124 Modena, Italy
* Corresponding author.
E-mail address: luca.richeldi@unimore.it

Clin Chest Med 33 (2012) 85–94
doi:10.1016/j.ccm.2011.11.005
0272-5231/12/$ – see front matter © 2012 Elsevier Inc. All rights reserved.

chestmed.theclinics.com

Table 1
Summary of current evidence-based recommendations on management of patients with IPF

	Recommendation				Number of Votes (As in Ref.[1])			
	For		Against					
	Strong	Weak	Weak	Strong	For	Against	Abstention	Absent
Pharmacologic Therapies in Stable IPF								
Corticosteroids alone				×	0	21	2	8
Colchicine				×	0	21	2	8
Cyclosporin A				×	0	21	2	8
Cyclophosphamide + corticosteroids				×	0	21	2	8
Azathioprine + corticosteroids				×	0	21	2	8
Prednisone + NAC + azathioprine			×		3	17	3	8
NAC alone			×		5	15	3	8
Interferon gamma-1b				×	0	17	6	8
Bosentan				×	0	10	13	8
Etanercept				×	0	18	4	9
Anticoagulation therapy			×		1	20	2	8
Pirfenidone			×		4	10	17	0
Pharmacologic Therapies in Acute Exacerbations of IPF								
Corticosteroids		×			14	5	1	11
Treatment of comorbidities								
Pulmonary hypertension			×		8	14	1	8
Gastroesophageal reflux		×			15	8	0	8
Nonpharmacologic Therapies								
Long-term oxygen therapy (in case of resting hypoxemia)	×				18	0	4	9
Rehabilitation		×			19	0	3	9
Mechanical ventilation			×		2	19	2	8
Lung Transplantation (Selected Patients)	×				21	0	1	9

Official recommendations are not available for sildenafil and imatinib because evidence on these drugs was published after the publication of the ATS/ERS/JRS/ALAT 2011 guideline document.[1] See text for details.
Abbreviations: NA, not applicable; NAC, N-acetylcysteine.

in which a strong recommendation against the use of corticosteroid monotherapy in IPF has been made. This important recommendation relies on the availability of very-low-quality evidence and places a high value on preventing treatment-related morbidity using long-term corticosteroid therapy. From the aforementioned results, steroids alone should never be used to treat IPF.

Low-quality evidence is also available for the use of nonsteroid immunomodulatory drugs in IPF, such as colchicine, cyclosporin A, cyclophosphamide, or azathioprine, either alone or in combination with corticosteroids[5]; as such, current guidelines[1] strongly recommend against the use of immunomodulatory agents in the treatment of patients with IPF. A weak recommendation against the use of a combination therapy with azathioprine, prednisone, and the antioxidant drug N-acetylcysteine has also been made.[1] Regarding this combination regimen only one randomized clinical trial is available, which evaluated the effect of N-acetylcysteine in patients already receiving combination therapy with prednisone and azathioprine.[6] The main points of criticism regarding the results of this trial are related to the substantial drop-out rate observed in the study (and the consequent statistical corrections needed) and to the lack of a true (ie, not taking any potentially effective drug) placebo group. Nonetheless, significant results supporting the use of the so-called triple therapy were observed in the change of vital capacity and diffusing capacity at 12 months; however, no difference was observed in mortality or in other secondary outcomes, such as dyspnea or quality-of-life scores. To further investigate the possible efficacy of N-acetylcysteine in the treatment of patients with IPF, a three-arm large trial sponsored by the IPFnet consortium (the PANTHER [Prednisone, Azathioprine, and N-acetylcysteine: A Study That Evaluates Response in IPF] trial) is currently recruiting patients in the United States. However, an interim results from this study showed that compared to placebo, those assigned to triple therapy had greater mortality, more hospitalizations, and more serious adverse events, while not showing any difference in lung function test changes. Therefore the National Heart, Lung, and Blood Institute (NHLBI) has recently stopped the triple-therapy arm of this study (NIH Release on October 21, 2011). The other two study arms of this IPF trial comparing NAC alone to placebo alone will continue. At present, N-acetylcysteine, neither alone nor in combination with prednisone and azathioprine, can be recommended for the routine treatment of IPF.

Antifibrotic and Antiproliferative Drugs

Over the last decade, the perspective on IPF pathogenesis has profoundly changed.[7] The cause of the disease has not been identified and the pathogenesis remains largely unknown. Recent findings suggest that the disease is likely the result of an aberrant reparative mechanism, following an injury that primarily targets the lung epithelium. Therefore, the disease appears to be characterized by the proliferation and accumulation of fibroblasts/myofibroblasts in the lungs, with excessive deposition of extracellular matrix, resulting in the fibrotic distortion of the lung architecture, typically observed by radiologists and pathologists in the lungs of patients with IPF. Several pathways of these processes are under investigation at present, aimed at identifying the key molecular mediators and the potential sources of myofibroblasts as well as the mechanisms responsible for the initial injury.

As such, recent randomized clinical trials on the treatment of IPF have shifted their attention to drugs with antifibrotic and antiproliferative effects. As a general observation, the rationale for using most of the drugs tested so far in clinical trials has been limited because of both the lack of a reliable animal model of the disease[8] and the relative scarcity of in vivo and ex vivo data. As a consequence, in some cases the background for conducting clinical trials is derived from post hoc analyses of previous studies, with the unavoidable risks related to no predefined statistical analyses on subgroups.[9]

Interferon gamma-1b has been one of the first agents evaluated in IPF for its antifibrotic as well as immunomodulatory properties. A first small pilot study[10] published in 1999 pioneered the era of the randomized controlled trial (RCT) in IPF, showing an unexpected and substantial improvement of lung function in the active treatment group, which prompted 2 subsequent large randomized, placebo-controlled clinical trials addressing the efficacy of this intervention.[11,12] Despite the promising initial results, both trials failed to meet the primary end points, and a recent meta-analysis on the efficacy of interferon gamma-1b failed to show any effect of this treatment on clinically relevant outcomes, such as overall survival, progression-free survival, or lung function.[5] Therefore, current guidelines include a strong recommendation against the use of interferon gamma-1b in the treatment of patients with IPF, based on high-quality evidence.[1] As a consequence, and notwithstanding the publication of small uncontrolled studies suggesting some effect in a minority of patients with IPF,[13,14] interferon gamma-1b is no longer a therapeutic option for patients with IPF.

Drugs already approved for other indications in different diseases, but with background for being effective in fibrotic disorders, have been evaluated in IPF clinical trials. Coming from the field of pulmonary hypertension (PH), the endothelin receptor A and B antagonist bosentan has been evaluated in 2 randomized placebo-controlled clinical trials. The IPF guidelines strongly recommend against the use of this drug in IPF based on the results of the first phase II trial,[15] which did not reach statistical significance in the primary outcome and only showed a positive trend toward a benefit for the drug in some secondary end points. Moreover, the results of the largest trial on bosentan in IPF[16] confirmed the lack of effect of this drug. More recently, a phase III, randomized, double-blind, placebo-controlled, multicenter study comparing ambrisentan (another endothelin receptor antagonist selective for type A receptor) to placebo in subjects with IPF (the ARTEMIS-IPF [Randomized, Placebo-Controlled Study to Evaluate Safety and Effectiveness of Ambrisentan in IPF] trial) was prematurely stopped after an interim analysis showed no efficacy of the study drug. Furthermore, a phase II trial evaluating efficacy and safety in patients with IPF of another endothelin receptor antagonist, macitentan, is active, but not recruiting patients.

Etanercept, an anti–tumor necrosis factor α drug widely used in rheumatology, has also been evaluated in IPF. A strong recommendation against its use in IPF has been made in the current guidelines.[1] In a single, well-conducted, randomized placebo-controlled trial,[17] this drug failed to show a statistically significant difference between treatment groups, although some effects on secondary outcomes were noted.

Several novel oncological agents have been tried in patients with IPF. Imatinib mesylate, a specific tyrosine kinase inhibitor with activity against Bcr-Abl, platelet-derived growth factor (PDGF) receptors, and c-kit, has also been studied in IPF. The inhibitory activity on PDGF receptors suggested a potential activity in IPF, through the suppression of the profibrotic and proliferative pathways mediated by PDGF. However, a recently published randomized clinical trial on imatinib in patients with IPF[18] failed to demonstrate an effect of this drug compared with placebo on any of the outcomes selected for this study, and in particular did not show a statistically significant difference between the treatment and the control group in progression-free survival or in the change of lung function over time. Also, a multiple kinase inhibitor (BIBF 1120) has been evaluated in a phase II trial in patients with IPF.[19] The encouraging results of this study[20] prompted the initiation of 2 parallel phase III studies, currently ongoing and aimed at demonstrating the efficacy of this drug in IPF.

Very low-quality evidence is available for the usage of anticoagulation therapy in IPF. In fact, only one small, unblinded, RCT performed in Japan has been published, showing a survival benefit in patients receiving anticoagulation, the effect being attributed to a reduced mortality during hospitalization for acute exacerbation or disease progression.[21] A larger trial on the efficacy of the use of anticoagulation therapy in IPF (the ACE-IPF [Anticoagulant Effectiveness in Idiopathic Pulmonary Fibrosis] trial), sponsored by the IPFnet network in the United States, was recently stopped based on a lack of efficacy at interim analysis.

Pirfenidone is a small synthetic nonpeptide molecule that has antifibrotic, anti-inflammatory, and antioxidant properties, with the ability to interfere with transforming growth factor β–induced collagen synthesis. Promising results from an open-label phase II study supported the use of this drug in the treatment of IPF.[22] Subsequently, the results of 2 multicenter trials performed in Japan and 2 large international multicenter clinical trials, all randomized and placebo-controlled, assessing the efficacy of pirfenidone compared with placebo in patients with IPF, have been published.[23–25] All these trials have been found to have a sufficient methodological quality, allowing their inclusion in a recent Cochrane systematic review.[5] Based on the results of this meta-analysis, pirfenidone appears to reduce the risk of disease progression (as measured by progression-free survival) by 30% and to provide a beneficial effect on the change of lung function from baseline, in comparison with placebo. Some limitations to the interpretation of these data still apply, mostly related to a certain degree of methodological heterogeneity across studies, mainly regarding the methodologies for reporting lung-function results. Current IPF guidelines, considering the cost of therapy and the potentially relevant side effects (such as gastrointestinal adverse events, liver laboratory abnormalities, photosensitivity, and rash), expressed a weak recommendation against the use of this drug. However, the majority of panel experts abstained from this voting. On the one hand, the Food and Drug Administration has denied approval for the use of the drug in the United States, requesting additional data. Consequently, a new study (the ASCEND [Assessment of Pirfenidone to Confirm Efficacy and Safety in IPF] trial), comparing pirfenidone and placebo in patients with IPF, is currently enrolling patients in North America, Central America, South America, Australia, and New Zealand. On the other hand, pirfenidone is approved and commercially available for the treatment of patients with IPF in India and Japan; in Europe the drug has been recognized as an orphan drug, and the European Medicines Agency has approved its use in the European Community for the treatment of patients with mild to moderate IPF. Part of these discrepancies can be explained by the fact that the trials assessing the efficacy of pirfenidone have been designed with lung function as the primary end point, whereas in a disease like IPF the reduction of mortality should be seen as the main goal of treatment. Although there is increasing evidence that a change (in particular a 10% decrease) in forced vital capacity is predictive of subsequent mortality,[26–28] lung function should be seen at best as a surrogate of mortality. In any case, pirfenidone will enter the European market over the next months and a named-patient program is currently ongoing. The administration of pirfenidone to all patients with IPF is still a matter of debate. Patients willing to receive pirfenidone should be fully informed on the available evidence for the efficacy of the drug and on the possible side effects.

MANAGEMENT OF COMORBIDITIES

IPF is often associated with morbidities (eg, PH and gastroesophageal reflux) and symptoms (eg, dyspnea, exercise limitation, fatigue, anxiety, mood disturbance, sleep disorders) that dramatically affect patients' lives.

PH affects most patients with IPF at the time of initial diagnosis, and ultimately many of them during the course of the disease.[29] Patients with IPF with concomitant PH (defined as a mean pulmonary artery pressure >25 mm Hg on right heart catheterization) have more dyspnea, greater impairment of their exercise capacity, and increased 1-year mortality in comparison with their counterparts without PH.[30] Once PH has been diagnosed, it is essential to exclude any causative or contributory comorbidity, such as obstructive sleep apnea, congestive heart failure, and pulmonary emboli; in addition, hypoxia should be sought and treated. Whether targeting of PH with medications approved for the treatment of pulmonary arterial hypertension has any utility in IPF remains unclear. In a small open-label trial, sildenafil, an oral phosphodiesterase-5 inhibitor, improved 6-minute walk distance (6MWD) and pulmonary hemodynamics without increasing shunt flow or worsening oxygenation.[31] However, a subsequent large multicenter, randomized, double-blind, placebo-controlled study did not meet the primary end point (change of 20% in 6MWD at 12 weeks), although statistically significant differences favoring sildenafil were observed in dyspnea, partial pressure of oxygen, diffusing capacity of lung for carbon monoxide, and quality of life.[32]

Bosentan, a dual endothelin receptor A and B antagonist, has been tested in a phase II RCT,[15] though in patients not evaluated for the presence of PH and thus more as an antifibrotic drug. Although the primary end point (change from baseline up to month 12 in exercise capacity, as measured by a modified 6MWD test) was not reached, the results of a post hoc analysis suggested that bosentan had a beneficial effect on time to disease progression or death and quality of life in patients who underwent surgical lung biopsy,[33] thus leading to a larger phase III study, which failed to demonstrate that bosentan delays IPF worsening or death, the primary end point.[16] As already mentioned, a phase III randomized, double-blind, placebo-controlled, multicenter study comparing ambrisentan (an endothelin receptor antagonist selective for type A receptor) with placebo in subjects with IPF (with or without associated PH) has been prematurely stopped after an interim analysis showing no efficacy of the study drug. Notwithstanding the disappointing results

from these studies, it is common practice for chest physicians and cardiologists to observe how the presence of PH affects patients' functional status and portends a worse outcome. Despite limited evidence of efficacy, current guidelines weakly recommend a trial of vasomodulatory agents in patients with moderate to severe PH, as documented by right heart catheterization (ie, mean pulmonary artery pressure >35 mm Hg).[1]

Acid gastroesophageal reflux (GER) is highly prevalent in patients with IPF, up to one-half of whom are asymptomatic.[34] Experimental animal studies and descriptive studies in humans suggest that chronic microaspiration caused by GER may cause subclinical injury leading to pulmonary fibrosis.[35,36] While the pathobiological significance of GER in IPF remains to be elucidated, there is evidence that treatment of GER, either medical or surgical, may stabilize lung function.[37,38] More recently, Lee and colleagues[39] reported in a large cohort of patients with IPF that use of GER medication, (ie, suppression of gastric content acidity with either proton-pump inhibitors (PPI) or H_2 blockers) was associated with lower high-resolution computed tomography (HRCT) fibrosis score and longer survival. These authors observed an additional survival benefit to Nissen fundoplication, a surgical intervention that reduces not only acid but also weakly acidic reflux and potential microaspiration, which may also contribute to the development of lung fibrosis.[40] At present, it is unclear whether aggressive treatment of GER disease may improve or halt disease progression. In addition, PPI only affect the acidity of the refluxate without preventing reflux or microaspiration of gastric contents. Furthermore, the use of PPI has been associated with an increased risk of hip fracture and community-acquired pneumonia.[41,42] Lifestyle modifications (small meals, raising the head of the bed) seem reasonable measures to suggest for symptomatic patients.

MANAGEMENT OF ACUTE EXACERBATION OF IPF

The clinical course of IPF is usually chronic and slowly progressive, although some patients experience rapidly progressive disease.[1] Acute worsening may occur as a consequence of multiple distinct causes, including respiratory infections, pulmonary embolism, pneumothorax, and heart failure; sometimes worsening cannot be linked to any identifiable cause, and this latter case is referred to as acute exacerbation of IPF (AE-IPF)[43] (see article elsewhere in this issue). The prognosis of AE-IPF is almost invariably poor; mortality during hospitalization is as high as 65% and those who survive have a greater than 90% mortality rate in the 6 months following discharge.[44]

If AF-IPF is suspected, the management should include chest HRCT, echocardiogram, bronchoalveolar lavage, and infection screen to rule out known and potentially treatable causes of disease progression. Many patients with AE-IPF require intensive care, particularly when respiratory failure is associated with hemodynamic instability, significant comorbidities, or severe hypoxemia requiring monitoring of arterial blood gases or mechanical ventilation.

A systematic review has been performed summarizing the current knowledge of acute exacerbations in IPF, including their treatment.[45] Treatment strategies varied in the different studies, but in almost all of them patients were administered broad-spectrum antibiotics and pulse doses of methylprednisolone (0.5–1 g/d) while the previous dose of oral steroids was also increased; in some studies, additional immunosuppression with cyclophosphamide and cyclosporine was used.

Two small studies showed that use of cyclosporine after treatment with pulse steroids can increase survival times.[46,47] Horita and colleagues[48] observed a higher survival ratio and longer survival duration in patients with AE-IPF treated with a combination therapy of tacrolimus and methylprednisolone pulse therapy. In the double-blind, prospective, placebo-controlled, randomized clinical trial by Azuma and colleagues[23] evaluating the effect of pirfenidone in patients with IPF, although statistical significance was not reached for the primary end point (ie, the change from baseline of the lowest oxygen saturation as measured by pulse oximetry during the 6-minute steady-state exercise test), the investigators observed a significant treatment effect on rates of AE-IPF, which occurred exclusively in the placebo group. As such, the study was then prematurely stopped on ethical grounds. Pirfenidone appeared also to favorably affect time to acute exacerbation and IPF-related death in the recent CAPACITY [Clinical Studies Assessing Pirfenidone in IPF: Research of Efficacy and Safety Outcomes] trials,[25] although the rate of AE-IPF was not a specific and separate end point in this study.

Kubo and colleagues[21] evaluated the effect of anticoagulant therapy on the survival of patients with IPF and found a beneficial effect on survival of combined anticoagulant and prednisolone therapy. This effect was largely driven by the reduced incidence of AE-IPF in the warfarin group.

Few nonrandomized small studies investigated the effect of polymyxin B–immobilized fiber column (PMX) hemoperfusion treatment, showing a potential beneficial effect of PMX treatment.

However, these results have largely been single-center and need confirmation before affecting clinical practice.[49–51]

Given the limited evidence, pharmacologic treatment of AE IPF is largely empiric and usually consists of intravenous corticosteroids up to 1 g/d, with or without immunosuppressive drugs. However, there are no controlled clinical trials to judge the efficacy of this therapeutic strategy, and substantial difference of opinion between clinicians exists regarding the appropriate treatment for patients suffering from this complication. Therefore, specific recommendations regarding dosage, route, and duration of corticosteroid therapy cannot be made at present.[1] Nonpharmacologic treatment of AE-IPF and progressive respiratory failure in patients with IPF are discussed below.

NONPHARMACOLOGIC TREATMENTS

Despite the lack of high-quality data demonstrating its benefit in patients with IPF, long-term oxygen therapy is commonly prescribed to patients showing resting hypoxemia or significant oxygen desaturation on exercise, and is strongly recommended by current guidelines.[1] Due to the progressive nature of IPF, higher flow rates than those commonly used in chronic obstructive pulmonary disease are likely to be required. Supplemental oxygen may improve symptoms, quality of life,[52] and endurance during rehabilitation training in selected patients without exercise-induced hypoxemia.[53] Conversely, long-term oxygen therapy does not affect survival.[54] Supplemental oxygen therapy is a critical component of the management of IPF, and recent guidelines recommend its use in patients with clinically significant resting hypoxemia.[1]

Lack of energy and fatigue is a common and disabling problem in IPF. Pulmonary rehabilitation (PR), defined as a multidisciplinary intervention for patients with chronic respiratory diseases who are symptomatic and often have reduced activities in daily life, is designed to alleviate symptoms and optimize functional status by stabilizing and/or reversing the extrapulmonary features of the disease. Typical PR programs include exercise training, nutritional modulation, occupational therapy, education, and psychosocial counseling, and consist of an initial intense component (usually 6–10 weeks) followed by a maintenance component.[55] At present, the most convincing evidence of a beneficial effect of PR on quality of life and functional mobility is derived from studies on patients with pulmonary emphysema, although it is conceivable that similar beneficial effects may be achieved in patients with comparable disability from other chronic respiratory diseases.[56] Previous studies, in which the physical training was compared with no physical training or other therapy, were not limited to patients with IPF, thus including conditions potentially more amenable to the beneficial effect of PR. In an RCT on the effect of 8 weeks of exercise-based PR in 57 patients with interstitial lung diseases, including 34 patients with IPF, Holland and colleagues[57] observed that the increase in 6MWD and the reduction in dyspnea and fatigue among patients with IPF were not as remarkable as among the non-IPF ones. In addition, these benefits were seen immediately following training but were not sustained 6 months after intervention. Patients with IPF tend with time to discontinue any routine exercise because of increasing dyspnea, which should be discouraged whenever possible. Indeed, exercise such as daily walks or the use of a stationary bicycle improves muscle strength and increases the sense of well-being.

The clinical course (progressive disease or associated with acute exacerbation) of IPF is often complicated by respiratory failure, and patients may be referred to the intensive care unit to receive ventilator support. However, mortality during the hospitalization is high.[58,59] In addition, patients with end-stage interstitial lung disease are difficult to ventilate and are rarely successfully weaned from mechanical ventilation.[58,60] Thus, while the decision not to ventilate a patient with IPF who also has acute respiratory failure is a tricky one, mechanical ventilation should be introduced only after carefully weighing up the patient's long-term prognosis and, whenever possible, the patient's wishes. The use of mechanical ventilation is discouraged by current guidelines.[1] Lung transplantation might be regarded as the last therapeutic option for patients with acute respiratory failure, in particular in younger patients with a firmly established diagnosis. In these patients, mechanical ventilation or extracorporeal life support (extracorporeal membrane oxygenation) may be used as a direct bridge to lung transplant.[61]

The outcome of life support as compared with palliative care should be discussed with patients and their families at an earlier stage. Palliative care should start when patients with a progressive disease become symptomatic, which means that in some patients with IPF this type of intervention should start as early as the diagnosis is established. In IPF, dyspnea can be extremely distressing, thus impairing physical activity and quality of life. In selected cases of particularly severe dyspnea, morphine could be considered. In a small case series, Allen and colleagues[62] reported that low-dose diamorphine reduces dyspnea, anxiety, and cough without significant decrease in oxygen saturation. Further, oxygen therapy may be useful for palliation of dyspnea in hypoxemic patients. With disease progression, patients may also experience fear, anxiety, and depression; psychological counseling and, in selected cases, pharmacologic treatment should therefore be considered. In a recent cross-sectional study of outpatients with interstitial lung disease, including IPF, Ryerson and colleagues[63] reported that dyspnea is strongly associated with depression score, functional status (as assessed by 4 minutes walk time), and pulmonary function. These investigators demonstrated that the relationship between dyspnea and depression is independent of other clinical variables, thus suggesting that treatment of depression (observed in as many as 23% of patients in this study) may improve dyspnea and quality of life. The poor prognosis and significantly impaired quality of life in patients with IPF make palliative care an urgent need in these patients.

LUNG TRANSPLANTATION

Pulmonary fibrosis represents the second most frequent disease for which lung transplantation is performed.[64] More recently the number of lung transplants performed for IPF has steadily increased, particularly in the United States, where IPF now represents the leading indication for lung transplantation.[65] Five-year survival rates after lung transplantation in IPF are estimated at 50% to 56%.[62,66,67] Additional evidence suggests that patients with pulmonary fibrosis undergoing lung transplantation have favorable long-term survival compared with other disease indications[67] (see article elsewhere in this issue).

SUMMARY

Despite more than a decade of efforts to show a definite effect on disease course in IPF, a treatment regimen that is unanimously recognized as a standard of care is still lacking. Current guidelines recommend enrollment in clinical trials as the standard of care for patients with IPF. However, given that one drug, pirfenidone, is currently approved for the treatment of IPF in parts of the world that are home to about 2 billion people, it is reasonable to say that a major step forward has been made with the identification of this drug. Nonetheless there is no global recognition of this fact, and it is fair to say that if pirfenidone can be seen as a starting point in the treatment of IPF, it cannot be seen as a point of arrival. Based on the current knowledge of IPF pathogenesis, it is easy to predict that the future treatment of IPF will be based on multiple drugs. Although this is discouraging on one hand, on the other hand identification of more milestone drugs is getting closer, and it seems likely that within a few years the first globally accepted standard of care will become a reality for the management of this deadly disease. The knowledge gained until now and the one that will be gained over the next few years are important and will also form the basis to approach the vast and heterogeneous spectrum represented by the other fibrotic interstitial lung diseases, for which a systematic attempt to discover an effective pharmacologic treatment is almost completely lacking. In this way, patients with IPF will lead the way in the discovery of therapies for lung fibrosis and, while achieving the important critical goal of the identification of the first effective treatment, will also help the large number of patients with non-IPF fibrotic lung disorders.

REFERENCES

1. Raghu G, Collard HR, Egan JJ, et al. Idiopathic pulmonary fibrosis: evidence based guidelines for diagnosis and management. Am J Respir Crit Care Med 2011;183(6):788–824.
2. Schunemann HJ, Jaeschke R, Cook DJ, et al. An official ATS statement: grading the quality of evidence and strength of recommendations in ATS guidelines and recommendations. Am J Respir Crit Care Med 2006;174(5):605–14.
3. Richeldi L, Davies HR, Ferrara G, et al. Corticosteroids for idiopathic pulmonary fibrosis. Cochrane Database Syst Rev 2003;3:CD002880. Edited; published in Issue 2, 2010.
4. Richeldi L, Davies HR, Spagnolo P, et al. Corticosteroids for idiopathic pulmonary fibrosis. Cochrane Database Syst Rev 2010;2:CD002880.
5. Spagnolo P, Del Giovane C, Luppi F, et al. Nonsteroid agents for idiopathic pulmonary fibrosis. Cochrane Database Syst Rev 2010;9:CD003134.
6. Demedts M, Behr J, Buhl R, et al. High-dose acetylcysteine in idiopathic pulmonary fibrosis. N Engl J Med 2005;353(21):2229–42.
7. King TE Jr, Pardo A, Selman M. Idiopathic pulmonary fibrosis. Lancet 2011;378(9807):1949–61.
8. Gauldie J, Kolb M. Animal models of pulmonary fibrosis: how far from effective reality? Am J Physiol Lung Cell Mol Physiol 2008;294(2):L151.
9. Noble PW, Richeldi L, Kaminski N. End of an ERA: lessons from negative clinical trials in idiopathic pulmonary fibrosis. Am J Respir Crit Care Med 2011;184(1):4–5.
10. Ziesche R, Hofbauer E, Wittmann K, et al. A preliminary study of long-term treatment with interferon gamma-1b and low-dose prednisolone in patients with idiopathic pulmonary fibrosis. N Engl J Med 1999;341(17):1264–9.
11. Raghu G, Brown KK, Bradford WZ, et al. A placebo-controlled trial of interferon gamma-1b in patients with idiopathic pulmonary fibrosis. N Engl J Med 2004;350(2):125–33.
12. King TE Jr, Albera C, Bradford WZ, et al. Effect of interferon gamma-1b on survival in patients with idiopathic pulmonary fibrosis (INSPIRE): a multicentre, randomised, placebo-controlled trial. Lancet 2009; 374(9685):222–8.
13. Luppi F, Losi M, D'Amico R, et al. Endogenous blood maximal interferon-gamma production may predict response to interferon gamma 1beta treatment in patients with idiopathic pulmonary fibrosis. Sarcoidosis Vasc Diffuse Lung Dis 2009; 26(1):64–8.
14. Casoni GL, Chilosi M, Romagnoli M, et al. Another "chance" for interferon gamma 1b? Sarcoidosis Vasc Diffuse Lung Dis 2011;28(1):79–80.
15. King TE Jr, Behr J, Brown KK, et al. BUILD-1: a randomized placebo-controlled trial of bosentan in idiopathic pulmonary fibrosis. Am J Respir Crit Care Med 2008;177(1):75–81.
16. King TE Jr, Brown KK, Raghu G, et al. BUILD-3: a randomized, controlled trial of bosentan in idiopathic pulmonary fibrosis. Am J Respir Crit Care Med 2011;184(1):92–9.
17. Raghu G, Brown KK, Costabel U, et al. Treatment of idiopathic pulmonary fibrosis with etanercept: an exploratory, placebo-controlled trial. Am J Respir Crit Care Med 2008;178(9):948–55.
18. Daniels CE, Lasky JA, Limper AH, et al. Imatinib treatment for idiopathic pulmonary fibrosis: Randomized placebo-controlled trial results. Am J Respir Crit Care Med 2010;181(6):604–10.
19. Richeldi L, Brown KK, Costabel U, et al. The oral triple kinase inhibitor BIBF 1120 reduces decline in lung function in patients with idiopathic pulmonary fibrosis (IPF): results from the tomorrow study. Am J Respir Crit Care Med 2011;183:A5303.
20. Richeldi L, Costabel U, Selman M, et al. Efficacy of a tyrosine kinase inhibitor in idiopathic pulmonary fibrosis. N Engl J Med 2011;365(12):1079–87.
21. Kubo H, Nakayama K, Yanai M, et al. Anticoagulant therapy for idiopathic pulmonary fibrosis. Chest 2005;128(3):1475–82.
22. Raghu G, Johnson WC, Lockhart D, et al. Treatment of idiopathic pulmonary fibrosis with a new antifibrotic agent, pirfenidone: Results of a prospective, open-label phase II study. Am J Respir Crit Care Med 1999;159(4 I):1061–9.
23. Azuma A, Nukiwa T, Tsuboi E, et al. Double-blind, placebo-controlled trial of pirfenidone in patients with idiopathic pulmonary fibrosis. Am J Respir Crit Care Med 2005;171(9):1040–7.
24. Taniguchi H, Ebina M, Kondoh Y, et al. Pirfenidone in idiopathic pulmonary fibrosis. Eur Respir J 2010; 35(4):821–9.

25. Noble PW, Albera C, Bradford WZ, et al. Pirfenidone in patients with idiopathic pulmonary fibrosis (CAPACITY): two randomised trials. Lancet 2011; 377(9779):1760–9.

26. King TE Jr, Safrin S, Starko KM, et al. Analyses of efficacy end points in a controlled trial of interferon-gamma1b for idiopathic pulmonary fibrosis. Chest 2005;127(1):171–7.

27. Collard HR, King TE Jr, Bartelson BB, et al. Changes in clinical and physiologic variables predict survival in idiopathic pulmonary fibrosis. Am J Respir Crit Care Med 2003;168(5):538–42.

28. du Bois RM, Weycker D, Albera C, et al. Ascertainment of individual risk of mortality for patients with idiopathic pulmonary fibrosis. Am J Respir Crit Care Med 2011;184(4):459–66.

29. Nathan SD, Shlobin OA, Ahmad S, et al. Serial development of pulmonary hypertension in patients with idiopathic pulmonary fibrosis. Respiration 2008;76(3):288–94.

30. Glaser S, Noga O, Koch B, et al. Impact of pulmonary hypertension on gas exchange and exercise capacity in patients with pulmonary fibrosis. Respir Med 2009;103(2):317–24.

31. Collard HR, Anstrom KJ, Schwarz MI, et al. Sildenafil improves walk distance in idiopathic pulmonary fibrosis. Chest 2007;131(3):897–9.

32. Zisman DA, Schwarz M, Anstrom KJ, et al. A controlled trial of sildenafil in advanced idiopathic pulmonary fibrosis. N Engl J Med 2010;363(7):620–8.

33. Raghu G, King TE Jr, Behr J, et al. Quality of life and dyspnoea in patients treated with bosentan for idiopathic pulmonary fibrosis (BUILD-1). Eur Respir J 2010;35(1):118–23.

34. Raghu G, Weycker D, Edelsberg J, et al. Incidence and prevalence of idiopathic pulmonary fibrosis. Am J Respir Crit Care Med 2006;174(7):810–6.

35. Lee JS, Collard HR, Raghu G, et al. Does chronic microaspiration cause idiopathic pulmonary fibrosis? Am J Med 2010;123(4):304–11.

36. Tobin RW, Pope CE 2nd, Pellegrini CA, et al. Increased prevalence of gastroesophageal reflux in patients with idiopathic pulmonary fibrosis. Am J Respir Crit Care Med 1998;158(6):1804–8.

37. Raghu G, Yang ST, Spada C, et al. Sole treatment of acid gastroesophageal reflux in idiopathic pulmonary fibrosis: a case series. Chest 2006;129(3):794–800.

38. Linden PA, Gilbert RJ, Yeap BY, et al. Laparoscopic fundoplication in patients with end-stage lung disease awaiting transplantation. J Thorac Cardiovasc Surg 2006;131(2):438–46.

39. Lee JS, Ryu JH, Elicker BM, et al. Gastroesophageal reflux therapy is associated with longer survival in idiopathic pulmonary fibrosis. Am J Respir Crit Care Med 2011 Jun 23. [Epub ahead of print].

40. Savarino E, Bazzica M, Zentilin P, et al. Gastroesophageal reflux and pulmonary fibrosis in scleroderma: a study using pH-impedance monitoring. Am J Respir Crit Care Med 2009;179(5): 408–13.

41. Gulmez SE, Holm A, Frederiksen H, et al. Use of proton pump inhibitors and the risk of community-acquired pneumonia: a population-based case-control study. Arch Intern Med 2007;167(9):950–5.

42. Yang YX, Lewis JD, Epstein S, et al. Long-term proton pump inhibitor therapy and risk of hip fracture. JAMA 2006;296(24):2947–53.

43. Collard HR, Moore BB, Flaherty KR, et al. Acute exacerbations of idiopathic pulmonary fibrosis. Am J Respir Crit Care Med 2007;176(7):636–43.

44. Hyzy R, Huang S, Myers J, et al. Acute exacerbation of idiopathic pulmonary fibrosis. Chest 2007;132(5): 1652–8.

45. Agarwal R, Jindal SK. Acute exacerbation of idiopathic pulmonary fibrosis: a systematic review. Eur J Intern Med 2008;19(4):227–35.

46. Inase N, Sawada M, Ohtani Y, et al. Cyclosporin A followed by the treatment of acute exacerbation of idiopathic pulmonary fibrosis with corticosteroid. Intern Med 2003;42(7):565–70.

47. Sakamoto S, Homma S, Miyamoto A, et al. Cyclosporin A in the treatment of acute exacerbation of idiopathic pulmonary fibrosis. Intern Med 2010; 49(2):109–15.

48. Horita N, Akahane M, Okada Y, et al. Tacrolimus and steroid treatment for acute exacerbation of idiopathic pulmonary fibrosis. Intern Med 2011;50(3): 189–95.

49. Enomoto N, Suda T, Uto T, et al. Possible therapeutic effect of direct haemoperfusion with a polymyxin B immobilized fibre column (PMX-DHP) on pulmonary oxygenation in acute exacerbations of interstitial pneumonia. Respirology 2008;13(3):452–60.

50. Seo Y, Abe S, Kurahara M, et al. Beneficial effect of polymyxin B-immobilized fiber column (PMX) hemoperfusion treatment on acute exacerbation of idiopathic pulmonary fibrosis. Intern Med 2006;45(18): 1033–8.

51. Yoshida T, Kodama M, Tamura Y, et al. [Direct hemoperfusion with a polymyxin B-immobilized fiber column eliminates neutrophils and improves pulmonary oxygenation–a comparison of two cases with acute exacerbation of idiopathic pulmonary fibrosis]. Nihon Kokyuki Gakkai Zasshi 2007;45(11):890–7 [in Japanese].

52. De Vries J, Kessels BL, Drent M. Quality of life of idiopathic pulmonary fibrosis patients. Eur Respir J 2001;17(5):954–61.

53. Ries AL, Bauldoff GS, Carlin BW, et al. Pulmonary rehabilitation: joint ACCP/AACVPR evidence-based clinical practice guidelines. Chest 2007;131(Suppl 5):4S–42S.

54. Douglas WW, Ryu JH, Schroeder DR. Idiopathic pulmonary fibrosis: Impact of oxygen and colchicine,

prednisone, or no therapy on survival. Am J Respir Crit Care Med 2000;161(4 Pt 1):1172–8.

55. Nici L, Donner C, Wouters E, et al. American Thoracic Society/European Respiratory Society statement on pulmonary rehabilitation. Am J Respir Crit Care Med 2006;173(12):1390–413.

56. Spruit MA, Janssen DJ, Franssen FM, et al. Rehabilitation and palliative care in lung fibrosis. Respirology 2009;14(6):781–7.

57. Holland AE, Hill CJ, Conron M, et al. Short term improvement in exercise capacity and symptoms following exercise training in interstitial lung disease. Thorax 2008;63(6):549–54.

58. Stern JB, Mal H, Groussard O, et al. Prognosis of patients with advanced idiopathic pulmonary fibrosis requiring mechanical ventilation for acute respiratory failure. Chest 2001;120(1):213–9.

59. Mallick S. Outcome of patients with idiopathic pulmonary fibrosis (IPF) ventilated in intensive care unit. Respir Med 2008;102(10):1355–9.

60. Saydain G, Islam A, Afessa B, et al. Outcome of patients with idiopathic pulmonary fibrosis admitted to the intensive care unit. Am J Respir Crit Care Med 2002;166(6):839–42.

61. Beckmann A, Benk C, Beyersdorf F, et al. Position article for the use of extracorporeal life support in adult patients. Eur J Cardiothorac Surg 2011;40(3):676–80.

62. Allen S, Raut S, Woollard J, et al. Low dose diamorphine reduces breathlessness without causing a fall in oxygen saturation in elderly patients with end-stage idiopathic pulmonary fibrosis. Palliat Med 2005;19(2).128–30.

63. Ryerson CJ, Berkeley J, Carrieri-Kohlman VL, et al. Depression and functional status are strongly associated with dyspnea in interstitial lung disease. Chest 2011;139(3):609–16.

64. Trulock EP, Edwards LB, Taylor DO, et al. The Registry of the International Society for Heart and Lung Transplantation: twentieth official adult lung and heart-lung transplant report—2003. J Heart Lung Transplant 2003;22(6):625–35.

65. Yusen RD, Shearon TH, Qian Y, et al. Lung transplantation in the United States, 1999-2008. Am J Transplant 2010;10(4 Pt 2):1047–68.

66. Mason DP, Brizzio ME, Alster JM, et al. Lung transplantation for idiopathic pulmonary fibrosis. Ann Thorac Surg 2007;84(4):1121–8.

67. Keating D, Levvey B, Kotsimbos T, et al. Lung transplantation in pulmonary fibrosis: challenging early outcomes counterbalanced by surprisingly good outcomes beyond 15 years. Transplant Proc 2009;41(1):289–91.

Genetic Interstitial Lung Disease

Megan Stuebner Devine, MD,
Christine Kim Garcia, MD, PhD*

KEYWORDS

- Genetics • Pulmonary fibrosis • Interstitial lung disease
- Mutations

The interstitial lung diseases (ILDs), or diffuse parenchymal lung diseases, are a heterogeneous collection of more than 100 different pulmonary disorders that affect the tissue and spaces surrounding the alveoli. For many of the ILDs, this delicate tissue is filled with inflammatory cells, proliferating fibroblasts, collagen, fibronectin, laminin, and other macromolecules, which cause irreversible architectural distortion and impaired gas exchange. Patients affected by ILD usually present with shortness of breath and cough; for many, there is evidence of pulmonary restriction, decreased diffusion capacity, and radiographic appearance of alveolar and/or reticulonodular infiltrates. This article reviews the inherited ILDs, with a focus on the diseases that may be seen by pulmonologists caring for adult patients. The authors conclude by briefly discussing the utility of genetic testing in this population.

Inherited ILDs are those that result from the transmission of genetic mutations from a parent or ancestor, subdivided into two major categories: systemic disorders affecting multiple organs and disorders that primarily affect the lung. For both of these groups, thorough medical and family histories provide essential clues about the exact nature of the ILD. First, the pattern of inheritance provides important information; for example, the inborn errors of metabolism that are associated with an ILD demonstrate an autosomal recessive pattern of inheritance. Second, some diseases show a predisposition for affecting a certain gender; for example, lymphangioleiomyomatosis (LAM) occurs exclusively in women. The age of onset of disease is yet another important hint. Younger and more severely affected individuals seen in later generations may reflect genetic anticipation, which can be seen in autosomal dominant kindreds with inherited telomerase mutations and progressively shortened telomere lengths. Finally, the spectrum of disease in the patient and related family members provides important clues to the etiology of ILD. If there is reduced penetrance and variable expressivity, the proband may demonstrate only a subset of all possible clinical findings.

GENETIC DISORDERS AFFECTING MULTIPLE ORGANS, INCLUDING THE LUNG

Table 1 lists the defined genetic disorders that are associated with ILDs, with the lung being only one of many different affected organs.

Dyskeratosis Congenita

Dyskeratosis congenita (DC) is a rare multisystem disorder characterized by the triad of lacy reticular pigmentation on the upper chest and neck, nail dystrophy, and mucosal leukoplakia. The prevalence is approximately 1 in 1,000,000, with death occurring at a median age of 16 years.[1] Patients are usually healthy at birth, then develop the mucocutaneous findings during infancy and bone marrow failure during the first or second decade, followed by various organ dysfunctions, including

Funding was provided by the NIH and the Doris Duke Charitable Foundation.
The authors have nothing to disclose.
Division of Pulmonary and Critical Care Medicine, Department of Internal Medicine, Eugene McDermott Center for Human Growth and Development, University of Texas Southwestern Medical Center, 5323 Harry Hines Boulevard, Dallas, TX 75390-8591, USA
* Corresponding author.
E-mail address: Christine.Garcia@utsouthwestern.edu

Clin Chest Med 33 (2012) 95–110
doi:10.1016/j.ccm.2011.11.001
0272-5231/12/$ – see front matter © 2012 Elsevier Inc. All rights reserved.

Table 1
Inherited interstitial lung disease: disorders with multiple organ pathology

Disease	Inheritance	Gene[a]	Pathogenesis	Presentation
Dyskeratosis congenita	XLR, AD, AR	DKC1 TERC TERT TINF2	Telomere shortening	ILD
Neurofibromatosis, type I	AD	NF1	Loss of function of tumor suppressor	ILD, bullae
Tuberous sclerosis/LAM	AD	TSC1 TSC2	Proliferation of LAM cells	Multiple cysts
Birt-Hogg-Dubé syndrome	AD	FLCN	Loss of folliculin	Multiple cysts
Hyper-IgE syndrome	AD	STAT3	Lack of T_H17	Pneumatoceles, bronchiectasis
Hermansky-Pudlak syndrome	AR	HPS1 HPS4	Defects of cytoplasmic organelles	ILD
Gaucher disease, type I	AR	GBA	Deficiency of acid β-glucosidase	ILD, PAH
Niemann-Pick disease, type B	AR	SMPD1	Deficiency of acid sphinogomyelinase	ILD
Lysinuric protein intolerance	AR	SLC7A7	Defect of cationic amino acid transport	PAP, ILD

Abbreviations: AD, autosomal dominant; AR, autosomal recessive; IgE, immunoglobulin E; ILD, interstitial lung disease; LAM, lymphangioleiomyomatosis; PAH, pulmonary arterial hypertension; PAP, pulmonary alveolar proteinosis; T_H17, T helper 17 cells; XLR, X-linked recessive.
[a] Mutations in these genes have been found in patients with the following disorders and an ILD.

pulmonary fibrosis and eye, tooth, gastrointestinal, endocrine, skeletal, urological, and immunologic abnormalities.[2,3] Because clinical features include premature graying, testicular atrophy, an increased predisposition to cancer, and a shortened life span, DC has been considered a syndrome of premature aging. There is wide variation in the mode of inheritance, severity, and spectrum of clinical findings, which is only partly explained by locus and allelic heterogeneity. Most patients in a large international registry are male with X-linked recessive inheritance.[2] For this subgroup of patients, the classic skin and nail findings are present in approximately 90% of affected males. Bone marrow failure is very common (>85%) and accounts for the leading cause of death. Pulmonary fibrosis develops in 20%. DC families with autosomal recessive and autosomal dominant patterns of inheritance are less common.

Telomeres are specialized nucleoprotein structures that protect chromosomal ends, and telomerase is the multi-subunit enzyme that extends telomeres to offset the shortening that accompanies DNA replication due to lagging strand synthesis. In the setting of insufficient telomerase, telomere shortening limits tissue renewal by impairing the function of tissue stem cells and progenitor cells.[4] Genetic anticipation, or the finding

of more severe and earlier onset of disease in later generations, has been described in DC kindreds with mutations in the genes encoding telomerase (TERC and TERT).[5,6] Inheritance of progressively shorter telomere lengths in each subsequent generation of mutation carriers provides a molecular explanation for the genetic anticipation.

ILD associated with DC has been characterized as a progressive restrictive lung disease with interstitial fibrosis, often with histopathologic lesions suggestive of hypersensitivity.[7,8] More than 30% of DC patients develop a rapidly progressive interstitial fibrosis following bone marrow transplantation.[9,10] Pulmonary disease was 2.2-fold more common and apparent at a younger age (14 vs 37 years) in patients who had undergone hematopoietic stem cell transplantation than in those who did not.[11] Clinical survival of DC patients after the development of ILD is poor, with death 12 to 40 months after the onset of dyspnea.[8] Some patients with mutations in dyskerin (DKC1), the gene encoding a nucleolar protein that copurifies with telomerase,[12] have evidence of pulmonary fibrosis.[13,14] Mutations in either of the telomerase genes (TERT, TERC) or TINF2, a component of the shelterin complex, have been found in patients with autosomal dominant DC and ILD.[6,11,15] Homozygous mutations in NOLA2, NOLA3, and

TCAB1 are rare causes of DC[16–18]; to date none of the affected individuals have been described with pulmonary fibrosis.

Neurofibromatosis Type 1

Type 1 neurofibromatosis (NF1) is an autosomal dominant disorder that affects all ethnic groups and is caused by heterozygous loss-of-function mutations in the gene encoding neurofibromin, *NF1*. It is characterized by multiple (>6) café-au-lait spots, axillary and inguinal freckling, multiple cutaneous neurofibromas, Lisch nodules, optic gliomas, and osseous lesions. The incidence of ILD in NF1 has been estimated at 6% to 12%,[19–21] and is characterized by lower-lobe predominant diffuse interstitial fibrosis and honeycombing. Thin-walled bullae are present in almost all patients with ILD, or may be seen in isolation; these are large, asymmetric, and typically involve the upper lobes.[21] Of interest, histologic evidence of an alveolitis and interstitial fibrosis has been found in patients with normal chest radiographs or those with only apical bullae.[20] Although there is near complete penetrance of the disease after childhood, the ILD is not observed until adulthood and is typically seen in patients older than 40 years.[20] The disease is often progressive, and may lead to pulmonary hypertension and right heart failure. The pathogenesis of NF1-associated ILD is unknown. Other manifestations of the disease include large-airway obstruction, mediastinal, bronchial, or intraparenchymal neurofibromas, abnormal curvature of the spine, and intercostal tumors.[22]

Lymphangioleiomyomatosis and Tuberous Sclerosis Complex

Pulmonary lymphangioleiomyomatosis (LAM) is a rare disease that almost exclusively affects women. LAM is caused by proliferating smooth muscle–like cells, the so-called LAM cells, which can involve small airways, the pulmonary vasculature, and intrathoracic and extrathoracic lymphatic structures. The hallmark of the disease is a radiographic pattern of diffuse, numerous, round, thin walled cysts, generally between 2 and 60 mm in diameter. Other pulmonary abnormalities include pneumothorax and pleural effusions. Eighty percent of patients develop a pneumothorax at some time during the course of their disease. Pleural effusions are almost always chylous. Both obstructive and mixed obstructive-restrictive ventilatory defects are observed in LAM.

LAM can occur as an isolated disorder or in 1% to 3% of patients with tuberous sclerosis complex (TSC), an autosomal dominant multisystem disorder characterized by hamartomas affecting brain, skin, heart, kidneys, and lungs. The pulmonary ILD of TSC patients is indistinguishable from LAM[23]; those affected are usually women older than 30 years with little or no mental retardation. Major and minor criteria exist to diagnose the disease; two major features (or one major plus two minor features) are needed for diagnosis.[24] The major features include facial angiofibromas, nontraumatic ungula or periungual fibromas, 3 or more hypomelanotic macules (which are most easily visualized with a Wood light), a rough, yellow thickening of skin over the lumbosacral area (known as a Shagreen patch), multiple retinal nodular hamartomas, cortical tubers, subependymal nodules or giant-cell astrocytomas, cardiac rhabdomyomas, and LAM and/or renal angiomyolipomas. TSC patients with LAM have a high incidence of renal angiomyolipomas (>90%) compared with those with isolated LAM (~30%).[25]

Although TSC is characterized by its autosomal dominant inheritance, about two-thirds of patients have new mutations. Mutations in *TSC1* are found in 15% to 30% of all families and 10% to 15% of sporadic cases, whereas mutations in *TSC2* occur more frequently, accounting for 75% to 80% of all sporadic cases.[24,26,27] Inactivation of both alleles of *TSC1* or *TSC2* through loss of heterozygosity is found in renal angiomyolipomas and supports Knudson's two-hit model of tumor suppressor pathogenesis.[28] Most sporadic LAM renal angiomyolipomas are characterized by two mutations in *TSC2*; a few are caused by *TSC1* mutations.[29–31] In contrast to TSC patients whose germline mutations are present in tumor and normal tissues, genetic mutations are found only in abnormal lung and kidney cells in LAM patients.

The proteins encoded by TSC1 and TSC2 regulate the mammalian target of rapamycin (mTOR) pathway. Inhibition of the mTOR complex causes shrinkage of renal or retroperitoneal angiomyolipomas and subependymal giant-cell astrocytomas in TSC patients.[32–34] In addition, sirolimus, an mTOR inhibitor, stabilizes lung function, reduces respiratory symptoms, and improves the quality of life of LAM patients.[35]

Birt-Hogg-Dubé Syndrome

Birt-Hogg-Dubé syndrome (BHDS) is a rare disorder initially described in 1977 by 3 dermatologists, characterized by the autosomal dominant inheritance of multiple benign skin tumors including fibrofolliculomas. Approximately 90% of affected individuals have evidence of lung cysts[36] and about 10% have renal malignancy, usually with hybrid oncocytic-chromophobe histology.[37]

The disease is caused by loss-of-function mutations in the folliculin (*FLCN*) gene.[38] Two different studies, one using whole-genome linkage analysis and the other a candidate gene approach, independently found that kindreds presenting solely with familial spontaneous pneumothorax and/or lung cysts have mutations in *FLCN* and represent a lung-limited form of BHDS.[39,40] Overall, 24% of patients have a history of spontaneous pneumothorax.[36] The pulmonary cysts are generally bilateral, are usually located in the mid-lung and lower-lung zones, are of varying sizes, and range in shape from round, oval, lentiform, to multiseptated.[41,42] Because the skin findings typically appear in the fourth decade and the renal malignancy can be a late finding (mean age of 48 years), a spontaneous pneumothorax may be the presenting manifestation of this disease.[37,40] Genetic testing is indicated for all individuals suspected of having BHDS, including those with multiple facial or truncal papules histologically characterized as fibrofolliculomas or angiofibromas, those with multiple or bilateral renal tumors, and those with a family history of autosomal dominant primary spontaneous pneumothorax.

Hyper–Immunoglobulin E Syndrome

Autosomal dominant hyper–immunoglobulin E (IgE) syndrome (AD-HIES) is an immune deficiency disorder characterized by the triad of recurrent staphylococcal skin abscesses, cyst-forming pneumonias, and extreme elevations of IgE (usually >2000 IU/mL). Survival is typically into adulthood and death is usually secondary to infection. Diagnosis requires a high level of suspicion, due to variability of phenotypic features.[43] A clinical scoring system has been developed that combines immunologic (elevated IgE, eosinophilia >700/μL, decreased T_H17 cells, recurrent infections) and nonimmune features (retained primary teeth, scoliosis, joint hyperextensibility, bone fractures following minimal trauma, a characteristic facial appearance, and vascular abnormalities).[44] Pneumatoceles and bronchiectasis, the result of frequent pneumonias, are seen in approximately 70% of patients.[45] The most common pathogens are *Staphylococcus aureus*, *Streptococcus pneumoniae*, and *Haemophilus influenzae*. Although purulent sputum may be present, most patients with pneumonia often lack systemic signs of inflammation. The pneumatoceles may be sites of fungal and gram-negative infections, which lead to the significant mortality.[46] Patients' purified native T cells are unable to differentiate in vitro into interleukin-17–producing (T_H17) T-helper cells, which play a critical role in the clearance of fungal and

extracellular bacterial infections of the lung and skin.[47] More than 95% of patients have heterozygous missense, splice-site, or intragenic deletions of the *STAT3* gene.[48] Most patients represent sporadic cases, but autosomal dominant transmission has been seen in some kindreds.

Hermansky-Pudlak Syndrome

Hermansky-Pudlak syndrome (HPS) is an autosomal recessive disease first described in 1959.[49] HPS is characterized by oculocutaneous albinism, a bleeding diathesis resulting from platelet storage pool deficiency, and other organ involvement, including pulmonary fibrosis.[50] Other clinical features of the disease include inflammatory bowel disease, cutaneous malignant melanomas, renal failure, and cardiomyopathy. It is now known that HPS is caused by defects of multiple cytoplasmic organelles, including melanosomes, platelet-dense granules, and lysosomes. At present the diagnosis is confirmed by the absence of dense bodies on whole-mount electron microscopy of platelets.[51] Mutations in 8 different genes cause this disease. Each of these genes functions in trafficking of vesicular cargo proteins to cytoplasmic organelles (*HPS2*)[52] or organelle biogenesis and maturation (*HPS1*, *HPS3*, *HPS4*, *HPS5*, *HPS6*, *HPS7*, and *HPS8*).[53–57] HPS is the most common single-gene disorder in Puerto Rico, with an estimated frequency of about 1 in 1800 and a carrier frequency of 1 in 21.[58] Mutations in *HPS1* and *HPS3* are found in 75% and 25% of Puerto Rican HPS patients, respectively.

The clinical, physiologic, and radiographic features of the pulmonary fibrosis associated with HPS are similar to those of idiopathic pulmonary fibrosis (IPF). Pulmonary fibrosis has been described most frequently in patients with *HPS1* mutations, and more rarely in patients with *HPS4* mutations.[59–63] In one of the largest studies to date, the mean age of onset was 35 years with a range of 15 to 53 years.[59] The variability of pulmonary findings was not attributable to prior environmental exposures (13% were prior smokers). More than 80% of patients had abnormalities on computed tomography (CT) scans, which were generally predictive of the degree of physiologic impairment and mortality. Most patients demonstrate a peripheral distribution of high-resolution CT (HRCT) reticulations with a trend toward increasing involvement of the central portions of the lungs. The amount of the interstitial reticulation, bronchiectasis, and peribronchial thickening seen by HRCT correlates well with patient age and extent of pulmonary dysfunction.[60] Surgical lung biopsies demonstrate lung remodeling, numerous chronic inflammatory cells, and distinctive clusters of clear vacuolated type II pneumocytes with florid foamy swelling and degeneration (giant lamellar body degeneration).[64,65]

Mice homozygous for both *HPS1* and *HPS2* mutations (double mutant) develop spontaneous pulmonary fibrosis.[66] The abnormalities begin with subpleural disease at 3 months and develop into extensive fibrosis by 9 months.[67] The histology of the mouse lung replicates the human phenotype with giant lamellar body degeneration of the type II cells, and demonstrates decreased phospholipid and surfactant protein B and C secretion.[66,68]

Gaucher Disease

Gaucher disease is an autosomal recessive lysosomal storage disease characterized by the accumulation of the glycolipid glucosylceramide, due to the deficiency of the enzyme acid β-glucosidase. Diagnosis relies on the demonstration of deficient enzyme activity in cells or the identification of 2 disease-causing mutations in the *GBA* gene. Patients can display a large variety of symptoms, ranging from patients who are completely asymptomatic to those who present with perinatal lethality. The usual clinical findings include hepatosplenomegaly, anemia, thrombocytopenia, and bone manifestations including ostopenia, lytic lesions, bone crisis, and skeletal deformities. Infiltration of Gaucher cells into the alveoli, interstitium, and pulmonary capillaries can lead to lung involvement. More than 65% of patients with type I disease have pulmonary function abnormalities, but only a fraction (<5%) have diffuse lower-lobe linear infiltrates, restrictive physiologic impairment, and a reduced diffusion capacity consistent with ILD.[69,70] Enzyme replacement therapy can reduce organ volumes and improve the hematologic parameters and bone pain, but are usually poorly effective in treating the lung manifestations of this disease.[71]

Niemann-Pick Disease

Niemann-Pick disease types A and B are caused by an inherited deficiency of acid sphingomyelinase activity. Patients demonstrate a range of phenotypes from infantile death (type A) to later-onset with survival to adulthood (type B). Nearly all type B patients have hepatosplenomegaly and lung disease.[72] By thin-section chest CT scans, 98% have evidence of a basal-predominant ILD, with thickened interlobular septa, interlobular lines, and ground-glass opacities; however, the radiographic appearance of the lung is not a good predictor of lung function.[73]

Lysinuric Protein Intolerance

Lysinuric protein intolerance (LPI) is an autosomal recessive disease caused by an inherited defect of cationic amino acid transport. Most patients present in infancy with failure to thrive, growth retardation, protein aversion, muscular hypotonia, hepatosplenomegaly, and osteoporosis. In one study, all patients who developed a fatal respiratory insufficiency were children younger than 15 years [74] Adult patients have evidence of an ILD on CT scans of the chest, with interlobular and intralobular septal thickening and subpleural cysts, but only a few are symptomatic.[74]

GENETIC DISEASES PRIMARILY AFFECTING THE LUNG

Table 2 lists the genetic disorders in which an ILD is the dominant clinical feature. Within the last decade a group of genetic disorders involving the production, processing, and clearance of surfactant has been recognized as an important cause of neonatal and pediatric respiratory illness. This group, collectively referred to as surfactant dysfunction disorders,[75] encompasses a variety of mutations involving the genes that encode surfactant protein B (*SFTPB*), surfactant protein C (*SFTPC*), the adenosine triphosphate (ATP)-binding cassette transporter A3 (*ABCA3*), and the receptor for granulocyte macrophage-colony stimulating factor (GM-CSF) (*CSF2R*). There are several good reviews of the surfactant dysfunction disorders in infants and children, and the reader is referred to these for more detail.[76–78]

Surfactant Metabolism Dysfunction Type 1, and Surfactant Protein B Deficiency

Surfactant protein B (SP-B) deficiency is inherited in an autosomal recessive manner, and the majority of affected patients develop respiratory failure in the neonatal period, with rapid progression of disease and death at 3 to 6 months.[79–83] Children with mutations associated with partial expression of the SP-B protein survive longer and go on to develop a chronic ILD.[84,85]

Surfactant Metabolism Dysfunction Type 2, and Surfactant Protein C Deficiency

Autosomal dominant lung disease due to mutations in the gene encoding surfactant protein C (SP-C), *SFTPC*, was first described by Nogee and colleagues[86] in a mother and infant with heterozygous splice-site mutations resulting in skipping of exon 4 and deletion of 37 amino acids. A large 5-generation kindred was later described with 14 affected family members, including 4 adults with

Table 2
Inherited ILD: disorders with primary lung pathology

Disease	Inheritance	Gene	Pathogenesis	Presentation
Surfactant metabolism dysfunction 1	AR	SFTPB	Absent SP-B	Neonatal respiratory failure
Surfactant metabolism dysfunction 2	AD	SFTPC	Lack of SP-C and ER stress	ILD, PAP
Surfactant metabolism dysfunction 3	AR	ABCA3	Defective transport of phospholipid into lamellar bodies	PAP, ILD
Surfactant metabolism dysfunction 4	AR	CSF2RA CSF2RB	Defective GM-CSF signaling	PAP
Familial pulmonary fibrosis	AD	TERT TERC	Telomere shortening	ILD
	AD	SFTPA2	ER stress of alveolar epithelium	ILD
Pulmonary alveolar microlithiasis	AR	SLC34A2	Reduced phosphate clearance from alveolar space	Micronodules

Abbreviations: ER, endoplasmic reticulum; GM-CSF, granulocyte macrophage-colony stimulating factor; SP-B, surfactant protein B; SP-C, surfactant protein C.

surgical lung biopsy evidence of usual interstitial pneumonitis (UIP) and 3 children with nonspecific interstitial pneumonitis (NSIP), with a rare heterozygous missense SP-C mutation (L188Q).[87] Many other mutations in SFTPC have been identified, including the I73T missense variant, which may be one of the more common abnormal alleles.[88–90] The lung disease associated with SFTPC mutations is characterized by marked phenotypic heterogeneity. Manifestations range from severe respiratory distress in infants to IPF in older adults. Mutations of SFTPC are rare in individuals without a family history of pulmonary fibrosis.[91,92] At present the disease phenotype is thought to be caused by aberrant surfactant protein folding, decreased endogenous SP-C secretion, endoplasmic reticulum (ER) stress, and apoptosis of alveolar epithelial cells.[93–96]

Surfactant Metabolism Dysfunction Type 3, and ABCA3 Mutations

There is a significant amount of phenotypic overlap between patients with SFTPB mutations and those with defects in ABCA3. This gene encodes for an ATP-binding cassette transporter that facilitates the translocation of phospholipids into lamellar bodies for the production of surfactant in type II epithelial cells.[97–100] Like SP-B deficiency, the disease is inherited in an autosomal recessive manner. Since the first mutation was discovered in 2004[101] more than 100 distinct mutations have been found, and mutations in ABCA3 may be the most common cause of inherited defects in

surfactant metabolism.[102,103] Initially the ABCA3 mutations were thought to cause only severe respiratory distress and death in infants. Recently it has been found that mutations in ABCA3 are associated with a wider continuum of disease. Some patients have a more indolent course, with the development of a chronic ILD in late childhood or during the adult years.[104–106] One particular mutation resulting in the substitution of a valine residue for glutamic acid at position 292 (E292V) has been found in multiple, unrelated patients with a milder phenotype.[103,104]

Surfactant Metabolism Dysfunction Type 4, and the GM-CSF Receptor Dysfunction

Pulmonary alveolar proteinosis (PAP) is a rare form of lung disease characterized by intra-alveolar overaccumulation of surfactant, which results in respiratory insufficiency. Histopathology specimens from affected patients demonstrate distal airspaces filled with foamy alveolar macrophages and a granular, eosinophilic material that stains positive with periodic acid-Schiff reagent. In general, the underlying lung architecture is normal unless altered by infection.[107] Approximately 90% of PAP cases are acquired (also referred to as primary) and are associated with the presence of antibodies against the GM-CSF receptor.[108–110] These antibodies block GM-CSF signaling in vivo, reduce alveolar macrophage surfactant catabolism, and impair surfactant clearance.[111–113] Secondary PAP occurs in several different clinical settings, such as in association with hematologic malignancies, immunosuppression, inhalation of inorganic dusts, and certain infections.

The GM-CSF receptor is composed of an α and a β chain, encoded by the CSF2RA and CSF2RB genes, respectively. The chains dimerize and activate downstream signaling via the signal transducer and activator of phosphorylation 5 (STAT5) protein. Mice with deletion of the gene encoding the GM-CSF receptor or GM-CSF itself demonstrate a phenotype very similar to adults with acquired PAP.[114,115] To date, mutations in both CSF2RA and CSF2RB have been identified in children with PAP.[78,116] In 2011 a case of adult-onset hereditary PAP was reported in a 36-year-old Japanese woman with a homozygous, single-base deletion at nucleotide 631 in exon 6 of CSF2RB.[117] Multiple hereditary PAP kindreds demonstrate an autosomal recessive pattern of inheritance.

Familial Adult-Onset Pulmonary Fibrosis

The prototype of the adult-onset ILDs is IPF. This disease preferentially affects older males of white and Hispanic ethnicities, and smokers.[118,119] The mean life expectancy is 2 to 3 years after diagnosis.[120] In 2000 Marshall and colleagues[121] published the first large collection of IPF kindreds, and estimated that 0.5% to 2.2% of IPF cases are familial. In 2005 Steele and colleagues[122] published an even larger number of kindreds with familial IPF, the largest of which demonstrated autosomal dominant inheritance with reduced penetrance. Multiple studies have been performed to investigate genetic associations with common single-nucleotide polymorphisms (SNPs).[120] The most significant result has been found for a variant located within the cluster of mucin genes on chromosome 11, which is present in approximately 35% of subjects with familial or sporadic IPF and in 9% of controls.[123]

Familial Pulmonary Fibrosis Associated with Telomerase Mutations

Both a candidate gene approach and a whole-genome linkage approach have led to the discovery of mutations in the genes encoding telomerase (TERT and TERC) in kindreds with familial pulmonary fibrosis (defined as kindreds with 2 or more cases of an idiopathic interstitial pneumonia or unclassified pulmonary fibrosis).[124,125] Heterozygous mutations in TERT are more common, and are found in approximately 18% of familial pulmonary fibrosis kindreds and in about 3% of patients with sporadic idiopathic interstitial pneumonia.[125–127] Mutations in TERC are rarer. As was seen in the DC patients with telomerase mutations, each of the TERT or TERC mutations is associated with short telomere lengths and decreased in vitro activity of telomerase.[125,126] The mutations are loss-of-function frameshift, splice-site, or missense changes that span the length of the gene; most are unique to the family in which they are found.[127]

The penetrance of pulmonary fibrosis in the TERT mutation carriers is age-dependent and gender-dependent (**Fig. 1**A).[127] Disease is rare in subjects younger than 40 years. However, the penetrance of pulmonary fibrosis increases with age and is higher in men than in women. Sixty percent of men older than 60 years have a self-reported diagnosis of ILD; for women of this age, 50% have pulmonary fibrosis.

The ILD subtype most commonly found in TERT mutation carriers is IPF. CT scans of the chest were evaluated for 39 different cases of TERT-associated pulmonary fibrosis.[127] For 74% of patients, their CT scan was typical of UIP and IPF, with reticulation concentrated at the periphery and bases accompanied by honeycombing (**Fig. 1**C). For 13% of cases the CT scans were consistent with UIP except for an absence of honeycombing. For the remaining cases (13%), the CT scans were atypical of UIP because the fibrosis was predominantly located in the mid-lung or upper-lung fields or it was located along the bronchi. The majority of surgical lung biopsy specimens (86%) had histologic features of UIP (**Fig. 1**D). Small, loosely formed nonnecrotizing granulomas were seen in 17%; these are not typically seen in IPF.

More than 95% of TERT mutation carriers with pulmonary fibrosis report past cigarette smoking or an exposure to a fibrogenic environmental or occupational agent, suggesting that alveolar epithelial damage in conjunction with the underlying inherited genetic predisposition leads to the lung disease.[127] Overall, the clinical course of the TERT-associated pulmonary fibrosis mirrored that of IPF, with a mean survival of 3 years after diagnosis (**Fig. 1**B).[127]

Familial Adult-Onset Pulmonary Fibrosis Due to Mutations in Surfactant Protein A

Whole-genome linkage analysis led to the mapping and identification of heterozygous mutations in the gene encoding surfactant protein (SP-)A2 (SFTPA2) in two kindreds with familial adult-onset pulmonary fibrosis and/or lung adenocarcinoma with features of bronchoalveolar cell carcinoma.[128] Both mutations (G231V and F198S) reside within the highly conserved carbohydrate-recognition domain of the protein and are predicted to disrupt protein structure. Recombinant

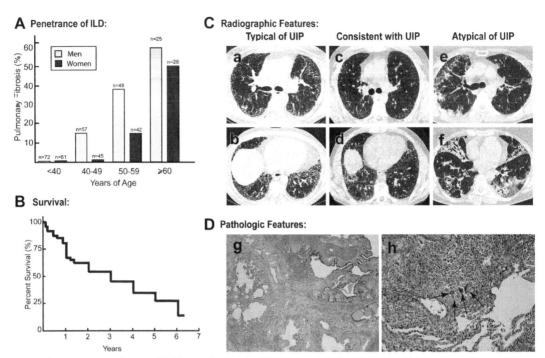

Fig. 1. Characteristics of interstitial lung disease (ILD) associated with telomerase (*TERT*) mutations. (*A*) Penetrance of self-reported pulmonary fibrosis is shown for men (*yellow bars*) and women (*blue bars*) of different ages. Penetrance of pulmonary fibrosis for men versus women 40 to 49, 50 to 59, and older than 60 years is 14% versus 2%, 38% versus 14%, and 60% versus 50%. (*B*) Kaplan-Meier survival curve of 47 different *TERT* mutation carriers with ILD demonstrate a mean survival of 3 years after diagnosis. (*C*) Computed tomography (CT) scans of 3 different *TERT* mutation carriers with ILD. Representative cases are shown with a pattern typical of usual interstitial pneumonia (UIP) with peripheral, basal-predominant fibrosis and moderate to severe honeycombing (*a, b*), a pattern consistent with UIP except for the absence of honeycombing (*c, d*), and a pattern atypical of UIP with fibrosis predominantly affecting the upper lobes and along the bronchi (*e, f*). Scans are shown at the level of the carina (*a, c, e*) and the lung base (*b, d, f*). The majority of carriers (74%) had a CT scan typical of UIP, 13% had a CT scan consistent with UIP except for the absence of honeycombing, and 13% had a CT scan atypical of UIP. (*D*) Histology of surgical lung biopsies from *TERT* mutation carriers with ILD. The majority of cases (86%) of *TERT* mutation carriers with lung specimens available for review had diagnostic histologic features of UIP. In this low-magnification view of UIP (*g*), typical variegated honeycomb areas are seen alternating with normal areas and scarred lung. The case shown in (*h*) shows increased inflammation and a small, loosely aggregated, nonnecrotizing granuloma (*arrows*) that is characterized by a cluster of epithelioid histiocytes and multinucleated giant cells surrounded by chronic inflammation in the interstitium (original magnification: *g*, ×40; *h*, ×100). (*Data from* Diaz de Leon A, Cronkhite JT, Katzenstein AL, et al. Telomere lengths, pulmonary fibrosis and telomerase (TERT) mutations. PLoS One 2010;5(5):e10680.)

proteins carrying these mutations are retained within the ER and are not secreted into the culture media. In addition, the mutant proteins form fewer intracellular oligomers, demonstrate greater sensitivity to proteolytic digestion, and increase markers of ER stress.[129] Family members with the heterozygous G231V mutation secrete comparable amounts of total surfactant protein A (encoded by two human paralogs, *SFTPA1* and *SFTPA2*) into the alveolar space, in comparison with control family members.[129] The mechanism of disease is likely not related to an overt lack of SP-A within the alveolar space, but instead is related to pathogenic effects to epithelial cells expressing the mutant protein.

Familial Pulmonary Alveolar Microlithiasis

Pulmonary alveolar microlithiasis (PAM) is a rare disorder characterized by laminated calcium-phosphate concretions within the alveoli. PAM is inherited in an autosomal recessive manner and is particularly prevalent in Turkey, Italy, the United States, and Japan.[130–132] The chest radiographs of patients with PAM show diffuse, bilateral, micro-nodular opacities, which obscure the heart border, mediastinum, and diaphragmatic surfaces. Despite the "sandstorm-like" appearance, the clinical presentation of PAM is variable.[130,131,133,134] Early in the disease course patients are often asymptomatic, but over time develop cough, dyspnea, and a restrictive defect with reduced diffusion. At present, treatment is supportive and the overall prognosis is poor.

In 2006 Corut and colleagues[135] reported the discovery of several mutations in the gene encoding the type IIb sodium-phosphate cotransporter protein (SCL34A2) in individuals with PAM. The group used linkage analysis of a large consanguineous family and ultimately identified 6 homozygous mutations in SCL34A2 that predict loss of protein function. Using genome-wide SNP association mapping, a Japanese group independently identified mutations in SCL34A2.[136] Two patients had homozygous frameshift mutations and 4 had splice-site mutations. None of the mutations were identified in normal controls. Since these initial discoveries, additional missense and frameshift mutations as well as intragenetic deletions have been identified.[137–139] The SCL34A2 gene is expressed in high levels in the lung, predominantly in type II epithelial cells.[140–142] Its hypothesized role is to remove phosphate from the alveolar space.[135,136]

Familial Sarcoidosis

Sarcoidosis is a multisystem granulomatous disorder of unknown etiology that affects the lungs in more than 90% of patients; lymph nodes, liver, bone, spleen, and other organs can also be involved.[143] The development and progression of the ILD appear to result from the complex interaction of various genetic and environmental factors. The importance of genetic predisposition is indicated by observation of familial clustering,[144] increased concordance in monozygotic twins compared with dizygotic or non-twin siblings,[145] and variations among different racial and ethnic groups.[146,147] In a twin study from Finland and Denmark, monozygotic twins had an 80-fold increased risk for developing sarcoidosis compared with a 7-fold increased risk among dizygotic twins.[145] Although there were statistically more concordant pairs among monozygotic twins than among dizygotic twins, the majority of monozygotic twins were actually discordant for the presence of disease. Strong genetic associations are found with polymorphisms within the major histocompatibility complex (MHC)[148]; some of these are also associated with disease phenotype and progression. For other, well-studied associations the reader is referred to the reviews by Grunewald[149] and Smith and colleagues.[150]

CLINICAL MANAGEMENT OF GENETIC INTERSTITIAL LUNG DISEASES

The ILDs are a clinically heterogeneous group of pulmonary disorders, and the genetic underpinnings of this group demonstrate that aberrations of multiple different pathways can lead to interstitial disease. Given the increasing volumes of data generated by novel genetic and genomic techniques, how does the clinician make sense of all these genetic discoveries? For all these various genetic polymorphisms and mutations, what information is clinically significant or will influence patient care?

The risk-to-benefit ratio for genetic screening is specific for each disorder, and is related to its pretest probability and the availability of therapeutic actions. Given the current cost of genetic screening for mutations or intragenic deletions and the possibility of identifying genetic variants of unknown clinical significance, this approach is generally reserved for those diseases that show low genetic locus heterogeneity and those diseases for which a particular genetic diagnosis would affect clinical care. The following case illustrates both of these points.

The proband of kindred F42 is a 37-year-old white woman who was referred for evaluation of familial spontaneous pneumothorax (**Fig. 2**). She had suffered 4 spontaneous pneumothoraces and underwent bilateral video-assisted thoracic surgery with bleb resection and mechanical pleurodesis. Her family history was significant for a great uncle who also had multiple spontaneous pneumothoraces. Because her CT scan of the chest showed multiple subpleural and intraparenchymal lung cysts, a diagnosis of BHDS was considered. Genetic sequencing of the FLCN gene of the proband revealed a heterozygous deletion of a coding nucleotide that predicts the premature termination of the protein; this variant has been previously described in families with BHDS.[37] Her available family members were screened for this deleterious variant, and 3 other mutation carriers were identified. Each individual underwent genetic counseling and screening for kidney cancer. Renal ultrasonography of the 35-year-old sister revealed a 3-cm right mass, and she was referred for partial nephrectomy.

This case illustrates how the pulmonary phenotype (here, familial spontaneous pneumothorax) may be the presenting symptom that provides the clue for the underlying disorder. This case also demonstrates that mutations in a single gene may result in a spectrum of clinical manifestations. The characteristic skin lesions for BHDS are frequently not seen until the fourth decade and were not apparent in the proband or her younger sister, who had also inherited the same FLCN mutation. Genetic analysis is recommended in the workup of BHDS because there is no locus

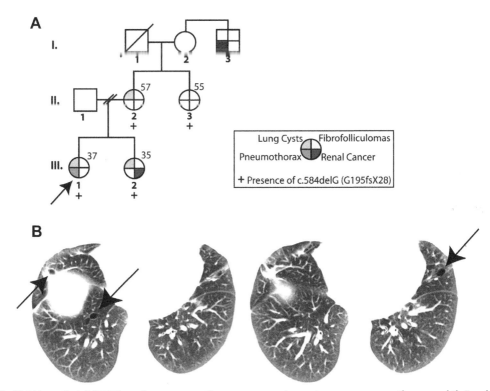

Fig. 2. Birt-Hogg-Dubé (BHD) syndrome presenting as recurrent spontaneous pneumothoraces. (*A*) Condensed pedigree of kindred F42 presenting with familial spontaneous pneumothorax. Circles represent females and squares represent males. Individuals with a pneumothorax, lung cysts as detected by high-resolution CT scans of the chest, fibrofolliculomas, and renal cancer are indicated by blue, green, yellow, and red symbols, respectively. The presence of a heterozygous frameshift mutation in the gene encoding folliculin (*FLCN*) predicting the premature termination of the protein is indicated by the plus signs. The sequence variant is described according to recommended guidelines.[151] Of the 4 mutation carriers, only the 2 elder family members had histopathologic evidence of multiple fibrofolliculomas, the characteristic skin lesion of BHD syndrome. The proband, her sister, and her mother have evidence of at least one pulmonary cyst by high-resolution CT (HRCT). A 3-cm renal mass was detected in the proband's sister, who was referred for partial nephrectomy. (*B*) HRCT scan of the proband reveals multiple subcentimeter cysts (*arrows*) within the lower lobes.

heterogeneity (only one culprit gene is known) and the presence of a mutation necessitates screening for renal cancer, which is found in approximately 10%. In this case, nephrectomy was curative.

Is genetic screening indicated for the other inherited ILDs? Certainly in many cases the identification of a genetic mutation clarifies the underlying diagnosis and may explain a variety of seemingly unrelated clinical phenotypes. However, in some cases genetic screening yields a rare variant of unknown clinical significance. The variant may be so rare that it has not been previously described or its functional effects on the resulting protein are unpredictable. Penetrance of clinical phenotypes is another key issue. Predictions of genetic risk for first-degree family members are tenuous for dominant genetic mutations of low penetrance. Genetic counseling of patients prior to mutation

analysis needs to be specific for each disease and clinical scenario.

The ultimate goal of genetic investigations is to identify the underlying molecular pathogenesis of the disease. The identification of new targets for therapeutic intervention may lead to successful treatments of the ILDs. The success of sirolimus in stabilizing lung function, reducing respiratory symptoms, and improving the quality of life of tuberous sclerosis/LAM patients is proof of concept that therapy targeting defective genetic and biochemical pathways can be successful.[35] Let us hope that other personalized medical therapies will be soon forthcoming for other inherited ILDs. Until that time, the genetic workup for some of these conditions may clarify the diagnosis for the proband and in some situations provide clinical predictions for related family members.

REFERENCES

1. Drachtman RA, Alter BP. Dyskeratosis congenita. Dermatol Clin 1995;13(1):33–9.
2. Dokal I. Dyskeratosis congenita in all its forms. Br J Haematol 2000;110(4):768–79.
3. Calado RT, Young NS. Telomere diseases. N Engl J Med 2009;361(24):2353–65.
4. Lee HW, Blasco MA, Gottlieb GJ, et al. Essential role of mouse telomerase in highly proliferative organs. Nature 1998;392(6676):569–74.
5. Vulliamy T, Marrone A, Szydlo R, et al. Disease anticipation is associated with progressive telomere shortening in families with dyskeratosis congenita due to mutations in TERC. Nat Genet 2004;36(5):447–9.
6. Armanios M, Chen JL, Chang YP, et al. Haploinsufficiency of telomerase reverse transcriptase leads to anticipation in autosomal dominant dyskeratosis congenita. Proc Natl Acad Sci U S A 2005;102(44):15960–4.
7. Paul SR, Perez-Atayde A, Williams DA. Interstitial pulmonary disease associated with dyskeratosis congenita. Am J Pediatr Hematol Oncol 1992;14(1):89–92.
8. Verra F, Kouzan S, Saiag P, et al. Bronchoalveolar disease in dyskeratosis congenita. Eur Respir J 1992;5(4):497–9.
9. Yabe M, Yabe H, Hattori K, et al. Fatal interstitial pulmonary disease in a patient with dyskeratosis congenita after allogeneic bone marrow transplantation. Bone Marrow Transplant 1997;19(4):389–92.
10. Rocha V, Devergie A, Socie G, et al. Unusual complications after bone marrow transplantation for dyskeratosis congenita. Br J Haematol 1998;103(1):243–8.
11. Giri N, Lee R, Faro A, et al. Lung transplantation for pulmonary fibrosis in dyskeratosis congenita: case report and systematic literature review. BMC Blood Disord 2011;11(1):3.
12. Cohen SB, Graham ME, Lovrecz GO, et al. Protein composition of catalytically active human telomerase from immortal cells. Science 2007;315(5820):1850–3.
13. Parry EM, Alder JK, Lee SS, et al. Decreased dyskerin levels as a mechanism of telomere shortening in X-linked dyskeratosis congenita. J Med Genet 2011;48(5):327–33.
14. Safa WF, Lestringant GG, Frossard PM. X-linked dyskeratosis congenita: restrictive pulmonary disease and a novel mutation. Thorax 2001;56(11):891–4.
15. Marrone A, Sokhal P, Walne A, et al. Functional characterization of novel telomerase RNA (TERC) mutations in patients with diverse clinical and pathological presentations. Haematologica 2007;92(8):1013–20.
16. Walne AJ, Vulliamy T, Marrone A, et al. Genetic heterogeneity in autosomal recessive dyskeratosis congenita with one subtype due to mutations in the telomerase-associated protein NOP10. Hum Mol Genet 2007;16(13):1619–29.
17. Vulliamy T, Beswick R, Kirwan M, et al. Mutations in the telomerase component NHP2 cause the premature ageing syndrome dyskeratosis congenita. Proc Natl Acad Sci U S A 2008;105(23):8073–8.
18. Zhong F, Savage SA, Shkreli M, et al. Disruption of telomerase trafficking by TCAB1 mutation causes dyskeratosis congenita. Genes Dev 2011;25(1):11–6.
19. Burkhalter JL, Morano JU, McCay MB. Diffuse interstitial lung disease in neurofibromatosis. South Med J 1986;79(8):944–6.
20. Massaro D, Katz S. Fibrosing alveolitis: its occurrence, roentgenographic, and pathologic features in von Recklinghausen's neurofibromatosis. Am Rev Respir Dis 1966;93(6):934–42.
21. Webb WR, Goodman PC. Fibrosing alveolitis in patients with neurofibromatosis. Radiology 1977;122(2):289–93.
22. Hirsch NP, Murphy A, Radcliffe JJ. Neurofibromatosis: clinical presentations and anaesthetic implications. Br J Anaesth 2001;86(4):555–64.
23. Lenoir S, Grenier P, Brauner MW, et al. Pulmonary lymphangiomyomatosis and tuberous sclerosis: comparison of radiographic and thin-section CT findings. Radiology 1990;175(2):329–34.
24. Curatolo P, Bombardieri R, Jozwiak S. Tuberous sclerosis. Lancet 2008;372(9639):657–68.
25. Avila NA, Dwyer AJ, Rabel A, et al. Sporadic lymphangioleiomyomatosis and tuberous sclerosis complex with lymphangioleiomyomatosis: comparison of CT features. Radiology 2007;242(1):277–85.
26. van Slegtenhorst M, de Hoogt R, Hermans C, et al. Identification of the tuberous sclerosis gene TSC1 on chromosome 9q34. Science 1997;277(5327):805–8.
27. The European Chromosome 16 Tuberous Sclerosis Consortium. Identification and characterization of the tuberous sclerosis gene on chromosome 16. Cell 1993;75(7):1305–15.
28. Henske EP, Wessner LL, Golden J, et al. Loss of tuberin in both subependymal giant cell astrocytomas and angiomyolipomas supports a two-hit model for the pathogenesis of tuberous sclerosis tumors. Am J Pathol 1997;151(6):1639–47.
29. Carsillo T, Astrinidis A, Henske EP. Mutations in the tuberous sclerosis complex gene TSC2 are a cause of sporadic pulmonary lymphangioleiomyomatosis. Proc Natl Acad Sci U S A 2000;97(11):6085–90.
30. Sato T, Seyama K, Fujii H, et al. Mutation analysis of the TSC1 and TSC2 genes in Japanese patients with pulmonary lymphangioleiomyomatosis. J Hum Genet 2002;47(1):20–8.

31. Smolarek TA, Wessner LL, McCormack FX, et al. Evidence that lymphangiomyomatosis is caused by TSC2 mutations; chromosome 16p13 loss of heterozygosity in angiomyolipomas and lymph nodes from women with lymphangiomyomatosis. Am J Hum Genet 1998;62(4):810–5.

32. Bissler JJ, McCormack FX, Young LR, et al. Sirolimus for angiomyolipoma in tuberous sclerosis complex or lymphangioleiomyomatosis. N Engl J Med 2008;358(2):140–51.

33. Morton JM, McLean C, Booth SS, et al. Regression of pulmonary lymphangioleiomyomatosis (PLAM)-associated retroperitoneal angiomyolipoma post-lung transplantation with rapamycin treatment. J Heart Lung Transplant 2008;27(4):462–5.

34. Krueger DA, Care MM, Holland K, et al. Everolimus for subependymal giant-cell astrocytomas in tuberous sclerosis. N Engl J Med 2010;363(19):1801–11.

35. McCormack FX, Inoue Y, Moss J, et al. Efficacy and safety of sirolimus in lymphangioleiomyomatosis. N Engl J Med 2011;364(17):1595–606.

36. Toro JR, Pautler SE, Stewart L, et al. Lung cysts, spontaneous pneumothorax, and genetic associations in 89 families with Birt-Hogg-Dubé syndrome. Am J Respir Crit Care Med 2007;175(10):1044–53.

37. Toro JR, Wei MH, Glenn GM, et al. BHD mutations, clinical and molecular genetic investigations of Birt-Hogg-Dubé syndrome: a new series of 50 families and a review of published reports. J Med Genet 2008;45(6):321–31.

38. Nickerson ML, Warren MB, Toro JR, et al. Mutations in a novel gene lead to kidney tumors, lung wall defects, and benign tumors of the hair follicle in patients with the Birt-Hogg-Dubé syndrome. Cancer Cell 2002;2(2):157–64.

39. Painter JN, Tapanainen H, Somer M, et al. 4-bp deletion in the Birt-Hogg-Dubé gene (FLCN) causes dominantly inherited spontaneous pneumothorax. Am J Hum Genet 2005;76(3):522–7.

40. Graham RB, Nolasco M, Peterlin B, et al. Nonsense mutations in folliculin presenting as isolated familial spontaneous pneumothorax in adults. Am J Respir Crit Care Med 2005;172(1):39–44.

41. Agarwal PP, Gross BH, Holloway BJ, et al. Thoracic CT findings in Birt-Hogg-Dubé syndrome. AJR Am J Roentgenol 2011;196(2):349 52.

42. Tobino K, Gunji Y, Kurihara M, et al. Characteristics of pulmonary cysts in Birt-Hogg-Dubé syndrome: thin-section CT findings of the chest in 12 patients. Eur J Radiol 2011;77(3):403–9.

43. Grimbacher B, Holland SM, Gallin JI, et al. Hyper-IgE syndrome with recurrent infections—an autosomal dominant multisystem disorder. N Engl J Med 1999;340(9):692–702.

44. Grimbacher B, Schaffer AA, Holland SM, et al. Genetic linkage of hyper-IgE syndrome to chromosome 4. Am J Hum Genet 1999;65(3):735–44.

45. Freeman AF, Holland SM. Clinical manifestations, etiology, and pathogenesis of the hyper-IgE syndromes. Pediatr Res 2009;65(5 Pt 2):32R–7R.

46. Freeman AF, Kleiner DE, Nadiminti H, et al. Causes of death in hyper-IgE syndrome. J Allergy Clin Immunol 2007;119(5):1234–40.

47. Milner JD, Brenchley JM, Laurence A, et al. Impaired T(H)17 cell differentiation in subjects with autosomal dominant hyper-IgE syndrome. Nature 2008;452(7188):773–6.

48. Minegishi Y, Saito M, Tsuchiya S, et al. Dominant-negative mutations in the DNA-binding domain of STAT3 cause hyper-IgE syndrome. Nature 2007;448(7157):1058–62.

49. Hermansky F, Pudlak P. Albinism associated with hemorrhagic diathesis and unusual pigmented reticular cells in the bone marrow: report of two cases with histochemical studies. Blood 1959;14(2):162–9.

50. Gahl WA, Brantly M, Kaiser-Kupfer MI, et al. Genetic defects and clinical characteristics of patients with a form of oculocutaneous albinism (Hermansky-Pudlak syndrome). N Engl J Med 1998;338(18):1258–64.

51. Witkop CJ, Krumwiede M, Sedano H, et al. Reliability of absent platelet dense bodies as a diagnostic criterion for Hermansky-Pudlak syndrome. Am J Hematol 1987;26(4):305–11.

52. Dell'Angelica EC, Shotelersuk V, Aguilar RC, et al. Altered trafficking of lysosomal proteins in Hermansky-Pudlak syndrome due to mutations in the beta 3A subunit of the AP-3 adaptor. Mol Cell 1999;3(1):11–21.

53. Morgan NV, Pasha S, Johnson CA, et al. A germline mutation in BLOC1S3/reduced pigmentation causes a novel variant of Hermansky-Pudlak syndrome (HPS8). Am J Hum Genet 2006;78(1):160–6.

54. Martina JA, Moriyama K, Bonifacino JS. BLOC-3, a protein complex containing the Hermansky-Pudlak syndrome gene products HPS1 and HPS4. J Biol Chem 2003;278(31):29376–84.

55. Suzuki T, Li W, Zhang Q, et al. The gene mutated in cocoa mice, carrying a defect of organelle biogenesis, is a homologue of the human Hermansky-Pudlak syndrome-3 gene. Genomics 2001;78(1–2):30–7.

56. Zhang Q, Zhao B, Li W, et al. Ru2 and Ru encode mouse orthologs of the genes mutated in human Hermansky-Pudlak syndrome types 5 and 6. Nat Genet 2003;33(2):145–53.

57. Li W, Zhang Q, Oiso N, et al. Hermansky-Pudlak syndrome type 7 (HPS-7) results from mutant dysbindin, a member of the biogenesis of lysosome-related organelles complex 1 (BLOC-1). Nat Genet 2003;35(1):84–9.

58. Wildenberg SC, Oetting WS, Almodovar C, et al. A gene causing Hermansky-Pudlak syndrome in

a Puerto Rican population maps to chromosome 10q2. Am J Hum Genet 1995;57(4):755–65.

59. Brantly M, Avila NA, Shotelersuk V, et al. Pulmonary function and high-resolution CT findings in patients with an inherited form of pulmonary fibrosis, Hermansky-Pudlak syndrome, due to mutations in HPS-1. Chest 2000;117(1):129–36.

60. Avila NA, Brantly M, Premkumar A, et al. Hermansky-Pudlak syndrome: radiography and CT of the chest compared with pulmonary function tests and genetic studies. AJR Am J Roentgenol 2002; 179(4):887–92.

61. Anderson PD, Huizing M, Claassen DA, et al. Hermansky-Pudlak syndrome type 4 (HPS-4): clinical and molecular characteristics. Hum Genet 2003; 113(1):10–7.

62. Bachli EB, Brack T, Eppler E, et al. Hermansky-Pudlak syndrome type 4 in a patient from Sri Lanka with pulmonary fibrosis. Am J Med Genet A 2004; 127A(2):201–7.

63. Gahl WA, Brantly M, Troendle J, et al. Effect of pirfenidone on the pulmonary fibrosis of Hermansky-Pudlak syndrome. Mol Genet Metab 2002;76(3): 234–42.

64. Nakatani Y, Nakamura N, Sano J, et al. Interstitial pneumonia in Hermansky-Pudlak syndrome: significance of florid foamy swelling/degeneration (giant lamellar body degeneration) of type-2 pneumocytes. Virchows Arch 2000;437(3):304–13.

65. Pierson DM, Ionescu D, Qing G, et al. Pulmonary fibrosis in Hermansky-Pudlak syndrome. a case report and review. Respiration 2006;73(3):382–95.

66. Lyerla TA, Rusiniak ME, Borchers M, et al. Aberrant lung structure, composition, and function in a murine model of Hermansky-Pudlak syndrome. Am J Physiol Lung Cell Mol Physiol 2003;285(3):L643–53.

67. Mahavadi P, Korfei M, Henneke I, et al. Epithelial stress and apoptosis underlie Hermansky-Pudlak syndrome-associated interstitial pneumonia. Am J Respir Crit Care Med 2010;182(2):207–19.

68. Guttentag SH, Akhtar A, Tao JQ, et al. Defective surfactant secretion in a mouse model of Hermansky-Pudlak syndrome. Am J Respir Cell Mol Biol 2005;33(1):14–21.

69. Kerem E, Elstein D, Abrahamov A, et al. Pulmonary function abnormalities in type I Gaucher disease. Eur Respir J 1996;9(2):340–5.

70. Miller A, Brown LK, Pastores GM, et al. Pulmonary involvement in type 1 Gaucher disease: functional and exercise findings in patients with and without clinical interstitial lung disease. Clin Genet 2003; 63(5):368–76.

71. Goitein O, Elstein D, Abrahamov A, et al. Lung involvement and enzyme replacement therapy in Gaucher's disease. QJM 2001;94(8):407–15.

72. McGovern MM, Wasserstein MP, Giugliani R, et al. A prospective, cross-sectional survey study of the natural history of Niemann-Pick disease type B. Pediatrics 2008;122(2):e341–9.

73. Mendelson DS, Wasserstein MP, Desnick RJ, et al. Type B Niemann-Pick disease: findings at chest radiography, thin-section CT, and pulmonary function testing. Radiology 2006;238(1):339–45.

74. Parto K, Svedstrom E, Majurin ML, et al. Pulmonary manifestations in lysinuric protein intolerance. Chest 1993;104(4):1176–82.

75. Deutsch GH, Young LR, Deterding RR, et al. Diffuse lung disease in young children: application of a novel classification scheme. Am J Respir Crit Care Med 2007;176(11):1120–8.

76. Nogee LM. Genetic basis of children's interstitial lung disease. Pediatr Allergy Immunol Pulmonol 2010;23(1):15–24.

77. Wert SE, Whitsett JA, Nogee LM. Genetic disorders of surfactant dysfunction. Pediatr Dev Pathol 2009; 12(4):253–74.

78. Suzuki T, Sakagami T, Young LR, et al. Hereditary pulmonary alveolar proteinosis: pathogenesis, presentation, diagnosis, and therapy. Am J Respir Crit Care Med 2010;182(10):1292–304.

79. Nogee LM, de Mello DE, Dehner LP, et al. Brief report: deficiency of pulmonary surfactant protein B in congenital alveolar proteinosis. N Engl J Med 1993;328(6):406–10.

80. Nogee LM, Garnier G, Dietz HC, et al. A mutation in the surfactant protein B gene responsible for fatal neonatal respiratory disease in multiple kindreds. J Clin Invest 1994;93(4):1860–3.

81. Andersen C, Ramsay JA, Nogee LM, et al. Recurrent familial neonatal deaths: hereditary surfactant protein B deficiency. Am J Perinatol 2000;17(4): 219–24.

82. Somaschini M, Wert S, Mangili G, et al. Hereditary surfactant protein B deficiency resulting from a novel mutation. Intensive Care Med 2000;26(1): 97–100.

83. Wegner DJ, Hertzberg T, Heins HB, et al. A major deletion in the surfactant protein-B gene causing lethal respiratory distress. Acta Paediatr 2007; 96(4):516–20.

84. Dunbar AE 3rd, Wert SE, Ikegami M, et al. Prolonged survival in hereditary surfactant protein B (SP-B) deficiency associated with a novel splicing mutation. Pediatr Res 2000;48(3):275–82.

85. Ballard PL, Nogee LM, Beers MF, et al. Partial deficiency of surfactant protein B in an infant with chronic lung disease. Pediatrics 1995;96(6): 1046–52.

86. Nogee LM, Dunbar AE 3rd, Wert SE, et al. A mutation in the surfactant protein C gene associated with familial interstitial lung disease. N Engl J Med 2001;344(8):573–9.

87. Thomas AQ, Lane K, Phillips J 3rd, et al. Heterozygosity for a surfactant protein C gene mutation

associated with usual interstitial pneumonitis and cellular nonspecific interstitial pneumonitis in one kindred. Am J Respir Crit Care Med 2002;165(9): 1322–8.

88. Cameron HS, Somaschini M, Carrera P, et al. A common mutation in the surfactant protein C gene associated with lung disease. J Pediatr 2005;146(3):370–5.

89. van Moorsel CH, van Oosterhout MF, Barlo NP, et al. Surfactant protein C mutations are the basis of a significant portion of adult familial pulmonary fibrosis in a Dutch cohort. Am J Respir Crit Care Med 2010;182(11):1419–25.

90. Guillot L, Epaud R, Thouvenin G, et al. New surfactant protein C gene mutations associated with diffuse lung disease. J Med Genet 2009;46(7): 490–4.

91. Lawson WE, Grant SW, Ambrosini V, et al. Genetic mutations in surfactant protein C are a rare cause of sporadic cases of IPF. Thorax 2004;59(11): 977–80.

92. Markart P, Ruppert C, Wygrecka M, et al. Surfactant protein C mutations in sporadic forms of idiopathic interstitial pneumonias. Eur Respir J 2007;29(1):134–7.

93. Bridges JP, Wert SE, Nogee LM, et al. Expression of a human surfactant protein C mutation associated with interstitial lung disease disrupts lung development in transgenic mice. J Biol Chem 2003;278(52):52739–46.

94. Mulugeta S, Nguyen V, Russo SJ, et al. A surfactant protein C precursor protein BRICHOS domain mutation causes endoplasmic reticulum stress, proteasome dysfunction, and caspase 3 activation. Am J Respir Cell Mol Biol 2005;32(6):521–30.

95. Mulugeta S, Maguire JA, Newitt JL, et al. Misfolded BRICHOS SP-C mutant proteins induce apoptosis via caspase-4- and cytochrome c-related mechanisms. Am J Physiol Lung Cell Mol Physiol 2007; 293(3):L720–9.

96. Lawson WE, Cheng DS, Degryse AL, et al. Endoplasmic reticulum stress enhances fibrotic remodeling in the lungs. Proc Natl Acad Sci U S A 2011;108(26):10562–7.

97. Weaver TE. Synthesis, processing and secretion of surfactant proteins B and C. Biochim Biophys Acta 1998;1408(2–3):173–9.

98. Serrano AG, Perez-Gil J. Protein-lipid interactions and surface activity in the pulmonary surfactant system. Chem Phys Lipids 2006;141(1–2):105–18.

99. Mulugeta S, Gray JM, Notarfrancesco KL, et al. Identification of LBM180, a lamellar body limiting membrane protein of alveolar type II cells, as the ABC transporter protein ABCA3. J Biol Chem 2002;277(25):22147–55.

100. Cheong N, Madesh M, Gonzales LW, et al. Functional and trafficking defects in ATP binding cassette A3 mutants associated with respiratory distress syndrome. J Biol Chem 2006;281(14): 9791–800.

101. Shulenin S, Nogee LM, Annilo T, et al. ABCA3 gene mutations in newborns with fatal surfactant deficiency. N Engl J Med 2004;350(13):1296–303.

102. Somaschini M, Nogee LM, Sassi I, et al. Unexplained neonatal respiratory distress due to congenital surfactant deficiency. J Pediatr 2007; 150(6):649–53, 653 e641.

103. Garmany TH, Wambach JA, Heins HB, et al. Population and disease-based prevalence of the common mutations associated with surfactant deficiency. Pediatr Res 2008;63(6):645–9.

104. Bullard JE, Wert SE, Whitsett JA, et al. ABCA3 mutations associated with pediatric interstitial lung disease. Am J Respir Crit Care Med 2005; 172(8):1026–31.

105. Young LR, Nogee LM, Barnett B, et al. Usual interstitial pneumonia in an adolescent with ABCA3 mutations. Chest 2008;134(1):192–5.

106. Yokota T, Matsumura Y, Ban N, et al. Heterozygous ABCA3 mutation associated with non-fatal evolution of respiratory distress. Eur J Pediatr 2008; 167(6):691–3.

107. Trapnell BC, Whitsett JA, Nakata K. Pulmonary alveolar proteinosis. N Engl J Med 2003;349(26): 2527–39.

108. Kitamura T, Tanaka N, Watanabe J, et al. Idiopathic pulmonary alveolar proteinosis as an autoimmune disease with neutralizing antibody against granulocyte/macrophage colony-stimulating factor. J Exp Med 1999;190(6):875–80.

109. Bonfield TL, Russell D, Burgess S, et al. Autoantibodies against granulocyte macrophage colony-stimulating factor are diagnostic for pulmonary alveolar proteinosis. Am J Respir Cell Mol Biol 2002;27(4):481–6.

110. Inoue Y, Trapnell BC, Tazawa R, et al. Characteristics of a large cohort of patients with autoimmune pulmonary alveolar proteinosis in Japan. Am J Respir Crit Care Med 2008;177(7):752–62.

111. Carey B, Trapnell BC. The molecular basis of pulmonary alveolar proteinosis. Clin Immunol 2010;135(2):223–35.

112. Uchida K, Nakata K, Trapnell BC, et al. High-affinity autoantibodies specifically eliminate granulocyte-macrophage colony-stimulating factor activity in the lungs of patients with idiopathic pulmonary alveolar proteinosis. Blood 2004;103(3):1089–98.

113. Uchida K, Beck DC, Yamamoto T, et al. GM-CSF autoantibodies and neutrophil dysfunction in pulmonary alveolar proteinosis. N Engl J Med 2007;356(6): 567–79.

114. Nishinakamura R, Nakayama N, Hirabayashi Y, et al. Mice deficient for the IL-3/GM-CSF/IL-5 beta c receptor exhibit lung pathology and impaired

immune response, while beta IL3 receptor-deficient mice are normal. Immunity 1995;2(3):211–22.

115. Stanley E, Lieschke GJ, Grail D, et al. Granulocyte/macrophage colony-stimulating factor-deficient mice show no major perturbation of hematopoiesis but develop a characteristic pulmonary pathology. Proc Natl Acad Sci U S A 1994;91(12):5592–6.

116. Suzuki T, Sakagami T, Rubin BK, et al. Familial pulmonary alveolar proteinosis caused by mutations in CSF2RA. J Exp Med 2008;205(12):2703–10.

117. Tanaka T, Motoi N, Tsuchihashi Y, et al. Adult-onset hereditary pulmonary alveolar proteinosis caused by a single-base deletion in CSF2RB. J Med Genet 2011;48(3):205–9.

118. Raghu G, Weycker D, Edelsberg J, et al. Incidence and prevalence of idiopathic pulmonary fibrosis. Am J Respir Crit Care Med 2006;174(7):810–6.

119. Olson AL, Swigris JJ, Lezotte DC, et al. Mortality from pulmonary fibrosis increased in the United States from 1992 to 2003. Am J Respir Crit Care Med 2007;176(3):277–84.

120. Raghu G, Collard HR, Egan JJ, et al. An official ATS/ERS/JRS/ALAT statement: idiopathic pulmonary fibrosis: evidence-based guidelines for diagnosis and management. Am J Respir Crit Care Med 2011;183(6):788–824.

121. Marshall RP, Puddicombe A, Cookson WO, et al. Adult familial cryptogenic fibrosing alveolitis in the United Kingdom. Thorax 2000;55(2):143–6.

122. Steele MP, Speer MC, Loyd JE, et al. Clinical and pathologic features of familial interstitial pneumonia. Am J Respir Crit Care Med 2005;172(9):1146–52.

123. Seibold MA, Wise AL, Speer MC, et al. A common MUC5B promoter polymorphism and pulmonary fibrosis. N Engl J Med 2011;364(16):1503–12.

124. Armanios MY, Chen JJ, Cogan JD, et al. Telomerase mutations in families with idiopathic pulmonary fibrosis. N Engl J Med 2007;356(13):1317–26.

125. Tsakiri KD, Cronkhite JT, Kuan PJ, et al. Adult-onset pulmonary fibrosis caused by mutations in telomerase. Proc Natl Acad Sci U S A 2007;104(18):7552–7.

126. Cronkhite JT, Xing C, Raghu G, et al. Telomere shortening in familial and sporadic pulmonary fibrosis. Am J Respir Crit Care Med 2008;178(7):729–37.

127. Diaz de Leon A, Cronkhite JT, Katzenstein AL, et al. Telomere lengths, pulmonary fibrosis and telomerase (TERT) mutations. PLoS One 2010;5(5):e10680.

128. Wang Y, Kuan PJ, Xing C, et al. Genetic defects in surfactant protein A2 are associated with pulmonary fibrosis and lung cancer. Am J Hum Genet 2009;84(1):52–9.

129. Maitra M, Wang Y, Gerard RD, et al. Surfactant protein A2 mutations associated with pulmonary fibrosis lead to protein instability and endoplasmic reticulum stress. J Biol Chem 2010;285(29):22103–13.

130. Sosman MC, Dodd GD, Jones WD, et al. The familial occurrence of pulmonary alveolar microlithiasis. Am J Roentgenol Radium Ther Nucl Med 1957;77(6):947–1012.

131. Ucan ES, Keyf AI, Aydilek R, et al. Pulmonary alveolar microlithiasis: review of Turkish reports. Thorax 1993;48(2):171–3.

132. Castellana G, Lamorgese V. Pulmonary alveolar microlithiasis. World cases and review of the literature. Respiration 2003;70(5):549–55.

133. Melamed JW, Sostman HD, Ravin CE. Interstitial thickening in pulmonary alveolar microlithiasis: an underappreciated finding. J Thorac Imaging 1994;9(2):126–8.

134. Helbich TH, Wojnarovsky C, Wunderbaldinger P, et al. Pulmonary alveolar microlithiasis in children: radiographic and high-resolution CT findings. AJR Am J Roentgenol 1997;168(1):63–5.

135. Corut A, Senyigit A, Ugur SA, et al. Mutations in SLC34A2 cause pulmonary alveolar microlithiasis and are possibly associated with testicular microlithiasis. Am J Hum Genet 2006;79(4):650–6.

136. Huqun, Izumi S, Miyazawa H, et al. Mutations in the SLC34A2 gene are associated with pulmonary alveolar microlithiasis. Am J Respir Crit Care Med 2007;175(3):263–8.

137. Wang H, Yin X, Wu D. Novel human pathological mutations. SLC34A2. Disease: pulmonary alveolar microlithiasis. Hum Genet 2010;127(4):471.

138. Dogan OT, Ozsahin SL, Gul E, et al. A frame-shift mutation in the SLC34A2 gene in three patients with pulmonary alveolar microlithiasis in an inbred family. Intern Med 2010;49(1):45–9.

139. Ishihara Y, Hagiwara K, Zen K, et al. A case of pulmonary alveolar microlithiasis with an intragenetic deletion in SLC34A2 detected by a genome-wide SNP study. Thorax 2009;64(4):365–7.

140. Feild JA, Zhang L, Brun KA, et al. Cloning and functional characterization of a sodium-dependent phosphate transporter expressed in human lung and small intestine. Biochem Biophys Res Commun 1999;258(3):578–82.

141. Traebert M, Hattenhauer O, Murer H, et al. Expression of type II Na-P(i) cotransporter in alveolar type II cells. Am J Physiol 1999;277(5 Pt 1):L868–73.

142. Hashimoto M, Wang DY, Kamo T, et al. Isolation and localization of type IIb Na/Pi cotransporter in the developing rat lung. Am J Pathol 2000;157(1):21–7.

143. Hunninghake GW, Costabel U, Ando M, et al. ATS/ERS/WASOG statement on sarcoidosis. American Thoracic Society/European Respiratory Society/World Association of Sarcoidosis and other

Granulomatous Disorders. Sarcoidosis Vasc Diffuse Lung Dis 1999;16(2):149–73.

144. Rybicki BA, Iannuzzi MC, Frederick MM, et al. Familial aggregation of sarcoidosis. A case-control etiologic study of sarcoidosis (ACCESS). Am J Respir Crit Care Med 2001;164(11):2085–91.

145. Sverrild A, Backer V, Kyvik KO, et al. Heredity in sarcoidosis: a registry-based twin study. Thorax 2008;63(10):894–6.

146. Rybicki BA, Major M, Popovich J Jr, et al. Racial differences in sarcoidosis incidence: a 5-year study in a health maintenance organization. Am J Epidemiol 1997;145(3):234–41.

147. Pietinalho A, Ohmichi M, Hiraga Y, et al. The mode of presentation of sarcoidosis in Finland and Hokkaido, Japan. A comparative analysis of 571 Finnish and 686 Japanese patients. Sarcoidosis Vasc Diffuse Lung Dis 1996;13(2):159–66.

148. Schurmann M, Lympany PA, Reichel P, et al. Familial sarcoidosis is linked to the major histocompatibility complex region. Am J Respir Crit Care Med 2000;162(3 Pt 1):861–4.

149. Grunewald J. Review: role of genetics in susceptibility and outcome of sarcoidosis. Semin Respir Crit Care Med 2010;31(4):380–9.

150. Smith G, Brownell I, Sanchez M, et al. Advances in the genetics of sarcoidosis. Clin Genet 2008;73(5):401–12.

151. den Dunnen JT, Antonarakis SE. Mutation nomenclature extensions and suggestions to describe complex mutations: a discussion. Hum Mutat 2000;15(1):7–12.

Nonspecific Interstitial Pneumonia

Brent Wayne Kinder, MD, MS[a,b,*]

KEYWORDS

- Nonspecific interstitial pneumonia
- Idiopathic interstitial pneumonia
- Undifferentiated connective tissue disease
- Autoimmune

The etiology and classification of interstitial lung diseases (ILDs) are a challenge for scientists and clinicians interested in respiratory diseases. ILD can occur in patients with an identifiable underlying cause of lung injury (such as an environmental exposure or a systemic disease such as rheumatoid arthritis) or in isolation where the disease is classified as idiopathic (unknown cause). Over the last few decades, pathologic classification of idiopathic interstitial pneumonias (IIP) has evolved.[1,2] In-depth histopathologic evaluation has shown the clinical diagnosis of IIP to be more heterogeneous than once believed.[3] The subclassification of IIPs, based on clinical-radiologic-pathologic criteria, has important therapeutic and prognostic implications. These prognostic and therapeutic differences have led to an increased interest and, subsequently, understanding of the IIPs.

THE CLINICAL ENTITY OF NONSPECIFIC INTERSTITIAL PNEUMONITIS

Before the turn of the century, a subset of the patients diagnosed as having idiopathic pulmonary fibrosis (IPF) had cellular infiltration on lung biopsy (prominent lymphoplasmacytic inflammation), bronchoalveolar lavage (BAL) lymphocytosis, a clinical response to steroids, and a better long-term prognosis.[4–7] On retrospective reevaluation of lung histopathology, most of these cases were classified as nonspecific interstitial pneumonia

(NSIP) (ie, their surgical lung biopsy showed a pattern, termed NSIP, distinct from usual interstitial pneumonia [UIP], the pattern characteristic of IPF).[8,9] Consequently, in 2002, a joint American Thoracic Society/European Respiratory Society International Consensus Panel for classification of ILD included idiopathic NSIP as a provisional clinical diagnosis and recommended further study and characterization of this condition.[10] The NSIP histopathologic pattern can be seen in a variety of other clinical scenarios, including connective tissue diseases (CTDs),[8,11–16] chronic hypersensitivity pneumonitis,[17] drug effect on the lung, and after acute lung injury.[11] Thus, the clinical context and features are critical in evaluating a patient with an NSIP pattern on surgical lung biopsy. A thorough history taking including detailed review of occupational endeavors, domiciliary environment, medication use (both current and prior), and a systematic review of symptoms for evidence of CTD are critical for appropriate diagnosis, classification, and treatment of any patient with an NSIP pattern of lung injury.

HISTORY OF THE NOMENCLATURE OF IIPS

In 1969, Liebow and Carrington[1] introduced 5 histopathologic subgroups of chronic IIP: UIP, bronchiolitis interstitial pneumonia, desquamative interstitial pneumonia (DIP), lymphoid interstitial pneumonia (LIP), and giant cell interstitial pneumonia. Liebow

Sources of support: Award Number K23HL094532 from the National Heart, Lung, and Blood Institute. The content is solely the responsibility of the author and does not necessarily represent the official views of the National Heart, Lung, And Blood Institute or the National Institutes of Health.
a Department of Medicine, Mercy Medical Associates, 2055 Hospital Drive, Suite 200, Batavia, OH 45103, USA
b Department of Medicine, Mercy Health Partners, Cincinnati, OH 45267, USA
* Department of Medicine, Mercy Medical Associates, 2055 Hospital Drive, Suite 200, Batavia, OH 45103.
E-mail address: bwkinder2011@gmail.com

Clin Chest Med 33 (2012) 111–121
doi:10.1016/j.ccm.2011.11.003
0272-5231/12/$ – see front matter © 2012 Elsevier Inc. All rights reserved.

believed that the most common or usual type of diffuse lung fibrosis occurring in older individuals was UIP. The investigators suggested that lung biopsy and histopathologic subclassification might help distinguish clinically distinct conditions with regard to prognosis. These subgroups identified by Liebow and Carrington formed the basis for subsequent classification schema used for IIP as described in 1998 by Katzenstein and Myers.[2] Their classification scheme included the following histopathologic distinct subgroups: UIP, DIP and a closely related pattern termed respiratory bronchiolitis–associated ILD (RBILD), acute interstitial pneumonia (AIP), and NSIP. The term NSIP was used for those IIPs that did not meet the criteria for UIP, DIP/RBILD, or AIP and thus began as a category defined but what it was not, rather than what it was. The introduction of the NSIP pattern in this classification scheme would have important implications for the prognosis and management of patients with IIP going forward. The LIP and giant cell interstitial pneumonia subgroups identified by Liebow and Carrington were removed because they were no longer idiopathic; the former being a lymphoproliferative disorder and the latter caused by cobalt resulting from exposure to tungsten carbide fumes from hard metal processing. Bronchiolitis interstitial pneumonia, subsequently known as bronchiolitis obliterans with organizing pneumonia, was also excluded because it is a predominantly intraluminal process.

In 2002, the American Thoracic Society and the European Respiratory Society revised the classification schema of Katzenstein and Myers by introducing an integrated clinical and pathologic approach to the diagnosis of IIP.[10] The classification of the American Thoracic Society and the European Respiratory Society combined the histopathologic pattern seen on lung biopsy (using Katzenstein and Myers' scheme) with clinical information to arrive at a final clinicopathologic diagnosis. This approach preserved the existing histopathologic and clinical terms while attempting to describe the relationship between them.[3] When the terms are the same for the histopathologic pattern and the clinical diagnosis (eg, DIP), it was recommended that the pathologist use the addendum "pattern" when referring to the appearance on lung biopsy (eg, DIP pattern) and reserve the initial term for the final clinicopathologic diagnosis.

NSIP HISTOPATHOLOGIC PATTERN

The NSIP histopathologic pattern is characterized by varying degrees of inflammation and fibrosis, with some forms primarily inflammatory (cellular

NSIP) and others primarily fibrotic (fibrotic NSIP).[8] In the original description by Katzenstein and Fiorelli,[8] 3 subgroups of NSIP were identified on the basis of whether the histology showed chronic interstitial inflammation only (group I), a mixture of inflammation and fibrosis (group II), or predominantly interstitial fibrosis with minimal inflammation (group III). When NSIP is predominantly cellular, chronic interstitial inflammation involves the alveolar walls.[18] Type II pneumocyte hyperplasia is often seen in areas of inflammation. The distribution of inflammatory lesions may be inconsistent, but, unlike UIP, little normal–appearing lung is usually present in biopsy specimens. The fibrotic form of NSIP may include advanced fibrosis with some focal areas of architectural distortion. However, in most cases, the fibrosis shows more diffuse involvement of the lung with relative preservation of the lung architecture. Tansey and colleagues[19] have suggested that some histologic findings in NSIP may be more suggestive of an underlying CTD including the following: follicular bronchiolitis, lymphoid follicles, or lymphoplasmacytic infiltration of the pleura.

Although NSIP may have a substantial amount of fibrosis, it is usually of temporal uniformity (ie, varying proportions of interstitial inflammation and fibrosis appear to have occurred over a single time span), and fibroblastic foci and honeycombing, if present, are rare (**Figs. 1–3**). The temporal uniformity is distinct from the temporal heterogeneity observed in UIP. Although the histopathologic

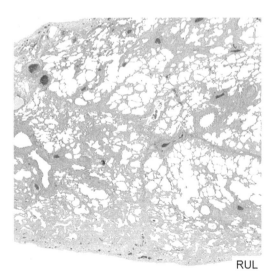

RUL

Fig. 1. A representative low-power view of a surgical lung biopsy specimen in a patient with NSIP. Temporally uniform fibrosis demonstrated is a key histopathologic feature of this disease (hematoxylin-eosin, original magnification ×30). (*Courtesy of* Dr Kathryn Wikenheiser-Brokamp, MD, PhD.)

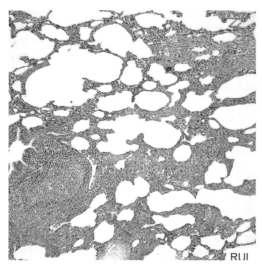

Fig. 2. Surgical lung biopsy specimen in a patient with NSIP. Interstitial expansion and a lymphoid aggregate with germinal center formation are demonstrated (hematoxylin-eosin, original magnification ×62.5). (*Courtesy of* Dr Kathryn Wikenheiser-Brokamp, MD, PhD.)

features of NSIP are now well established in the literature, the practical separation of NSIP from other IIPs, particularly UIP, is challenging.[5,20] Nicholson and colleagues[21] evaluated the level of interobserver agreement using the κ coefficient of agreement between 10 expert thoracic pathologists in the United Kingdom. The diagnosis of NSIP was present in more than half of conflicting cases, and the overall κ coefficient for a diagnosis of NSIP was only 0.32 (considered to be fair).

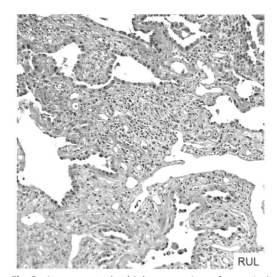

Fig. 3. A representative high-power view of a surgical lung biopsy specimen in a patient with NSIP. The interstitium is expanded by fibrosis and chronic inflammation (hematoxylin-eosin, original magnification ×100). (*Courtesy of* Dr Kathryn Wikenheiser-Brokamp, MD, PhD.)

THE AMERICAN THORACIC SOCIETY WORKING GROUP ON IDIOPATHIC NSIP

In early 2001, an American Thoracic Society working group was convened with the following goal: to define the clinical, radiologic, and pathologic features of idiopathic NSIP based on a pooled dataset of cases with surgical lung biopsy, high-resolution chest computed tomography (HRCT), and clinical data.[22] In addition, the group sought to determine what critical questions needed to be answered related to NSIP. The assembly identified 67 cases as definite (N = 17) or probable (N = 50) NSIP after detailed clinical-radiographic-pathologic review and completed their report in 2008. This multidisciplinary workshop showed that there is a consensus among experts that idiopathic NSIP is a distinct clinical entity with characteristic clinical, radiologic, and pathologic features that differ from other IIPs. The typical clinical presentation was breathlessness and cough of approximately 6 to 7 months' duration, predominantly in women, in never-smokers, and in the sixth decade of life. These patients with NSIP often had positive serology test results for collagen vascular disease. Most patients had a restrictive ventilatory defect on lung function testing. The key features on HRCT were bilateral, symmetric, predominantly lower lung reticular opacities with traction bronchiectasis and lower lobe volume loss that was usually diffuse or subpleural in the axial dimension but sometimes spared the subpleural lung. The key histopathologic features of the NSIP pattern were the uniformity of interstitial involvement with a spectrum from a cellular to a fibrosing process. The group revised the histopathologic features for the diagnosis of NSIP (**Box 1**). Most patients with idiopathic NSIP had a good prognosis, with a 5-year mortality rate estimated at less than 18%.

CLINICAL PRESENTATION

The clinical manifestations of NSIP are in many ways akin to that of the other IIPs. Indeed, the similarity in presentation among the IIPs is responsible for their grouping as the syndrome known as IPF until 2 decades ago. Idiopathic NSIP seems to be most common among women in their 40s to 50s who are nonsmokers.[22–25] However, these demographic trends are not universal, and NSIP can be seen in a wide range of ages and amongst men or smokers.[11] The most common respiratory symptoms are dyspnea on exertion and a cough, which is typically dry or nonproductive. The chest examination reveals bilateral inspiratory crackles in most patients, with a tendency to be heard best at the lung bases. Digital clubbing is much may show a higher percentage of lymphocytes,[4–7] but this is not universally the case.[26] In our practice we consider a BAL lymphocytosis of greater than 20% to be suggestive, but not diagnostic, of NSIP. Importantly, other diseases in the differential diagnosis, such as chronic hypersensitivity pneumonitis and drug-induced pneumonitis, also frequently display a lymphocytosis on BAL cellular studies.

RADIOGRAPHY

Plain film chest radiography in patients with NSIP typically reveals bilateral interstitial opacities in a lower lobe distribution.[8] However, HRCT scans provide a much more detailed evaluation of the radiographic features of NSIP. The most common features include diffuse ground-glass opacification (GGO) associated with reticular opacities and occasionally traction bronchiectasis (**Figs. 4** and **5**). These features tend to have a basilar predominance. Honeycomb cystic changes are less common and can be predictive of IPF when found in the absence of significant GGO.[27–29] The HRCT findings of idiopathic NSIP and connective tissue–associated NSIP are similar.[23,25]

The recent American Thoracic Society project provided detailed description of the HRCT features seen in 61 patients with a consensus diagnosis of NSIP.[22] Ninety-two percent of patients had lower lobe predominance. In the axial distribution, approximately half of the patients were predominantly peripherally distributed and half were diffusely distributed; a minority was predominantly centrally distributed. The most common characteristics observed included reticulation, traction bronchiectasis, lobar volume loss, and GGO. The finding of subpleural sparing of the lung opacities was seen in only 21%. Airspace consolidation was observed in 13%, whereas honeycomb change was only observed in 5%.

less common in patients with NSIP than in those with IPF.[22,23] Systemic/inflammatory symptoms are also frequently observed, including arthralgia and esophageal abnormalities[23]; fever may be present in up to one-third of cases.[20] Pulmonary function tests usually show a restrictive ventilatory defect with impairment in gas transfer. Reports have suggested that BAL in patients with NSIP

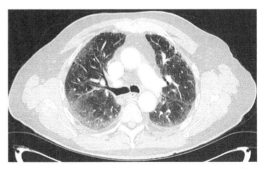

Fig. 4. A representative computed tomography of the chest from a patient with NSIP. The key features seen are ground-glass opacity, reticular changes, and traction bronchiectasis.

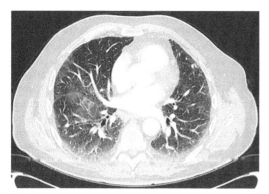

Fig. 5. A representative computed tomography of the chest from a patient with NSIP. The findings tend to be basilar predominant and bilateral.

A recent cross-sectional study evaluated the findings on HRCT that were most predictive of a surgical biopsy diagnosis of chronic hypersensitivity pneumonitis, NSIP, or IPF.[30] The features that best differentiated NSIP from the other diagnoses were relative subpleural sparing, absence of lobular areas with decreased attenuation, and lack of honeycombing. A confident diagnosis was made in 70 (53%) of 132 readings. This diagnosis was correct in 66 (94%) of 70 readings. A correct first diagnosis of NSIP was observed in 90% of NSIP cases. The accuracy for the entire cohort was reported as 80%. Interobserver agreement among readers for a confident diagnosis was in the good to excellent range ($\kappa = 0.77$–0.96).

Somewhat akin to histopathology interpretation, HRCT reading is subject to substantial interobserver disagreement.[31] In another cross-sectional study of HRCT as a diagnostic study in ILD, HRCT images of 131 patients with diffuse lung disease (from a tertiary referral hospital [N = 66] and regional teaching centers [N = 65]) were reviewed by 11 thoracic radiologists. The investigators found that the κ statistic was 0.51 for a diagnosis of NSIP, considered to be a moderate level of agreement. These data suggest that HRCT findings alone cannot definitively diagnose NSIP. However, it is unknown if the combination of characteristic clinical features (age, gender, smoking status, and so forth) and specific HRCT findings could obviate surgical lung biopsy in some patients.

DIAGNOSTIC APPROACH

A comprehensive medical, environmental, and occupational history taking is the critical first step in the evaluation of all patients with a potential diagnosis of ILD. Specific attention should be given to environmental organic antigen exposures (such as domiciliary birds or water damage in the home), and connective tissue signs and symptoms, such as hypersensitivity pneumonitis and CTDs, have many overlapping findings on radiography and histopathologic examination with NSIP. The initial testing of patients with a potential diagnosis of NSIP includes HRCT and pulmonary function testing (spirometry, lung volumes and diffusing capacity for carbon monoxide [DLCO]). These tests are used to determine the extent and severity of disease and the magnitude of impairment in lung function and to rule out other diseases with specific HRCT patterns such as IPF.[29] In addition, it is important to establish a baseline for these radiographic and functional parameters before initiating therapy.

We regularly send a comprehensive panel of serum autoantibodies and inflammatory markers when evaluating patients with incipient ILD, including antinuclear antibody, rheumatoid factor, anti-Scl-70, anti–transfer RNA synthetase antibodies (eg, Jo-1, PL-7, PL-12, EJ, OJ), anti-Ro (SS-A), anti-La (SS-B), antiribonucleoprotein, aldolase, creatine kinase, erythrocyte sedimentation rate, C-reactive protein, and anti–cyclic citrullinated peptide. These test results when positive are supportive, although not necessarily diagnostic, of a CTD diagnosis and should be interpreted in the context of the symptoms and signs of CTD.

BAL is controversial and not necessarily regularly warranted except to rule out infection. BAL is more likely to show lymphocytosis in patients with NSIP than those with IPF[32] and thus can be a clue to the diagnosis if present and surgical lung biopsy is not possible. Bronchoscopy with transbronchial lung biopsy is of limited utility in the diagnosis of NSIP because of the small tissue sample and difficulty in pathologic diagnosis.

We routinely recommend surgical lung biopsy for definitive diagnosis of NSIP. There are no data available in the literature to suggest that NSIP can be diagnosed definitively without histopathologic confirmation; however, demographic and clinical characteristics can be suggestive.[23] The underlying histopathologic features may provide some prognostic and therapeutic benefits. For instance, if multiple fibroblastic foci and microscopic honeycombing are observed, the prognosis is likely worse and response to immunosuppressive treatment may be less likely. Decrements in serial pulmonary function tests, particularly forced vital capacity (FVC) or DLCO, are likely the best indicators of progressive disease and a worse prognosis (see the section "Prognosis").[33] We use these parameters predominantly based on extrapolation from evidence in IPF.[34] We do not routinely follow serial chest computed tomographies because of the cumulative radiation exposure risks and the potential for lengthy survival with effective treatment.

PROGNOSIS

Most data regarding clinical outcomes in patients with NSIP are from retrospective cohort studies of heterogeneous patient populations that were previously classified as having IPF or cryptogenic fibrosing alveolitis (CFA). Most of these patients had been treated with immunosuppressive agents. There are no prospective cohort studies of patients with NSIP who were not treated. Thus, the natural history of NSIP is unknown. However, these retrospective cohort studies suggest that the prognosis, and possibly response to immunosuppressive therapy, of patients with NSIP is much better than that of IPF/CFA.[4,7,28,35] In a study of 104 patients, Latsi and colleagues[36] found that patients with NSIP had an approximately 2-year increase in median survival compared with subjects with IPF.

Several studies of fibrotic ILD have demonstrated that change in pulmonary function parameters have important implications for prognosis.[34,36–38] In a retrospective cohort study of 83 Korean subjects with NSIP, a reduction in FVC at 12 months was a predictor of mortality.[39] In another retrospective cohort study, 29 patients with undifferentiated connective tissue disease–associated ILD (UCTD-ILD, see section later), the majority of which were previously classified as having idiopathic NSIP, were followed up for a median of 8 months with baseline and follow-up pulmonary function tests. During follow-up, 38% of the patients with UCTD-ILD improved ($\geq$5% increase in percent predicted FVC), 34% stabilized, and 28% declined ($\geq$5% decrease in percent predicted FVC) in lung function.[24] This study showed that patients with UCTD-ILD had a more favorable short-term clinical course than did patients with IPF (as measured by change in FVC), a parameter associated with increased mortality in patients with IPF.[40] It should be noted that almost all subjects with UCTD-ILDs had received immunomodulatory agents (cyclophosphamide, azathioprine, or mycophenolate mofetil) and/or corticosteroids. There are no available controlled data to determine if the natural course of NSIP is such that there are some individuals with spontaneous improvement in lung function without therapy or if immunomodulatory therapy is necessary.

UCTD

Rheumatologic studies have estimated that up to one-fourth of patients with features of a systemic autoimmune disease do not fulfill American College of Rheumatology classification criteria for CTD.[41–45] These patients are considered to have diffuse or UCTD. Most such patients (65%–94%) after years of follow-up do not develop a differentiated CTD (such as rheumatoid arthritis, lupus, systemic sclerosis, mixed CTD, and so forth).[41–46] Consequently, it has been proposed that UCTD represents a distinct clinical entity with the following criteria: signs and symptoms suggestive of a connective tissue disease, positive serologic results, and disease duration of at least 1 year.[46–48] The most common clinical manifestations of UCTD in rheumatologic populations include Raynaud phenomenon, arthritis/arthralgias, pleuritis/pericarditis, sicca symptoms, cutaneous involvement (photosensitivity, rash), esophageal involvement, fever, and myositis.[41] The specific pulmonary manifestations of UCTD in a population with respiratory disease have only recently been studied.[23] In this study it was shown that many patients presenting with idiopathic NSIP often have features suggestive of CTD and meet criteria for UCTD (**Table 1**). A more recent Italian study demonstrated that most patients initially diagnosed as having idiopathic NSIP developed evidence of autoimmune diseases within 2 years.[49] A retrospective Japanese study of idiopathic NSIP found that approximately half of the patients included met criteria for UCTD-ILD, despite the absence of prospectively collected symptom or laboratory assessment.[50] Vij and colleagues[51] performed a study of patients with idiopathic ILD and comprehensive laboratory evaluation and found that all subjects without a known cause for ILD who had an NSIP pattern on lung biopsy met criteria for UCTD similar to those we described.

The pulmonary manifestations of CTD occasionally precede the more typical systemic manifestations by months or years and are considered forme frustes of CTD (especially in rheumatoid arthritis, systemic lupus erythematosus, and polymyositis/dermatomyositis).[52] Consequently, one could expect that some of the patients initially diagnosed as having UCTD-ILD will go on to develop sufficient criteria to be classified as having another disease entity. However, if patients with ILD behave similarly to those with UCTD, in general, this is likely to be a minority of patients (eg, 25%).[41–46] Furthermore, among those patients with UCTD in whom another disorder evolve, the majority do so within the first year of follow-up.[46] Another study suggested that vitamin D deficiency in patients with UCTD may play a role in the subsequent progression into well-defined CTDs.[53] There are no prospective data published regarding the rate of evolution to another CTD among patients with UCTD-ILD. Patients with scleroderma sine scleroderma and amyopathic dermatomyositis might also meet criteria for UCTD-ILD. The study

Table 1
Diagnostic criteria for patients with UCTD

Diagnostic Criteria	Symptoms
Symptoms associated with CTD	Presence of at least 1 of the following symptoms: 1. Raynaud phenomenon 2. Arthralgias/multiple joint swelling 3. Photosensitivity 4. Unintentional weight loss 5. Morning stiffness 6. Dry mouth or dry eyes (sicca features) 7. Dysphagia 8. Recurrent unexplained fever 9. Gastroesophageal reflux 10. Skin changes (rash) 11. Oral ulceration 12. Nonandrogenic alopecia 13. Proximal muscle weakness
Evidence of systemic inflammation in the absence of infection	At least 1 of the follow positive: 1. Antinuclear antigen 2. Rheumatoid factor 3. Anti-SCL-70 antibody 4. SS-A or SS-B 5. Jo-1 antibody, 6. Sedimentation rate (>2 times normal), C-reactive protein

From Kinder BW, Collard HR, Koth L, et al. Idiopathic nonspecific interstitial pneumonia: lung manifestation of undifferentiated connective tissue disease? Am J Respir Crit Care Med 2007;176(7):691–7; with permission; and *Data from* Liebow AA, Carrington DB. The interstitial pneumonias. In: Simon M, Potchen EJ, LeMay M, editors. Frontiers of pulmonary radiology. New York: Grune & Stratteon; 1969. p. 102–41.

of UCTD-ILD is an evolving field, and, as such, there are limited published data available. However, if tertiary referral center estimates of prevalence are correct,[23,51] UCTD-associated ILD is either the first or second most common CTD-associated ILD.

Controversy Regarding Definition of UCTD-ILD

As no consensus criteria for UCTD are universally agreed on, several different schema have been used in the published literature, some by rheumatologists[42,47,54] and others primarily by pulmonologists.[23,49,50] There are no direct empirical data available in the literature to compare the performance characteristics (eg, sensitivity, specificity) of the alternative definitions. When our criteria for UCTD-ILD were applied to existing cohorts of well-characterized patients, they have been shown to be associated with specific radiologic and histopathologic patterns,[23] short-term functional outcomes,[24] and even mortality.[50]

In choosing among diagnostic criteria for a given condition, the clinician needs to consider contextual features. In screening tests, one often seeks to maximize the sensitivity of the test to avoid missing cases that may benefit from intervention. In doing so, one may be willing to compromise

some degree of specificity. This is particularly true if alternative diagnoses do not have particularly effective therapies (such as IPF). Misclassifying a patient as having IPF instead of NSIP (or UCTD-ILD) commits the patient to a pessimistic prognosis and may prevent some clinicians from offering potentially effective therapy. In contrast, a patient incorrectly diagnosed as having UCTD-ILD instead of IPF may be exposed to ineffective therapy but is unlikely to experience substantial harm if monitored carefully.

Our initial criteria did not necessarily represent the best possible diagnostic definition of UCTD-ILD. Indeed, they were chosen for a specific study based on the types of data available in the dataset and were intentionally more sensitive at the cost of some specificity. However, future iterations of diagnostic criteria for UCTD-ILD (or ILD with autoimmune features) should be rigorously compared with our prior definition with empirical data that considers important clinical outcomes.

MANAGEMENT AND TREATMENT

Most of the information available in the literature regarding treatment of NSIP is somewhat dated and from patients who were treated as having

IPF and subsequently reclassified as having NSIP.[4,7,8,11,22,28,39,50] The majority of these patients were treated with corticosteroids with or without cytotoxic agents such as cyclophosphamide or azathioprine. The treatment regimens were also varied in duration. The decision to begin treatment in a given patient is complex and must take into account several factors. The disease course of NSIP is believed to be heterogeneous, with some patients improving with treatment and others who do not have and have progressive disease. There are no high-quality data available to identify which patients are most likely to respond to therapy.

Patient Selection

A careful risk-benefit analysis for each patient is necessary when making decisions about who to treat because few ILD treatments have been rigorously studied in randomized controlled trials and the available treatments are potentially toxic. Generally, we recommend treatment of those patients who have mild to moderate symptomatic and physiologic impairment. Based on our clinical experience, we believe that this population is likely to progress and have not yet reached the end stage of fibrosis when treatment with immunomodulators is unlikely to reverse the process. In patients who are discovered incidentally (and asymptomatic) to have ILD, the decision to begin treatment is more complicated because some patients may not necessarily progress to symptomatic disease.

Treatment Regimen

There are several different regimens that have been used in patients with NSIP. We present the most common of these in our experience and in the published literature. Some ILD experts advocate corticosteroid monotherapy. However, in our experience most patients on high-dose corticosteroids will develop substantial toxic effects of the medicine if continued at even moderate doses (>15 mg/d) for the usual treatment duration of greater than 6 months. Consequently, we generally start a steroid-sparing cytotoxic agent at the initiation of therapy.

Corticosteroids and azathioprine

When used in conjunction with azathioprine, the typical starting dose of prednisone (or an equivalent dose of prednisolone) is 0.5 mg/kg/d given as a single daily oral dose (based on the patient's ideal body weight and not exceeding 40 mg/d). If the patient continues to remain stable or improves, the dose is progressively reduced over months 3 through 6 to 10 mg/d. This dose is maintained for as long as the treatment seems indicated. For azathioprine, we recommend beginning with 0.5 mg/kg/d and gradually increasing to a target dose of 2 to 3 mg/kg/d given orally as a single dose. A discernible response to therapy may not be evident until the patient has received 3 to 6 months of treatment.

Cyclophosphamide ± corticosteroids

Cyclophosphamide has been well studied in CTD-associated ILDs, which typically have an NSIP pattern on surgical lung biopsy. A National Institutes of Health–sponsored multicenter clinical trial (the Scleroderma Lung Study) assessed the efficacy and safety of oral cyclophosphamide in scleroderma-associated ILD.[55] This was a randomized placebo-controlled trial of 162 patients with early scleroderma-associated ILD (defined by the presence of ground-glass opacities on HRCT or BAL fluid with elevated neutrophils or eosinophils) to receive either oral cyclophosphamide (initial dose of 1 mg/kg/d increased to a maximum of 2 mg/kg/d as tolerated) or placebo. The concurrent use of glucocorticoids (up to 10 mg/d prednisone) was permitted. At the end of 12 months of therapy, the mean change in FVC, the primary outcome measure, showed a significantly smaller decline in patients who received cyclophosphamide compared with those on placebo (−1.4% vs −3.2%). There were more adverse events (hematuria, leukopenia, neutropenia, and pneumonia) in the cyclophosphamide-treated group. There are concerns about the long-term adverse events in the cyclophosphamide-treated group, such as bladder malignancy, that may not become clinically evident until years after treatment. Treatment with high cumulative cyclophosphamide doses has been shown to lead to a substantial risk of late-occurring serious malignancies in patients with granulomatosis with polyangiitis (GPA, formerly called Wegener). In a large population-based Danish study, patients treated with the equivalent of 100 mg of cyclophosphamide per day for longer than 1 year had a 20-times increased risk of acute myeloid leukemia and 3.5-times increased risk of bladder cancer within 7 to 19 years after therapy compared with the general population.[56] In a United States–based study of patients with GPA treated with cyclophosphamide, the estimated incidence of bladder cancer after the first exposure to cyclophosphamide was 5% at 10 years and 16% at 15 years.[57] The lack of direct clinical trial evidence, side effect profile, and potential increase in long-term risk of malignancy coupled with the modest observed clinical benefit of the intervention in CTD-ILD argue against the routine use of this regimen in patients with NSIP.

Mycophenolate mofetil ± corticosteroids

There are no controlled trials published with this regimen in patients with ILD. However, recently several major academic clinical centers have been using mycophenolate mofetil with or without corticosteroids in the treatment of CTD-associated ILD.[58] In a retrospective study of 28 patients with CTD-associated ILD, side effects occurred in 6 patients but improved with dose reduction.[59] In addition, the patients had modest improvements in lung function (average change in FVC of 2.3% predicted, total lung capacity [TLC] of 4.0% predicted, DLCO of 2.6% predicted). It should be noted that there is also a theoretical increased risk of malignancy associated with the use of mycophenolate; however, this has not been well established in the literature.

Assessing the Response to Therapy

The response to therapy should be assessed 3 to 6 months after its initiation. A favorable response to therapy is often defined by:

- A decrease in symptoms, especially dyspnea and cough
- Physiologic improvement assessed by FVC, TLC, DLCO, and both resting and exercise gas exchange
- Stabilization of lung function, radiographic abnormalities, and symptoms.

Frequently, some parameters improve, whereas others decline or are unchanged. Subjective improvement can occur in some patients who have no objective signs of improvement. In general, the subjective response should not be the only factor in determining whether to continue treatment.

The following findings are considered to represent failure of therapy and are an indication to modify the treatment regimen:

- A reduction in FVC or TLC by 10% or more
- Worsening of radiographic opacities, especially with development of honeycombing or signs of pulmonary hypertension
- Decreased gas exchange at rest or with exercise.

Clinical deterioration is most frequently caused by disease progression. However, disease-associated complications and adverse effects of therapy should also be considered.

REFERENCES

1. Liebow AA, Carrington DB. The interstitial pneumonias. In: Simon M, Potchen EJ, LeMay M, editors. Frontiers of pulmonary radiology. New York: Grune & Stratteon; 1969. p. 102–41.
2. Katzenstein AL, Myers JL. Idiopathic pulmonary fibrosis. Clinical relevance of pathologic classification. Am J Respir Crit Care Med 1998;157:1301–15.
3. Collard HR, King TE Jr. Demystifying idiopathic interstitial pneumonias. Arch Intern Med 2003;163:17–29.
4. Bjoraker JA, Ryu JH, Edwin MK, et al. Prognostic significance of histopathologic subsets in idiopathic pulmonary fibrosis. Am J Respir Crit Care Med 1998; 157:199–203.
5. Nicholson AG, Colby TV, Dubois RM, et al. The prognostic significance of the histologic pattern of interstitial pneumonia in patients presenting with the clinical entity of cryptogenic fibrosing alveolitis. Am J Respir Crit Care Med 2000;162:2213–7.
6. Daniil ZD, Gilchrist FC, Nicholson AG, et al. A histologic pattern of nonspecific interstitial pneumonia is associated with a better prognosis than usual interstitial pneumonia in patients with cryptogenic fibrosing alveolitis. Am J Respir Crit Care Med 1999;160:899–905.
7. Nagai S, Kitaichi M, Itoh H, et al. Idiopathic nonspecific interstitial pneumonia/fibrosis: comparison with idiopathic pulmonary fibrosis and BOOP. Eur Respir J 1998;12:1010–9.
8. Katzenstein AL, Fiorelli RF. Nonspecific interstitial pneumonia/fibrosis. Histologic features and clinical significance. Am J Surg Pathol 1994;18:136–47.
9. Katzenstein AL. Idiopathic interstitial pneumonia: classification and diagnosis. In: Katzenstein AL, Askin FB, editors. Surgical pathology of non-neoplastic lung disease. Philadelphia: W.B. Saunders; 1997. p. 1–31.
10. American Thoracic Society/European Respiratory Society International Multidisciplinary Consensus classification of the idiopathic interstitial pneumonias. Am J Respir Crit Care Med 2002;165:277–304.
11. Cottin V, Donsbeck AV, Revel D, et al. Nonspecific interstitial pneumonia. Individualization of a clinicopathologic entity in a series of 12 patients. Am J Respir Crit Care Med 1998;158:1286–93.
12. Fujita J, Yamadori I, Suemitsu I, et al. Clinical features of non-specific interstitial pneumonia. Respir Med 1999;93:113–8.
13. Douglas WW, Tazelaar HD, Hartman TE, et al. Polymyositis-dermatomyositis-associated interstitial lung disease. Am J Respir Crit Care Med 2001;164: 1182–5.
14. Bouros D, Wells AU, Nicholson AG, et al. Histopathologic subsets of fibrosing alveolitis in patients with systemic sclerosis and their relationship to outcome. Am J Respir Crit Care Med 2002;165:1581–6.
15. Kim DS, Yoo B, Lee JS, et al. The major histopathologic pattern of pulmonary fibrosis in scleroderma is nonspecific interstitial pneumonia. Sarcoidosis Vasc Diffuse Lung Dis 2002;19:121–7.

16. Ito I, Nagai S, Kitaichi M, et al. Pulmonary manifestations of primary Sjögren's syndrome: a clinical, radiologic and pathologic study. Am J Respir Crit Care Med 2005;171:632–8.

17. Vourlekis JS, Schwarz MI, Cool CD, et al. Nonspecific interstitial pneumonitis as the sole histologic expression of hypersensitivity pneumonitis. Am J Med 2002;112:490–3.

18. Leslie KO. Historical perspective: a pathologic approach to the classification of idiopathic interstitial pneumonias. Chest 2005;128:513S–9S.

19. Tansey D, Wells AU, Colby TV, et al. Variations in histological patterns of interstitial pneumonia between connective tissue disorders and their relationship to prognosis. Histopathology 2004;44:585–96.

20. Flaherty KR, Martinez FJ. Nonspecific interstitial pneumonia. Semin Respir Crit Care Med 2006;27:652–8.

21. Nicholson AG, Addis BJ, Bharucha H, et al. Interobserver variation between pathologists in diffuse parenchymal lung disease. Thorax 2004;59:500–5.

22. Travis WD, Hunninghake G, King TE Jr, et al. Idiopathic nonspecific interstitial pneumonia: report of an American Thoracic Society project. Am J Respir Crit Care Med 2008;177:1338–47.

23. Kinder BW, Collard HR, Koth L, et al. Idiopathic nonspecific interstitial pneumonia: lung manifestation of undifferentiated connective tissue disease? Am J Respir Crit Care Med 2007;176:691–7.

24. Kinder BW, Shariat C, Collard HR, et al. Undifferentiated connective tissue disease-associated interstitial lung disease: changes in lung function. Lung 2010;188:143–9.

25. Fujita J, Ohtsuki Y, Yoshinouchi T, et al. Idiopathic nonspecific interstitial pneumonia: as an "autoimmune interstitial pneumonia". Respir Med 2005;99:234–40.

26. Veeraraghavan S, Latsi PI, Wells AU, et al. BAL findings in idiopathic nonspecific interstitial pneumonia and usual interstitial pneumonia. Eur Respir J 2003;22:239–44.

27. Flaherty KR, Thwaite EL, Kazerooni EA, et al. Radiological versus histological diagnosis in UIP and NSIP: survival implications. Thorax 2003;58:143–8.

28. Flaherty KR, Toews GB, Travis WD, et al. Clinical significance of histological classification of idiopathic interstitial pneumonia. Eur Respir J 2002;19:275–83.

29. Hunninghake GW, Lynch DA, Galvin JR, et al. Radiologic findings are strongly associated with a pathologic diagnosis of usual interstitial pneumonia. Chest 2003;124:1215–23.

30. Silva CI, Muller NL, Lynch DA, et al. Chronic hypersensitivity pneumonitis: differentiation from idiopathic pulmonary fibrosis and nonspecific interstitial pneumonia by using thin-section CT. Radiology 2008;246:288–97.

31. Aziz ZA, Wells AU, Hansell DM, et al. HRCT diagnosis of diffuse parenchymal lung disease: interobserver variation. Thorax 2004;59:506–11.

32. Flaherty KR, King TE Jr, Raghu G, et al. Idiopathic interstitial pneumonia: what is the effect of a multidisciplinary approach to diagnosis? Am J Respir Crit Care Med 2004;170:904–10.

33. Flaherty KR, Andrei AC, Murray S, et al. Idiopathic pulmonary fibrosis: prognostic value of changes in physiology and six-minute-walk test. Am J Respir Crit Care Med 2006;174:803–9.

34. Collard HR, King TE Jr, Bartelson BB, et al. Changes in clinical and physiologic variables predict survival in idiopathic pulmonary fibrosis. Am J Respir Crit Care Med 2003;168:538–42.

35. Travis WD, Matsui K, Moss J, et al. Idiopathic nonspecific interstitial pneumonia: prognostic significance of cellular and fibrosing patterns: survival comparison with usual interstitial pneumonia and desquamative interstitial pneumonia. Am J Surg Pathol 2000;24:19–33.

36. Latsi PI, du Bois RM, Nicholson AG, et al. Fibrotic idiopathic interstitial pneumonia: the prognostic value of longitudinal functional trends. Am J Respir Crit Care Med 2003;168:531–7.

37. Flaherty KR, Mumford JA, Murray S, et al. Prognostic implications of physiologic and radiographic changes in idiopathic interstitial pneumonia. Am J Respir Crit Care Med 2003;168:543–8.

38. Jegal Y, Kim DS, Shim TS, et al. Physiology is a stronger predictor of survival than pathology in fibrotic interstitial pneumonia. Am J Respir Crit Care Med 2005;171:639–44.

39. Park IN, Jegal Y, Kim DS, et al. Clinical course and lung function change of idiopathic nonspecific interstitial pneumonia. Eur Respir J 2009;33:68–76.

40. King TE Jr, Safrin S, Starko KM, et al. Analyses of efficacy end points in a controlled trial of interferon-{gamma}1b for idiopathic pulmonary fibrosis. Chest 2005;127:171–7.

41. Bodolay E, Csiki Z, Szekanecz Z, et al. Five-year follow-up of 665 Hungarian patients with undifferentiated connective tissue disease (UCTD). Clin Exp Rheumatol 2003;21:313–20.

42. Williams HJ, Alarcon GS, Joks R, et al. Early undifferentiated connective tissue disease (CTD). VI. An inception cohort after 10 years: disease remissions and changes in diagnoses in well established and undifferentiated CTD. J Rheumatol 1999;26:816–25.

43. Danieli MG, Fraticelli P, Salvi A, et al. Undifferentiated connective tissue disease: natural history and evolution into definite CTD assessed in 84 patients initially diagnosed as early UCTD. Clin Rheumatol 1998;17:195–201.

44. Mosca M, Tavoni A, Neri R, et al. Undifferentiated connective tissue diseases: the clinical and serological profiles of 91 patients followed for at least 1 year. Lupus 1998;7:95–100.

45. Clegg DO, Williams HJ, Singer JZ, et al. Early undifferentiated connective tissue disease. II. The frequency of

circulating antinuclear antibodies in patients with early rheumatic diseases. J Rheumatol 1991;18:1340–3.

46. Mosca M, Tani C, Neri C, et al. Undifferentiated connective tissue diseases (UCTD). Autoimmun Rev 2006;6:1–4.

47. Mosca M, Neri R, Bombardieri S. Undifferentiated connective tissue diseases (UCTD): a review of the literature and a proposal for preliminary classification criteria. Clin Exp Rheumatol 1999;17:615–20.

48. Doria A, Mosca M, Gambari PF, et al. Defining unclassifiable connective tissue diseases. Incomplete, undifferentiated, or both? J Rheumatol 2005; 32:213–5.

49. Romagnoli M, Nannini C, Piciucchi S, et al. Idiopathic NSIP: an interstitial lung disease associated with autoimmune disorders? Eur Respir J 2011; 38(2):384–91.

50. Suda T, Kono M, Nakamura Y, et al. Distinct prognosis of idiopathic nonspecific interstitial pneumonia (NSIP) fulfilling criteria for undifferentiated connective tissue disease (UCTD). Respir Med 2010;104:1527–34.

51. Vij R, Noth I, Strek ME. Autoimmune-featured interstitial lung disease: a distinct entity. Chest 2011; 140(5):1292–9.

52. King TE Jr. Connective tissue disease. In: Schwarz MI, King TE Jr, editors. Interstitial lung diseases. 3rd edition. Hamilton: B.C. Decker, Inc.; 1998. p. 451–505.

53. Zold E, Szodoray P, Gaal J, et al. Vitamin D deficiency in undifferentiated connective tissue disease. Arthritis Res Ther 2008;10:R123.

54. Danieli MG, Fraticelli P, Franceschini F, et al. Five-year follow-up of 165 Italian patients with undifferentiated connective tissue diseases. Clin Exp Rheumatol 1999;17:585–91.

55. Tashkin DP, Elashoff R, Clements PJ, et al. Cyclophosphamide versus placebo in scleroderma lung disease. N Engl J Med 2006;354:2655–66.

56. Faurschou M, Sorensen IJ, Mellemkjaer L, et al. Malignancies in Wegener's granulomatosis: incidence and relation to cyclophosphamide therapy in a cohort of 293 patients. J Rheumatol 2008;35: 100–5.

57. Talar-Williams C, Hijazi YM, Walther MM, et al. Cyclophosphamide-induced cystitis and bladder cancer in patients with Wegener granulomatosis. Ann Intern Med 1996;124:477–84.

58. Zamora AC, Wolters PJ, Collard HR, et al. Use of mycophenolate mofetil to treat scleroderma-associated interstitial lung disease. Respir Med 2008;102: 150–5.

59. Swigris JJ, Olson AL, Fischer A, et al. Mycophenolate mofetil is safe, well tolerated, and preserves lung function in patients with connective tissue disease-related interstitial lung disease. Chest 2006;130:30–6.

Interstitial Lung Disease in the Connective Tissue Diseases

Danielle Antin-Ozerkis, MD[a],*, Ami Rubinowitz, MD[b],
Janine Evans, MD[c], Robert J. Homer, MD, PhD[d],
Richard A. Matthay, MD[e]

KEYWORDS

- Connective tissue • Interstitial lung disease • Inflammation
- Immunity

The connective tissue diseases (CTDs) are a group of inflammatory, immune-mediated disorders in which a failure of self-tolerance leads to autoimmunity and subsequent tissue injury. Involvement of the respiratory system, particularly interstitial lung disease (ILD), is common and is an important contributor to morbidity and mortality. The CTDs in which ILD is most commonly observed include rheumatoid arthritis (RA), systemic sclerosis/scleroderma (SSc), polymyositis (PM)/dermatomyositis (DM), Sjögren syndrome, and systemic lupus erythematosus (SLE).

When clinically apparent, CTD-associated interstitial lung disease (CTD-ILD) most often presents with the gradual onset of cough and dyspnea, although rarely it may present with fulminant respiratory failure. ILD may be the first manifestation of systemic rheumatic disease in a previously healthy patient. Before making a diagnosis of ILD, other causes of parenchymal abnormalities, such as drug toxicity or opportunistic infection, must be ruled out. Among patients with known CTD, subclinical disease is common and raises difficult questions regarding screening, diagnosis, treatment, and the ability to tolerate planned therapies to address other systemic manifestations of disease.

The radiographic findings and histopathologic appearance of ILD among the CTDs closely resembles those of the idiopathic interstitial pneumonias. However, close examination of radiographs and pathologic tissue may offer clues to a diagnosis of underlying CTD. The diagnosis of idiopathic ILD should never be made without a careful clinical search for evidence of CTD, and long-term follow-up of patients with idiopathic disease should include repeated rheumatologic evaluation as new symptoms evolve.

Few controlled trials address primary therapy for the lung disease, although corticosteroids and immunosuppressive agents are often used. Response to therapy and prognosis varies with the underlying CTD as well as with the histopathologic pattern, although further study on these issues is needed because data are limited.

[a] Yale Interstitial Lung Disease Program, Pulmonary & Critical Care Medicine Section, Department of Internal Medicine, Yale University School of Medicine, 15 York Street, LLCI 101B, New Haven, CT 06510, USA
[b] Department of Diagnostic Radiology, Yale University School of Medicine, PO Box 208042, Tompkin's East 2, New Haven, CT 06520-8042, USA
[c] Rheumatology Section, Department of Internal Medicine, Yale University School of Medicine, PO Box 208031, 300 Cedar Street, TAC S-425D, New Haven, CT 06520-8031, USA
[d] Yale University School of Medicine, PO Box 208023, 310 Cedar Street, LH 108, New Haven, CT 06520-8023, USA
[e] Pulmonary & Critical Care Medicine Section, Department of Internal Medicine, Yale University School of Medicine, PO Box 208057, 300 Cedar Street, New Haven, CT 06520-8057, USA
* Corresponding author.
E-mail address: danielle.antin-ozerkis@yale.edu

Clin Chest Med 33 (2012) 123–149
doi:10.1016/j.ccm.2012.01.004
0272-5231/12/$ – see front matter © 2012 Elsevier Inc. All rights reserved.

GENERAL APPROACH
Respiratory Symptoms

Patients with CTD-ILD are often asymptomatic early in the disease course and symptoms are usually nonspecific. Many patients present with dyspnea on exertion, fatigue, or cough. However, CTD-ILD in an asymptomatic patient may be discovered incidentally through radiographic abnormalities. Once lung function is significantly impaired, progressive dyspnea often develops. In time, diffusion defects lead to exertional hypoxemia. Increased dead space ventilation may also contribute to breathlessness. Ultimately, progressive fibrosis leads to increased work of breathing caused by high static recoil of the lung.[1]

The diagnosis of CTD-ILD may be delayed if patients attribute mild dyspnea to deconditioning and age. Limited functional status in patients with severe joint disease or significant muscle weakness may also contribute to delays in diagnosis. Conversely, the early onset of cough may lead to an earlier pulmonary evaluation. Other symptoms referable to the respiratory system include pleuritic chest pain secondary to serositis and other pleural involvement, or, rarely, the development of pneumothorax.[2,3] With advanced pulmonary fibrosis, pulmonary hypertension may develop, leading to symptoms of cor pulmonale, such as lower extremity edema and exertional chest discomfort or syncope.

Other Systems

In the patient with longstanding CTD, the underlying diagnosis is usually certain. However, in the patient with recent-onset ILD without a known CTD diagnosis, a detailed clinical history can uncover symptoms that suggest underlying CTD. For example, careful questioning regarding skin rashes may lead to the discovery of a heliotrope rash, Gottron papules, or so-called mechanic's hands in DM.[4] A history of skin thickening, telangiectasias, or digital nail pitting may suggest SSc.[5] Symptoms of acid reflux or regurgitation of food, or a history of dysphagia, may reflect underlying esophageal dysmotility and dysfunction, as seen in SSc and PM.[4,5] Musculoskeletal system complaints such as joint pain, swelling, and inflammation, as well as morning stiffness, may lead to a diagnosis of RA.[6] Swollen, tight skin on the fingers may be observed in SSc and PM, and a history of Raynaud phenomenon suggests underlying SSc, mixed CTD (MCTD), SLE, or PM.[5,7,8]

Physical Examination

Physical examination findings are often nonspecific but may include bibasilar fine, dry, velcro crackles in the patient with underlying lung fibrosis.[9] Late signs of CTD-ILD may include digital clubbing and evidence of right heart failure. Dermatologic and musculoskeletal signs of CTD, including skin rashes, sclerodactyly, skin thickening, mechanic's hands, synovitis, joint deformities, Raynaud phenomenon, and telangiectasias, may assist in uncovering primary or mixed diagnoses.

Serologic Testing

Serologic testing in patients with idiopathic ILD has historically been limited to antinuclear antibodies (ANA) and rheumatoid factor (RF). The most recent American Thoracic Society (ATS) guidelines on idiopathic pulmonary fibrosis cite only weak evidence in supporting recommendations to test ANA, RF, and anti–cyclic citrullinated peptide (anti-CCP) antibodies, but nonetheless recommend serologic testing in most patients.[10] This is recommended because it is clinically important to distinguish idiopathic from CTD-associated fibrotic lung disease. When careful evaluation for subtle historical and physical examination features is undertaken, it is estimated that at least 15% of patients have evidence of underlying CTD.[11] Nearly one-quarter of patients in one series who presented with presumed idiopathic interstitial pneumonia and negative ANA, but who had clinical findings of antisynthetase syndrome, were found to have antisynthetase antibodies.[12] Although not evidence based, some centers that specialize in the evaluation of patients with ILD routinely test for autoantibodies to Ro (anti-SSA) and La (anti-SSB), topoisomerase antibodies (anti–Scl-70), antisynthetase antibodies, antiribonucleoprotein (anti-RNP) antibodies, and anti-CCP antibodies, in addition to ANA and RF (**Table 1**).[13]

Pulmonary Function Tests

Typical pulmonary function test (PFT) abnormalities include restrictive physiology and diffusion impairment, the latter often predating other defects.[14,15] Exercise testing is an important, if underused, modality of testing patients with ILD, frequently unmasking exertional desaturation in the patient with a normal resting arterial saturation. Desaturation with exercise may be predicted by abnormalities in lung function,[16,17] and can be explained by a combination of inadequate pulmonary capillary recruitment with reduced time available for gas exchange, as well as reduced mixed venous oxygen content caused by areas of V/Q mismatch and intrapulmonary shunt.[18,19] In more advanced fibrosis, pulmonary vascular obliteration

Table 1
Autoantibody testing in the evaluation of ILD

Autoantibody	Type	Association with CTD
ANA	ANA	May be seen in various CTDs (SLE, SSc, SS, PM/DM) Nucleolar staining suggests SSc
dsDNA	Anti–dsDNA antibody	Highly specific for SLE
SSA	Anti-Ro antibody	SLE, SS, myositis associated
SSB	Anti-La antibody	Common in SS, 15% in SLE
Scl-70	Anti-DNA topoisomerase 1	Common in SSc (70% prevalence); high association with ILD
RF	RF	Sensitivity 60%–80% and specificity 60%–85% for RA
CCP	Anti-CCP antibody	Sensitivity 68% and specificity 96% for RA
RNP	Anti-U1 small nuclear RNP	High titers seen in MCTD
Jo-1, EJ, PL7, PL12, OJ	Anti-tRNA synthetases	Seen in DM/PM/antisynthetase syndrome

Abbreviations: ANA, antinuclear antibody; CCP, cyclic citrullinated peptide; dsDNA, double-stranded DNA; MCTD, mixed CTD; RF, rheumatoid factor; RNP, ribonucleoprotein; SSc, systemic sclerosis; SS, Sjogren syndrome.
   Data from Refs.[13,283–285]

leads to resting arterial hypoxemia and profound exertional desaturation. It is crucial to identify exertional desaturation, because the use of supplemental oxygen and correction of exertional hypoxemia improves exercise endurance.[20]

Chest Imaging

The first suggestion of underlying ILD may arise from an abnormal chest radiograph, typically showing basilar, peripheral reticular, or reticulonodular opacities.[21] However, particularly in early disease, the chest radiograph may be normal.[22] High-resolution computed tomography (HRCT) of the chest is more sensitive than the chest radiograph, particularly in the evaluation of CTD-ILD. In some cases of CTD-ILD, the pattern and distribution of radiographic abnormalities observed on HRCT accurately predict the pathologic findings.[23]

Common features that may be present on HRCT include ground-glass opacities (hazy areas of increased parenchymal density that do not obscure the underlying lung markings), reticulation (a series of crisscrossing lines resulting in a weblike pattern), bronchiectasis, and micronodules.[21,24,25] The abnormalities in CTD-ILD occur predominantly at the periphery of the lung and are often associated with architectural distortion, traction bronchiectasis, and honeycombing. HRCT findings in CTD-ILD are indistinguishable from those of the idiopathic interstitial pneumonias.[26] The radiographic differential diagnosis most often includes usual interstitial pneumonia (UIP), nonspecific interstitial pneumonia (NSIP), desquamative interstitial pneumonia (DIP), and organizing

pneumonia (OP) (**Table 2**). Mixed or unclassifiable patterns may also occur. Mosaic, heterogeneous lung attenuation caused by small airway obstruction with air trapping, as seen with bronchiolitis obliterans, can also be seen.

Among patients with idiopathic ILD, certain HRCT features predict the histopathologic findings of UIP, which is the pathologic equivalent of idiopathic pulmonary fibrosis (IPF).[24,27] In particular, the characteristic radiographic UIP pattern consists of peripheral, subpleural, basilar-predominant, reticular opacities in combination with basilar honeycombing, but without features, such as ground-glass opacities, that might suggest another form of ILD (**Fig. 1**). When present, these features have been shown to confidently predict the presence of pathologic UIP when surgical biopsy is obtained in idiopathic ILD.[28–30] The same correlation between radiographic and pathologic UIP likely occurs in patients with CTD-ILD.[31]

A radiographic NSIP pattern has also been described, in which the ILD is lower lobe predominant, often sparing the immediate subpleural area, and consisting of bilateral, patchy areas of ground-glass opacity with reticulation, architectural distortion, and traction bronchiectasis but without significant honeycombing (**Fig. 2**).[32–35] Correlation between this radiographic pattern and the histopathologic pattern of NSIP is not reliable.[33] Some characteristics in the inflammatory forms of CTD-ILD may suggest underlying abnormality, such as the peripheral, patchy alveolar opacities in OP, but the radiographic appearance in such cases is not specific and tissue may be required for diagnosis.[36] In CTD, it is common to see multiple

Table 2
Features of the common radiographic and pathologic patterns observed in CTD-ILD

	Distribution on HRCT	Typical Radiographic Features	Typical Pathologic Features
UIP	Peripheral, subpleural Basilar Bilateral	Reticular markings Traction bronchiectasis Honeycombing Minimal ground-glass opacities	Fibrosis with microscopic honeycombing Fibroblastic foci Heterogeneous lung involvement Subpleural distribution Absence of features suggesting alternative diagnosis
NSIP	Peripheral, subpleural Basilar Bilateral	Ground-glass opacities Reticular markings NSIP line Minimal or no honeycombing	Homogeneous interstitial fibrosis and/or inflammation Rare honeycombing
OP	Diffuse Often peripheral and patchy Occasionally peribronchovascular	Patchy ground-glass opacity and consolidation Sometimes nodular	Plugs of connective tissue in small airways Patchy distribution Little or no fibrosis Preservation of lung architecture Mild interstitial chronic inflammation
DAD	Diffuse	Ground-glass opacities Alveolar consolidation	Hyaline membranes Edema Diffuse distribution Uniform temporal appearance
LIP	Diffuse	Ground-glass opacities Centrilobular nodules Septal and bronchovascular thickening Thin-walled cysts	Diffuse interstitial infiltration by T lymphocytes, plasma cells, macrophages Alveolar septal distribution Lymphoid hyperplasia

Abbreviations: DAD, diffuse alveolar damage; LIP, lymphoid interstitial pneumonia.
Data from American Thoracic Society/European Respiratory Society International Multidisciplinary Consensus Classification of the Idiopathic Interstitial Pneumonias. Am J Respir Crit Care Med 2002;165(2):277–304.

radiographic patterns simultaneously. When observed over time, HRCT manifestations in CTD-ILD typically show progressive reticular and honeycomb change, with occasional acute exacerbations of disease, in which diffuse ground-glass opacities are superimposed on underlying fibrotic lung disease.[37] Progressive fibrosis on HRCT is associated with worse prognosis.[38] Despite the inability to clearly predict histology through the use of HRCT in all cases, many patients with CTD do not undergo surgical lung biopsy, because histopathologic diagnosis is thought unlikely to change management. It is only when clinical or radiographic features are atypical that biopsy is pursued.

Bronchoalveolar Lavage

Bronchoalveolar lavage (BAL) has long been advocated in the evaluation of CTD-ILD because it offers a noninvasive way to sample the cellular and protein composition of the lower respiratory tract in the absence of lung biopsy. Saline is instilled into the distal airways with the bronchoscope wedged in a subsegmental bronchus. Aliquots of fluid are then aspirated, forming the BAL fluid sample. The cellular differential in healthy adults consists predominantly of alveolar macrophages. Other leukocytes are present in smaller numbers, usually less than 15% lymphocytes, less than 3% neutrophils, and less than 2% eosinophils.[39] Research has focused on correlations between fluid characteristics and clinical features, including the presence or absence of ILD, the severity of ILD, progression of disease, and overall prognosis, as well as response to therapy.

Although BAL fluid analysis has been performed in all of the CTDs, it has received particular attention in SSc. In particular, the presence or absence of alveolitis has been described to reflect local

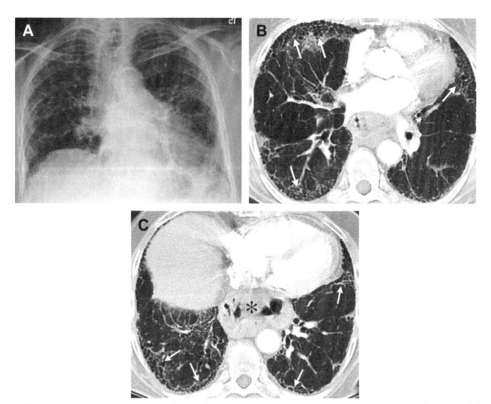

Fig. 1. A 73-year-old woman with a radiographic pattern of RA and UIP. Frontal chest radiograph (*A*) shows reduced lung volumes with lower lobe–predominant coarse interstitial markings compatible with pulmonary fibrosis. High-resolution (1.25-mm thick sections) computed tomography (CT) images at the level of the midthorax (*B*) and lower thorax (*C*) show peripheral reticular markings with architectural distortion and small subpleural cysts/honeycombing (*arrows*). The patient also has a large hiatal hernia (*asterisk*).

inflammation, in which neutrophils and eosinophils are predominant. Despite the correlation between BAL alveolitis and severity of lung disease in SSc, BAL cytology has not been consistently shown to correlate well with prognosis or response to therapy.[40] Similarly, in many of the other CTD-ILDs, BAL neutrophilia seems to correlate with poorer lung function but has not consistently proved useful for diagnosis or assessing prognosis and response to therapy.[41–44] Multiple biomarkers in BAL fluid have been proposed to give prognostic information, but no individual finding has been adequately replicated in larger studies.

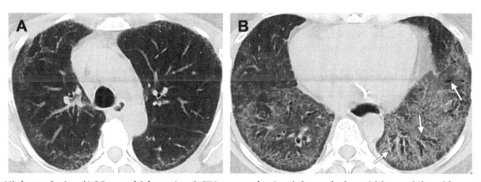

Fig. 2. High-resolution (1.25-mm thick sections) CT images obtained through the midthorax (*A*) and lower thorax (*B*) in a 57-year-old woman with scleroderma who presented with cough and shortness of breath. There are bilateral areas of ground-glass opacity with a peripheral distribution in (*A*) and lower lobe predominance (*B*), as well as reticular markings and traction bronchiectasis (*arrows*), all compatible with a nonspecific interstitial pneumonia (NSIP) pattern.

The promise of BAL sampling to give clinical information is likely limited by several issues. The largest constraint is a lack of standardization in the performance of the procedure. Some of the many variables between operators include the amount of fluid instilled, the pressure with which the fluid is aspirated, the location sampled and whether this is guided by HRCT abnormalities, which aliquots are examined and whether the first is discarded, and the skill of the technician examining the fluid.[45,46] Despite published guidelines, wide variability continues to exist and likely explains much of the inconsistent data that have resulted.[47,48] Another major factor in the inconsistent interpretation of BAL fluid results is that there are other explanations relevant to the CTD-ILD population for alterations in BAL cellularity, including infection, smoking, and recurrent aspiration.[46]

Despite these issues, BAL is an important adjunct in the evaluation of radiographic abnormalities, primarily in ruling out alternative diagnoses to CTD-ILD, including eosinophilia observed in some drug reactions, diffuse alveolar hemorrhage, and opportunistic infection.[49–51] Bronchoscopy with BAL should be considered in the evaluation of new air space opacities in any patient receiving immunosuppressive therapy.

Pathology

The major pathologic patterns recognized in CTD-ILD are the same as those recognized by the 2002 European Respiratory Society (ERS)/ATS reclassification of the idiopathic interstitial pneumonias (see **Table 2**).[52] UIP may be more common than NSIP in RA.[53] In other CTDs, particularly SSc and PM/DM, the NSIP pattern is the most common form (**Fig. 3**).[54,55] OP is more commonly observed in RA and PM/DM but may be present in SLE, Sjögren syndrome, and SSc (**Fig. 4**).[23] Diffuse alveolar damage (DAD), lymphoid interstitial pneumonia (LIP), and follicular bronchiolitis are less commonly observed patterns, but can complicate CTD.[2] Other findings, such as lymphoid hyperplasia and plasma cell infiltration, are more common in CTD-ILD and, when present pathologically, should suggest the diagnosis if CTD has not previously been suspected.[56] Another notable feature of CTD-ILD is that several pathologic patterns may be present in the same biopsy specimen.[2,57]

Prognosis in the idiopathic interstitial pneumonias is tightly linked with histopathologic pattern. UIP (IPF) carries a poor prognosis, whereas NSIP in general carries a significantly better prognosis.[16,30,58] Despite similar radiographic and

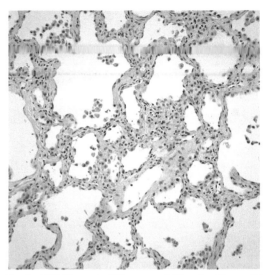

Fig. 3. NSIP. There is diffuse septal fibrosis with a mild mononuclear infiltrate, as well as mild diffuse type II cell hypertrophy. No organizing pneumonitis or fibroblast foci are seen. No granulomas or eosinophilic infiltrate are present. Honeycombing is absent. There is a mild accumulation of alveolar macrophages in the alveoli. 20× objective.

pathologic characteristics to the idiopathic interstitial pneumonias, most forms of CTD-ILD have been shown to carry a better prognosis than idiopathic ILD.[26,59,60] Among the CTD-ILDs, however,

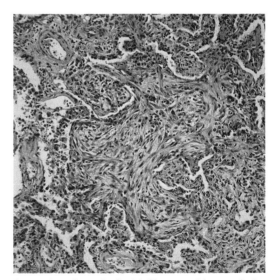

Fig. 4. OP. There is florid fibromyxoid granulation tissue within alveolar ducts and a moderate lymphoplasmacytic infiltrate. No hyaline membranes, necrosis, neutrophilic or eosinophilic infiltrate, or granulomas are seen. Established collagen fibrosis is not present, including lack of honeycombing. 10× objective.

RA may be the exception to this finding. Recent data suggest that the course of UIP in RA-ILD may be similar to that of IPF.[61]

Treatment of CTD-ILD

Immunosuppressive therapy
Many forms of CTD-ILD show responsiveness to immunosuppression. The decision to initiate immunosuppressive therapy should include an assessment of the likelihood of response as well as the risks and side effects of the medications. Corticosteroids have many potential toxicities, including glucose intolerance, bone loss, cataract development, delirium, and mood instability.[62] Underlying clinical characteristics, such as the patient's age and comorbidities (diabetes mellitus, osteoporosis, psychiatric disease) should be strongly considered. Frequently in CTD-ILD, a more prolonged course of therapy is warranted and the early addition of steroid-sparing medications can allow for lower doses of corticosteroids. Severity of disease, or particular CTD (such as SSc), may dictate the use of cytotoxic agents such as cyclophosphamide. These medications should only be prescribed by physicians familiar with their use and potential toxicities. Measures of objective improvement, including PFTs, exercise oximetry, and radiographic studies should be used; this is particularly true with the use of corticosteroids, which lead to an increase in energy level and mood, making subjective measures of patient assessment problematic. When patients either show progression despite ongoing therapy or show no improvement in the rate of decline in lung function after 6 months of therapy, discontinuation should be considered to avoid toxicity without the likelihood of benefit.

Supportive therapy
Measures intended to improve quality of life and decrease respiratory symptoms should be considered in all patients with CTD-ILD. Pulse oximetry testing can uncover resting and exertional hypoxemia. Even simple ambulation in the hallway can unmask exertional desaturation and the need for supplemental oxygen. The use of oxygen in the ILD population has not been studied in controlled trials in ILD, but is recommended to maintain saturations greater than 90% at rest or with exercise.[63] Similarly, nocturnal oxygen is used, based on data showing the negative impact nocturnal hypoxemia has on quality of life.[64] A wide variety of options are available to provide convenient, portable systems.

A large body of evidence shows that a structured form of exercise such as pulmonary rehabilitation improves muscle strength and endurance in chronic obstructive pulmonary disease (COPD).[65,66] Compelling data supporting the use of pulmonary rehabilitation in ILD are now increasing.[67–71] In addition to the benefits of improved exercise tolerance, patients with ILD may also benefit from education regarding oxygen use, breathing and pacing techniques, and social support.[65] Pulmonary rehabilitation can assist in the identification of anxiety and depression, a common problem for patients with chronic lung disease.[72]

Treatment of comorbidities
Patients with CTD-ILD frequently have comorbid conditions that need to be addressed concomitant with the ILD. Particularly in dyspneic patients, investigations for the presence of ischemic heart disease should be undertaken in patients with other cardiovascular risk factors. The risk for ischemic heart disease is increased among patients with ILD, and patients with SLE and RA are at risk for premature atherosclerosis.[73–75] Patients should also be counseled regarding smoking cessation. In particular, patients with some forms of pulmonary fibrosis have an increased risk of developing lung cancer, and CTD itself may carry some risk for malignancy.[63,76,77] The prevalence of obstructive sleep apnea may be high among patients with ILD, even in the absence of excessive sleepiness or obesity, and polysomnography should be considered.[78–80] Patients with ILD may be at increased risk for development of thromboembolic disease, and particularly patients with CTD such as SLE should have new complaints of leg swelling or shortness of breath evaluated with this in mind.[81,82]

There is a high prevalence of gastroesophageal reflux disease (GERD), often asymptomatic, among patients with IPF.[83,84] Some data suggest that GERD may be linked to the development of IPF and is correlated with worsening of disease.[85] Close ties between SSc lung disease and GERD are also suspected and many forms of CTD may be strongly associated with GERD.[86,87] The question of when to seek evidence of and to treat asymptomatic GERD is less clear.[63]

Pulmonary hypertension develops in a significant proportion of patients with ILD, often caused by the effects of chronic hypoxia and the destruction of capillaries by the fibrotic process.[88] In addition, pulmonary arterial hypertension (PAH) may complicate several of the CTDs, particularly scleroderma, MCTD, SLE, PM/DM, and more rarely RA.[89] Pulmonary hypertension contributes to diffusion impairment and symptoms. Right heart catheterization may be needed to further characterize the nature of the pulmonary hypertension, as well as to assess for any role of left heart dysfunction.[88,90] Therapy for the combination of

ILD and pulmonary hypertension is controversial but may be considered.[91,92]

Lung transplantation

Lung transplantation should be considered for patients with advanced, progressive CTD-ILD. Data suggest that carefully selected patients with CTD may have equivalent survival to other patients undergoing lung transplantation, particularly if esophageal dysfunction is addressed.[93–95] The Lung Allocation Score (LAS) tends to prioritize patients with advanced ILD.[96] Decisions regarding whether and when to list are difficult in CTD-ILD, because the rate of progression is difficult to predict, and a sudden, unanticipated exacerbation of disease may occur.[97] In the idiopathic interstitial lung diseases, fibrotic lung disease with a severely impaired diffusion capacity (DL_{CO}) (<39% predicted) predicts poor survival because of the underlying disease and this measure is often used to prompt evaluation for listing.[98] Lung transplantation requires the emotional and physical ability to tolerate a complex medical regimen of immunosuppressive therapy.[99]

RA

RA is a chronic inflammatory disease affecting the synovial lined joints and symmetrically involves the small joints of the hands and feet.[6] The diagnosis of RA has typically been made with the use of criteria proposed by the American Rheumatism Association in 1987.[6] However, the use of newer molecular markers such as anti-CCP antibodies has led to earlier diagnosis, reflected in the criteria proposed in 2010 by the American College of Rheumatology (ACR) and European League Against Rheumatism (EULAR) (Box 1).[100,101] RA occurs most commonly in women between the ages of 35 and 50 years, although men are also affected.[102,103]

Pulmonary disease is a major source of morbidity and mortality in RA, manifesting most commonly as ILD, obstructive airways disease, rheumatoid nodules, and pleural involvement.[102] RA-associated ILD (RA-ILD) is often diagnosed in the setting of longstanding RA, but may present before or at the same time as arthritis and other rheumatologic complaints.[104] In general, RA-ILD tends to be slowly progressive; however, some patients may experience periods of sudden deterioration and approximately 10% of patients die of progressive respiratory failure.[37,105,106] Hospitalization for a respiratory cause predicts high mortality over the subsequent 5 years.[107] Risk factors for the development of RA-ILD include older age, male sex, and a history of cigarette smoking.[108]

Box 1
2010 ACR/EULAR criteria for the diagnosis of RA

1. Presence of synovitis in at least 1 joint
2. Absence of an alternative diagnosis to explain the synovitis
3. Score of at least 6 out of 10 from table given later
4. Evidence of longstanding or inactive disease with previous fulfillment of criteria

1. Joints
   2–10 large joints (shoulder, elbow, hip, knee, ankle) — 1 point
   1–3 small joints — 2 points
   4–10 small joints — 3 points
   More than 10 joints (at least 1 small joint) — 5 points
2. Serology
   Low positive RF or anti-CCP — 2 points
   High positive RF or anti-CCP — 3 points
3. Acute phase reactants
   Increased CRP or ESR — 1 point
4. Duration of symptoms
   At least 6 weeks — 1 point

Abbreviations: CRP, C-reactive protein; RF, rheumatoid factor.
Adapted from Aletaha D, Neogi T, Silman AJ, et al. 2010 Rheumatoid arthritis classification criteria: an American College of Rheumatology/European League Against Rheumatism collaborative initiative. Arthritis Rheum 2010;62(9):2574.

Early reports prompted increased awareness of ILD in RA.[109–112] Estimates of its prevalence vary, largely because of variations in the sensitivity of the modalities used. For example, ILD identified by chest radiograph alone in patients with RA was present in fewer than 5% of patients.[22] Studies using PFTs identified ILD in 33% to 41% of patients with RA and HRCT identified abnormalities in 20% to 63%, which has been confirmed by autopsy studies.[14,15,105,106,113–115] Retrospective population-based studies have estimated a lower rate of clinically significant ILD among patients with RA (6.3%–9.4%).[116,117] Although it is possible that HRCT and PFT identify abnormalities without clinical significance, it is also likely that significant ILD is underrecognized in this population.

Clinical Features

Generally, ILD occurs in patients with well-established RA.[118] However, up to 20% of patients have onset of ILD before the diagnosis of RA.[108] Patients with idiopathic ILD are often found to have RA-related autoantibodies such as RF and anti-CCP but no articular findings of RA; some may eventually develop clinical RA.[119] The delay between presentation of lung disease and subsequent joint symptoms can be as long as 6 years.[108,120]

RA-ILD typically presents with progressive dyspnea, although cough and pleuritic chest pain may occur.[3] Physical examination findings are often nonspecific and may include bibasilar fine, dry, velcro crackles. Digital clubbing and evidence of right heart failure are late signs of RA-ILD.

Like other forms of CTD-ILD, PFTs in RA-ILD typically show restrictive physiology and diffusion impairment. A defect in DL_{CO} is often the earliest PFT finding in RA-ILD.[14,15] Exertional arterial oxygen desaturation may be present despite normal resting saturations and is predicted by abnormalities in lung function.[16,17]

Radiographic Features

The most common features on HRCT in RA-ILD are glass opacities, reticulation, bronchiectasis (**Fig. 5**), and micronodules.[21,24,25] In particular, the findings in RA-ILD have been grouped into 4 main patterns: a UIP pattern consisting of bibasilar subpleural reticulations and honeycombing; an NSIP pattern consisting of predominantly lower lobe reticulation and ground-glass opacities; a bronchiolitis pattern showing centrilobular micronodules and bronchiectasis or bronchiolectasis; and an OP pattern consisting of largely peripheral airspace consolidation and ground-glass opacities.[24] Based on several small studies, it is likely that the radiographic UIP pattern in RA-ILD predicts a pathologic finding of UIP.[31,53] It is not clear that the radiographic NSIP pattern similarly predicts its pathologic correlate.[33,121] Patients with a ground-glass–predominant pattern may have a better prognosis than those with well-established fibrosis.[37] On serial HRCT, RA-ILD may manifest radiographically with acute exacerbations of disease characterized by the onset of diffuse ground-glass opacities, or with progressive reticulation, traction bronchiectasis, and honeycombing.[37] Care should be taken with the interpretation of ground-glass opacities when present in a mosaic pattern. High-resolution inspiratory and expiratory images are needed to distinguish ground-glass opacities from small airways obstruction, in which the denser areas reflect normal lung adjacent to radiolucent areas of air trapping. This finding is observed in RA-associated bronchiolitis obliterans (**Fig. 6**).

Pathologic Features

In contrast with the other CTD-ILDs, the pathology of RA-ILD shows a preponderance of UIP.[53] Certain features, such as lymphoid hyperplasia and plasma cell infiltration, as well as the presence of more than 1 pathologic process in the same biopsy specimen, are common in RA-ILD and should suggest the diagnosis (**Fig. 7**).[2,56,57] Some less common histopathologic patterns observed in RA include OP, follicular bronchiolitis, LIP, and DAD.[2] RA-ILD may not share the favorable prognosis that some other forms of CTD-ILD seem to carry.[122] Recent data suggest that the course of UIP in RA-ILD may be inexorable and fatal, as seen in IPF (idiopathic UIP).[61]

Diagnostically, the differentiation between infection, drug reaction, and underlying RA-ILD can be difficult, because many of the drugs used to treat RA can cause pulmonary toxicity

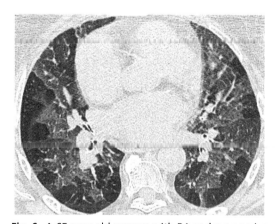

Fig. 6. A 65-year-old woman with RA and progressive shortness of breath secondary to bronchiolitis obliterans. High-resolution (1.25-mm sections) CT images performed during expiration at the level of the mid-thorax show multifocal lucent areas of moderate to severe air trapping. The greyer areas are normal lung at expiration.

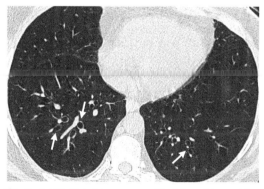

Fig. 5. A 56-year-old woman with RA and bronchiectasis. High-resolution (1.25-mm thick sections) CT image through the lower thorax shows mild, cylindrical bronchiectasis (*arrows*) in both lower lobes.

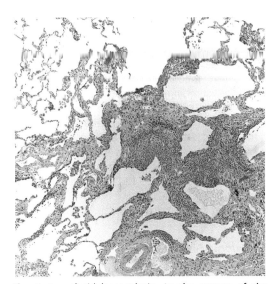

Fig. 7. Lymphoid hyperplasia. In the center of the image, there is a lymphoid follicle with a germinal center. Fibroblast foci and organizing pneumonitis are not present. There is established fibrosis. Although lymphoid hyperplasia in end-stage lung is nonspecific, in areas away from end-stage lung, this finding suggests collagen vascular disease. 4× objective.

(eg, methotrexate, leflunomide, and the TNF-α inhibitors etanercept, infliximab, and adalimumab) and can also predispose to opportunistic infection.[123–129] The diagnosis of RA-ILD should take into consideration the clinical features, the radiographic appearance, the pathology, and the temporal correlation with drug initiation.[130,131] Several different pathologic patterns may be consistent with drug toxicity, including cellular interstitial infiltrates, granulomas, tissue eosinophilia, and a DAD pattern with perivascular inflammation.[123,132]

Treatment

There are many unanswered questions pertaining to RA-ILD, in particular whether to treat subclinical disease and which therapies should be used. However, progressive lung disease is typically treated aggressively because response has been reported with corticosteroids, azathioprine, cyclosporine, and cyclophosphamide.[9,133,134] If there is no response, therapy can be discontinued to avoid toxicity without hope of benefit. Mycophenolate mofetil (MMF)has been reported to have a beneficial effect on CTD-ILD and may be considered in RA-ILD.[135,136] Data for the use of rituximab in RA-ILD are lacking. Some reports suggest that tumor necrosis factor α (TNF-α) inhibitors may be effective in RA-ILD, but others report cases of

pulmonary toxicity in patients with underlying ILD.[127,128,137] Lung transplant referral should be considered in patients with severe fibrotic lung disease.

SYSTEMIC SCLEROSIS (SCLERODERMA)

SSc is a multisystem disorder characterized by endothelial and epithelial cell injury, fibroblast dysregulation, and immune system abnormalities that ultimately lead to systemic inflammation, fibrosis, and vascular injury.[138,139] Clinically, the disease is heterogeneous and may involve multiple organ systems, most commonly the respiratory system, the skin, and the digestive system. Pulmonary involvement is the leading cause of morbidity and mortality among patients with SSc.[140] ILD is exceptionally common among patients with SSc, historically found in 28% of patients, and with the use of HRCT in more than 65% of all patients with SSc and up to 93% of patients with abnormal PFT results.[141,142] Clinically significant ILD is found in at least 40% of patients, and is a major contributor to morbidity and mortality.[143] At autopsy, most patients have microscopic evidence of lung fibrosis.[144] Clinically significant ILD is more commonly observed in diffuse SSc than in the limited form, but all types of SSc, including SSc sine scleroderma (SSc without skin involvement) may be complicated by ILD.[145,146]

PFTs

Early ILD in SSc is often asymptomatic and is detected only by PFT and HRCT abnormalities. In particular, the earliest sign of SSc-associated ILD (SSc-ILD) on PFT is a decrement in DL_{CO}, which correlates better than other lung function parameters with extent of radiographically evident ILD by HRCT.[147] In particular with SSc, decrements in DL_{CO} can reflect concomitant pulmonary vascular disease and evaluation should be undertaken to distinguish between ILD and pulmonary arterial hypertension.[148] Declines in both forced vital capacity (FVC) and DL_{CO} at diagnosis correlate well with severity of disease and with overall prognosis.[149] In particular, an FVC less than 80% predicted at diagnosis strongly predicts both the severity of decline in FVC percent predicted over the subsequent 5 years, as well as time to decline in DL_{CO} less than 70% predicted.[150] In addition, among patients with early SSc, FVC less than 50% strongly predicts mortality.[151] Most of the deterioration in FVC seems to occur in the first 2 years after diagnosis, making initial screening and follow-up PFTs particularly important during that period.[152] Patients with antitopoisomerase antibodies (anti–Scl-70) may be at higher risk for this more rapid decline.[153] Low 6-minute walk distance correlates with functional impairment in SSc-ILD, but may not be a reliable outcome measure for use in clinical trials, because it can be affected by musculoskeletal issues, including pain, weakness, and vascular insufficiency, as well as by concomitant PAH.[154]

Radiographic Features

As with all CTD-ILD, HRCT is more sensitive than the chest radiograph at identifying ILD in SSc as well as in characterizing the extent of fibrosis.[155] Radiographic features in SSc-ILD typically resemble those described in NSIP, characterized by subpleural ground-glass opacities and fine reticular markings with traction bronchiectasis, but little or no honeycombing (**Fig. 8**).[156] The presence of ground-glass opacities on initial computed tomography (CT) is a predictor for progression to more advanced fibrosis, whereas an initial CT without ground-glass opacities predicts a lack of progression for most patients.[157] Despite long-held presumptions that ground-glass opacities represent active alveolitis and inflammation, their presence may often reflect fine fibrosis and be irreversible despite therapy in SSc-ILD.[158] Intraobserver and interobserver variability has hampered the use of HRCT data for research and clinical assessment; however, computer-aided models may offer some improvement in reliability.[159,160] Combined staging systems, incorporating simple measurements of radiographic lung involvement with PFT data, may improve predictions of disease progression and mortality but also require further study.[161]

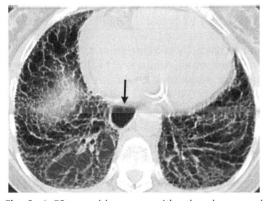

Fig. 8. A 58-year-old woman with scleroderma and fibrotic NSIP. Axial CT image through the lower thorax shows reticular markings, architectural distortion, and extensive traction bronchiectasis compatible with pulmonary fibrosis. A dilated distal esophagus (*arrow*) is also present.

Other clues to the presence of scleroderma that can be detected on chest CT include a dilated esophagus and the presence of soft tissue calcification.[162] Because esophageal dysmotility is common in these patients, they are also at increased risk of aspiration pneumonia, which can be seen at imaging as dependent areas of consolidation and ground-glass opacity, as well as small, clustered centrilobular nodules.[86]

Pathologic Features

The most common histopathologic pattern in SSc-ILD is NSIP, with a minority of biopsies showing UIP or end-stage fibrosis.[149] Unlike the marked contrast in survival seen between idiopathic UIP (IPF) and idiopathic NSIP, there seems to be little difference in mortality based on histopathologic subsets in SSc.[54,149] For this reason, surgical biopsy is generally not obtained in SSc-ILD unless atypical features are present. More recently, a central distribution of radiographic abnormalities on CT has been associated with the pathologic finding of centrilobular fibrosis and clinical evidence of esophageal reflux in SSc.[87] This finding suggests that there may be a causal link between subclinical aspiration and some forms of SSc-ILD. Abnormal esophageal motility, decreased lower esophageal sphincter pressure, and gastroparesis can all contribute to reflux in SSc and chronic aspiration may occur.[163] Among patients with more severe esophageal dysfunction, PFT parameters are more severely impaired, and there is an increased frequency of radiographically apparent ILD.[164–167] Over time, these patients seem to have more rapid progression of lung impairment.[167] It is not clear whether this association is causal for most patients or whether simultaneous worsening of lung and gastrointestinal (GI) disease reflects progression of fibrosis in multiple organ systems.

Treatment

Treatment in SSc-ILD has typically been targeted at the inflammatory component of the disease, although with only modest improvement in outcomes. Prednisone and other corticosteroids were used in the past but, with the discovery of a link between high-dose steroid use and scleroderma renal crisis, this has fallen out of favor.[168] Most studies of other immunosuppressive agents have included low dose of prednisone and, for this reason, it is often included in treatment regimens.

Multiple small, uncontrolled trials have suggested a beneficial effect of cyclophosphamide on symptoms, lung function, radiographic abnormalities, and survival.[169–171] The Sclero-derma Lung Study I was the first randomized, placebo-controlled trial to evaluate the effect of oral cyclophosphamide on lung function in SSc-ILD.[172] Cyclophosphamide had a statistically significant, although modest (2.53%), positive effect on the primary outcome of difference in FVC percent predicted at 1 year.[172] Some important secondary outcomes such as dyspnea, skin thickening, and health-related quality of life were also improved. Cyclophosphamide was associated with increased short-term toxicity in the study, and is known to have long-term risks including increased risk for bladder cancer and other malignancies.[173] Subset analysis has suggested that the group most likely to benefit from treatment includes those patients with more severe restriction and fibrosis at baseline, although this remains unproven.[172,174] Long-term follow-up showed that the beneficial effects of cyclophosphamide on lung function were lost by 24 months.[174] Despite the small absolute change in FVC percent predicted, it has been suggested that the stability of lung function attained in treated patients may represent the true success in SSc-ILD and that immunosuppressive therapy to prevent progression of disease may be required long-term.[175]

Methods to diminish the toxicity of treatment include alteration in the administration of cyclo-phosphamide from daily oral administration to monthly infusions, which minimize the cumulative dose; switching from cyclophosphamide after 6 to 12 months to another, less toxic agent such as azathioprine or MMF; or replacing cyclophospha-mide by initiating therapy with such agents.[175–177] MMF has shown some early promising results in small studies and further data are awaited.[178,179] The Scleroderma Lung Study II, which is ongoing, is examining the role of MMF as primary therapy for SSc-ILD compared with cyclophosphamide. Azathioprine has similarly been used when less severe disease is present, or when the side effects of cyclophosphamide are prohibitive. This agent may offer some efficacy but is not well studied and is limited by side effects in a substantial minority of patients.[180] It is more frequently used for maintenance after cyclophosphamide and seems to offer some usefulness in this regard.[181]

Other agents have been evaluated as potential alternatives to cyclophosphamide; however, none has fulfilled its promise. The endothelin-1 inhibitor bosentan was proposed for its antifibrotic effects in SSc skin and lungs, but failed to show treatment efficacy in SSc-ILD.[182] Imatinib mesylate, a tyro-sine kinase inhibitor, interferes in several profi-brotic pathways and has been proposed for use in SSc. Uncontrolled trials suggest improvement in skin scores with modest improvement in FVC as well.[183] Further study is needed to assess the role of imatinib in SSc-ILD; however, no effect was seen in a recent study in IPF.[184] Rituximab, an inhibitor of B-cell proliferation, has been shown in a small study of patients with SSc-ILD to improve FVC and DL_{CO}.[185] Other biologic agents and newer therapies require further study, including pirfeni-done and anti–connective tissue growth factor antibodies. Early data have supported the role of stem cell transplantation in SSc, with improvement in ground-glass opacities on HRCT as well as FVC.[186] Trials in the United States and Europe are enrolling patients to examine this high-risk strategy more fully.[187]

Lung transplantation may be considered for advanced fibrotic lung disease but has been controversial. SSc is considered a systemic disease that may increase overall morbidity and mortality after transplantation. In particular, concern has been raised about the role of gastro-esophageal reflux caused by motility issues in SSc that may predispose to chronic graft dysfunction. However, among carefully selected patients, early (1-year) and late (4-year) mortality seems to be similar to that of other groups, and patients with severe fibrotic lung disease without concomitant advanced GI or renal disease should be referred for evaluation.[93,95,188]

IDIOPATHIC INFLAMMATORY MYOPATHIES

The idiopathic inflammatory myopathies (IIMs) are autoimmune disorders typically affecting the skel-etal muscle, leading to inflammation and proximal muscle weakness.[189,190] Systemic involvement, including inflammation of the skin, lung, joints, and GI tract may be present.[191] In particular, the pres-ence of ILD has long been recognized and contrib-utes significantly to morbidity and mortality.[192–194] There are several subtypes of the IIMs, all of which may be complicated by ILD, including PM, DM, amyopathic DM (ADM), and the antisynthetase syndrome.

Criteria for classification of the IIMs are still in evolution. Initial diagnostic criteria proposed by Bohan and Peter[189,190] included the presence of symmetric proximal muscle weakness in combina-tion with increased serum muscle enzymes, typical electromyography and muscle biopsy find-ings, and typical rash; these criteria continue to be clinically useful. However, evolving immunohisto-chemical and pathologic features, as well as the discovery of myositis-related autoantibodies such as the anti-tRNA synthetase Jo-1, have led to the proposal of other classification schemes, although none is universally accepted.[195,196]

Clinical Features

The clinical presentation of PM/DM typically involves the subacute onset of proximal muscle symptoms, which may include myalgias, muscle fatigue, or frank weakness, in which patients complain of difficulty rising from a chair or lifting objects. In cases of DM, skin manifestations are present and may include the heliotrope rash, a violaceous discoloration of the eyelids; peri-orbital edema; Gottron papules, maculopapular erythematous lesions present on the extensor surface of the metacarpophalangeal and proximal interphalangeal joints of the hands; the shawl sign, poikilodermatous macules on the shoulders, arms, or upper back; and mechanic's hands, a scaly, cracked, hyperkeratotic erythema found on the lateral and palmar surfaces of hands and fingers, which has specific histopathologic features.[197,198]

Several pulmonary manifestations may be seen in the IIMs and are a major contributor to morbidity and mortality.[199,200] Primary muscle weakness may lead to hypoventilation and respiratory failure, and may be complicated by pneumonia caused by weak cough and poor airway clearance.[201–203] Aspiration pneumonia may occur because of respiratory muscle weakness but most commonly reflects the presence of skeletal muscle dysfunction in the pharynx and upper esophagus.[202]

Interstitial lung disease is the most common pulmonary complication of the IIMs, although, like other CTD-ILDs, the incidence of myositis-associated ILD (MA-ILD) is greatly affected by the mode of ascertainment, with high rates observed with the combined use of PFTs and HRCT. In a recent prospective study of patients with a new diagnosis of PM or DM, many of whom had no respiratory symptoms, 78% of patients were shown to have some lung involvement as defined by radiographic evidence (chest radiograph or HRCT abnormalities) or restrictive physiology and diffusion impairment on PFTs (total lung capacity and DL_{CO} <80% predicted).[204] Among a population of patients with anti–Jo-1 antibodies, 86% were shown to have ILD.[205] These numbers may be overestimates based on the lack of HRCT evidence of ILD for all patients, but they do suggest that parenchymal involvement is common and should be aggressively sought.

MA-ILD may occur concomitantly with the onset of myositis or skin rash but may precede the diagnosis of IIM.[194,206] Cases of DM with typical skin rash in association with ILD may occur without biochemical evidence for muscle involvement,

and is known as ADM.[207] The clinical course of MA-ILD is variable, ranging from a total lack of symptoms to fulminant hypoxemic respiratory failure, although many patients present subacutely and experience chronic, progressive disease.[199] Dyspnea and cough are the most common symptoms reported in MA-ILD. Almost one-third of patients with MA-ILD are asymptomatic, showing the need for evaluation of these patients with PFTs and chest imaging.[208] DM, and particularly ADM, may be more associated with an acute and fatal presentation, which is characterized by histopathologic findings of DAD, and resistance to treatment.[207,209,210] The strongest predictor for the onset of ILD in IIM is the presence of antisynthetase antibodies, particularly anti–Jo-1.[208,211]

The antisynthetase syndrome has been described to include ILD, myositis, arthritis, fever, Raynaud phenomenon, and mechanic's hands.[212] In many cases, only a few features are present, and, in many, the lung manifestations may predominate. In addition to anti–Jo-1, other antisynthetase antibodies (such as anti-PL7, anti-PL12, anti-EJ) have been associated with the development of ILD with IIM.[213] Particular antibodies may be more or less strongly associated with the development of ILD or myositis and subtypes based on antibody specificity may predict clinical course.[214,215] Among the myositis-associated antibodies, the presence of anti-SSA in conjunction with anti–Jo-1 has been associated with more severe and progressive ILD.[216,217]

Pulmonary Function Testing

PFTs are important in the assessment of MA-ILD and help assess disease severity and response to therapy. They also help to distinguish between the role of MA-ILD and diaphragmatic weakness, although this may not be straightforward.[218] Like other forms of ILD, PFTs in MA-ILD show restrictive physiology and reduced DL_{CO}. However, respiratory muscle insufficiency is also characterized by reductions in FVC and total lung capacity as well as reduction in other tests such as the maximum voluntary ventilation (MVV) and maximal inspiratory pressure (MIP) and expiratory pressure (MEP).[203] Reductions in the DL_{CO} may also be the result of pulmonary hypertension, which can coexist with ILD, or be caused by atelectasis from diaphragmatic weakness.[218]

Radiographic Features

HRCT findings are similar to those in other forms of CTD-ILD. In MA-ILD, the most common abnormalities are ground-glass opacities, reticular markings, and alveolar airspace opacities

(**Fig. 9**).[219] Honeycombing is less common. The radiographic findings suggest the underlying disorder (ie, dense consolidation reflecting DAD and OP; honeycombing reflecting UIP); however, these findings are not specific.[219] Micronodules, linear opacities, and traction bronchiectasis may also be observed.[219] Some studies have suggested that dense, peripheral consolidation in a pattern consistent with OP is associated with a better prognosis, whereas ground-glass opacities predict a worse outcome.[220,221]

Pathologic Features

Surgical lung biopsy is not typically obtained in the diagnosis of MA-ILD, and the role of pathologic diagnosis remains controversial. In studies reporting pathologic findings in MA-ILD, most patients have NSIP, with UIP and OP as the next most frequent possibilities, and DAD in a minority of patients.[218] Although some studies have suggested that DAD carries a poorer prognosis than either OP or cellular NSIP, it is not clear that pathologic pattern alters treatment choice, and other studies have not confirmed an impact of histopathologic pattern on overall survival.[54,194,199,222] In the setting of rapid-onset ILD, surgical biopsy may not be clinically feasible and may lead to postoperative complications in a patient who will likely receive high-dose corticosteroids and other immunosuppressive agents.

Treatment

All treatment is empiric in MA-ILD, because no controlled studies exist to guide treatment decisions. MA-ILD seems responsive to corticosteroids, but high doses may be required.[192,223] Corticosteroids continue to be the most common and widely accepted therapy for MA-ILD.[224] In acute, life-threatening disease, pulse dose regimens (1 g/d) of methylprednisolone may be required. Additional therapy is often needed in MA-ILD and may be added either for either steroid-sparing effect or for additional efficacy. In particular, some forms of MA-ILD with low creatine kinase levels may respond poorly to corticosteroids alone and require treatment with other agents.[225] Choice of agent often depends on clinician familiarity as well as on the severity of illness.

Azathioprine, an inhibitor of purine synthesis, is efficacious in treating myositis in the IIMs.[224] It is a commonly used agent in many CTD-ILDs and is often used in MA-ILD, although with few reports in the literature.[54,226] Cyclophosphamide is typically chosen for rapidly progressive or severe MA-ILD, either via monthly intravenous pulse infusions or oral therapy.[227] Pulse dosage between 300 and 800 mg/m^2 has been described to improve MA-ILD in treatment-resistant disease.[228] Methotrexate has long been used in the treatment of myositis in the IIMs and has been used in the treatment of MA-ILD.[224] However, the known pulmonary toxicity that may occur with this drug can be difficult to distinguish from progressive MA-ILD, making this agent less ideal.[229] Other agents such as cyclosporine, tacrolimus, MMF, intravenous immune globulin, and rituximab have all been used in small numbers of patients with refractory disease, and may be used in select situations.[225,230–235]

SJÖGREN SYNDROME

Sjögren syndrome is characterized by lymphocytic infiltration of the exocrine glands and marked B-cell hyperreactivity.[236] In particular, the salivary and lacrimal glands are affected, leading to the sicca syndrome characterized by dry eye (keratoconjunctivitis sicca) and dry mouth (xerostomia), often accompanied by arthritis.[237] When Sjögren syndrome is seen in isolation, it is called primary Sjögren syndrome. Secondary Sjögren syndrome may accompany other CTDs such as RA, SSc, SLE, and PM/DM.[238] In addition to the main sicca symptoms of Sjögren syndrome, involvement of the stomach, pancreas, kidney, and peripheral nervous system may occur.[238,239] Middle-aged women are most commonly affected.[240] The diagnosis depends on a combination of ocular and oral symptoms of dryness, objective testing for xerophthalmia and xerostomia, histopathologic features on minor salivary gland biopsy, and autoantibodies to Ro (anti-SSA) and/or La (anti-SSB).[241]

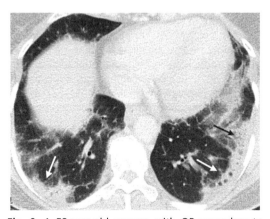

Fig. 9. A 58-year-old woman with OP secondary to PM. Axial images at the level of the lower thorax show peripheral, subpleural areas of consolidation, as indicated by the arrows.

Clinical Features

Like other forms of CTD-ILD, the prevalence of lung involvement in Sjögren syndrome depends on the methodology used to determine active disease and varies between 9% and 60%.[242] Although radiographic abnormalities observed on HRCT may be common, the prevalence of clinically significant pulmonary disease was 11% in a large cohort of patients with Sjögren syndrome.[243] Many patients are asymptomatic and lung involvement is mild and only slowly progressive.[242,244,245] Most commonly, lung involvement is manifested by both upper and lower airways disease, ILD, and lymphoproliferative disorders. Many patients complain of a dry cough (sicca cough), which is a result of xerosis of the airways caused by involvement of the submucosal glands.[246]

Symptoms of ILD most often include dyspnea and cough, with a minority complaining of chest pain and wheezing.[247] Sicca symptoms are present in most patients.[247] Inspiratory crackles are commonly found, although wheezing may also be present. Clubbing is rare.[247] PFTs are most often normal in patients with Sjögren syndrome but, among those with ILD, restriction and diffusion abnormalities predominate.[236,247,248] Care must be taken with interpretation, because airways obstruction is common in Sjögren syndrome and may lead to mixed obstructive and restrictive physiology.[249]

Radiographic Features

HRCT is abnormal in more than one-third of unselected patients with Sjögren syndrome.[250] Multiple abnormalities may be observed and include findings of large airways disease (bronchiectasis, bronchial wall thickening), small airways disease (air trapping, bronchiolectasis, centrilobular nodules, and tree-in-bud opacities), and interstitial disease (ground-glass opacities, air space consolidation, interlobular septal thickening, honeycombing, cysts and micronodules).[237,250,251] The presence of thin-walled cysts suggests the diagnosis of LIP, which is a lymphoproliferative disorder common in Sjögren syndrome (**Fig. 10**).[252,253] LIP is considered to be a steroid-responsive lung disease but may rarely evolve into lymphoma.[252,253] Findings that may suggest lymphoma include nonresolving air space consolidation, nodules greater than 1 cm in size, and enlarging lymph nodes.[254] If these features are present, biopsy should be considered. The presence of air trapping on expiratory films may be helpful in distinguishing small airways disease from ILD, and may be present in the absence of PFT abnormalities.[255] In general, in

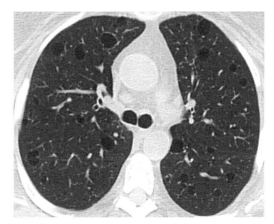

Fig. 10. A 63-year-old woman with Sjögren syndrome and lymphocytic interstitial pneumonia. Axial CT images through the upper thorax show multiple thin-walled cysts of varying sizes scattered throughout the lungs.

Sjögren syndrome–associated ILD (SS-ILD), HRCT features, and histopathology tend to correlate well, particularly for NSIP.[247,256]

Pathologic Features

Older studies of histologic pattern in Sjögren syndrome reported LIP as the most common ILD.[257] More recent studies, using the newer ERS/ATS classification of ILD, describe a higher frequency of NSIP, although with UIP, OP, and LIP also observed.[247,256] Rarely, primary pulmonary lymphoma and amyloidosis are found.[247] When CT features are typical for NSIP, biopsy need not be pursued but, when features that suggest lymphoma are present, tissue sampling is advisable.

Treatment

Treatment in SS-ILD is most often initiated with corticosteroids, although little is known about the optimal treatment. In some milder cases of LIP, observation without therapy may be reasonable.[247] In more advanced fibrotic lung disease, it is less clear that immunosuppressive therapy reverses the underlying injury, and it may expose the patient to excessive risk without significant benefit. In general, SS-ILD seems to be treatment responsive. When SS-ILD is treated, symptoms can improve rapidly, although objective treatment response may occur over months and may be incomplete.[247] The addition of steroid-sparing agents, such as azathioprine, may improve lung function but has not been rigorously studied and use of these agents is largely anecdotal.[257] Early data suggest that B-cell depletion with rituximab may play some role in the treatment of SS-ILD and deserves further study.[258,259]

SLE

SLE is an immune-mediated disease that most commonly occurs in younger women.[260] It typically presents with malar, discoid, and photosensitivity rashes, oral ulcers, nonerosive arthritis, glomerulonephritis, and hematologic abnormalities.[261] Autoantibodies including ANA, anti–double-stranded DNA (dsDNA), and anti-Smith are commonly detected and are part of the diagnostic criteria.[261] The most common form of pulmonary involvement in SLE is pleuritis, but parenchymal lung disease, pulmonary vascular disease, airways disease, and respiratory muscle dysfunction may all occur.[260] Diffuse parenchymal lung disease in SLE may have either acute or chronic presentation.

Acute Lupus Pneumonitis

One of the less common complications of SLE is acute lupus pneumonitis, which occurs in 1% to 12% of patients and may be the presenting feature of SLE.[262] Patients present with acute onset of fever, cough, dyspnea, and hypoxemia.[262] Acute respiratory failure requiring mechanical ventilatory support may occur. Physical examination may show bibasilar rales, and radiographic findings are significant for diffuse ground-glass and alveolar filling patterns on chest radiograph and HRCT.

In all forms of acute parenchymal lung disease in SLE, there is significant overlap in terms of presentation, with similar clinical history, radiographic findings, and progression. The most important piece of the clinical evaluation is to rule out infection. In particular, patients with SLE are at high risk for both bacterial and opportunistic infection. In addition to the common use of immunosuppressive medications, SLE itself is associated with innate immune dysfunction resulting from complement deficiency, immunoglobulin deficiency, defects in chemotaxis and phagocytosis, as well as functional asplenia.[263] Empiric antibiotics are typically begun in an acutely ill patient and bronchoalveolar lavage should be performed if clinically feasible, particularly in the patient already receiving immunosuppressive drugs.

Surgical lung biopsy is not always feasible or warranted in acute lupus pneumonitis, but, when performed, is nonspecific and commonly shows DAD characterized by hyaline membranes and type II pneumocyte proliferation and inflammation. Capillary inflammation and fibrin thrombi may be present, and immunofluorescence studies have shown immune complement deposition.[264]

Prognosis for acute lupus pneumonitis is generally thought to be poor, with older studies reporting mortalities of 50% and residual lung impairment among the survivors.[262] Newer data are not available to assess whether alterations in supportive care have changed these outcomes. Treatment is largely anecdotal, with emphasis on empiric antibiotics accompanied by a careful search for opportunistic infection, followed by corticosteroids. High doses are used for critically ill patients and include a 3-day pulse of methylprednisolone (1 g per day) followed by 1 to 2 mg/kg/d depending on clinical response. Additional cytotoxic therapies such as cyclophosphamide and azathioprine have been reported to improve lung function, but no well-controlled studies are available to guide practice.[265,266]

Diffuse Alveolar Hemorrhage

Diffuse alveolar hemorrhage (DAH) is also rare but, when it occurs, it contributes to high mortality and may be recurrent among survivors.[267,268] The clinical presentation is similar to that of acute lupus pneumonitis with the abrupt onset of dyspnea, cough, and hypoxemia. Fever may be present and hemoptysis may occur; however, at least half of patients may present without this feature.[267,269] Lupus nephritis or other active SLE involvement may be concomitant.

An acute drop in hematocrit may suggest the diagnosis. Radiographic findings may be initially unimpressive but can progress to diffuse ground-glass opacities and alveolar consolidation and can be indistinguishable from acute lupus pneumonitis, infectious pneumonia, or the acute respiratory distress syndrome (ARDS).[269] BAL is a crucial diagnostic step in the evaluation of these patients, both for the exclusion of infection, as well as for the diagnosis of DAH, which can be made with the observation of progressively bloody lavage fluid and hemosiderin-laden macrophages in the fluid. Among more clinically stable patients, DL_{CO} measurements obtained within the first 48 hours after the hemorrhage have been reported to show an increase of 30% more than baseline values while the erythrocytes are still within the alveoli.[269] Surgical lung biopsies are not typically performed in acutely ill patients. Histopathologic findings in DAH most commonly show bland hemorrhage, but some cases of capillaritis with immune complex deposition as well as small vessel vasculitis and microangiitis have been reported.[263,268,270]

DAH may be triggered by infection and initial treatment consists of empiric antibiotics, which may significantly improve survival.[269] High-dose corticosteroids are generally combined with intravenous cyclophosphamide.[267] Plasmapheresis may also improve survival.[271–273] MMF has been reported to be efficacious in maintaining remission from DAH episodes.[274]

Chronic ILD in SLE

Chronic ILD may be observed in SLE and has been reported as being less common than in other CTDs, with a reported prevalence of 3% to 13%.[275] However, subclinical disease is likely common, based on HRCT studies that estimate the prevalence of ILD at 38% among patients with lupus without previously diagnosed lung disease.[276] In some cases, an association is seen between ILD and anti-SSA antibodies, but it is unclear whether this is pathogenic and whether such findings describe an overlap with Sjögren syndrome.[277,278]

Like other forms of ILD, SLE-associated ILD (SLE-ILD) commonly presents with the insidious onset of dyspnea and occasional nonproductive cough. ILD may present acutely, as in acute lupus pneumonitis, and chronic lung disease may result from prior episodes of lupus pneumonitis.[262] ILD onset is associated with longer disease duration, male gender, older age, as well as later onset of SLE.[279]

HRCT findings in SLE-ILD are similar to those of other chronic ILD and show bibasilar-predominant reticulations and ground-glass with progression to traction bronchiectasis with some honeycombing. The most typical histopathologic patterns are NSIP, UIP, and LIP; however, surgical biopsy is rarely obtained.[60,280]

Treatment of SLE-ILD is not standardized and the choice to treat is an individualized decision based on clinical progression and radiographic findings. In particular, the presence of ground-glass opacities might suggest a more active alveolar inflammatory process with the possibility of treatment responsiveness. Corticosteroids are often used and, when chronic therapy is anticipated, steroid-sparing agents such as azathioprine and MMF are added. MMF has been shown to have a good safety profile in patients with CTD-ILD.[135,281] Cyclophosphamide has been used for refractory disease.[266] Rituximab has been reported to have controlled progressive and refractory ILD in 1 case.[282]

SUMMARY

Lung disease is a common manifestation of the CTDs and may be a presenting feature. Subclinical disease is common. Clinically apparent disease is often slowly progressive but may present in an acute fashion, contributing to high morbidity and mortality. Infection and drug reaction may share clinical features with CTD-ILD and should be considered when evaluating the patient with dyspnea and abnormal radiographic findings. Treatment of CTD-ILD is not well studied but typically includes corticosteroid therapy and immunosuppressive agents, as well as careful supportive care. Further study is needed for the many unanswered questions in this field.

REFERENCES

1. O'Donnell DE, Ora J, Webb KA, et al. Mechanisms of activity-related dyspnea in pulmonary diseases. Respir Physiol Neurobiol 2009;167(1):116–32.
2. Leslie KO, Trahan S, Gruden J. Pulmonary pathology of the rheumatic diseases. Semin Respir Crit Care Med 2007;28(4):369–78.
3. Roschmann RA, Rothenberg RJ. Pulmonary fibrosis in rheumatoid arthritis: a review of clinical features and therapy. Semin Arthritis Rheum 1987;16(3):174–85.
4. Khan S, Christopher-Stine L. Polymyositis, dermatomyositis, and autoimmune necrotizing myopathy: clinical features. Rheum Dis Clin North Am 2011; 37(2):143–58, v.
5. Hachulla E, Launay D. Diagnosis and classification of systemic sclerosis. Clin Rev Allergy Immunol 2010;40(2):78–83.
6. Arnett FC, Edworthy SM, Bloch DA, et al. The American Rheumatism Association 1987 revised criteria for the classification of rheumatoid arthritis. Arthritis Rheum 1988;31(3):315–24.
7. Katzap E, Barilla-LaBarca ML, Marder G. Antisynthetase syndrome. Curr Rheumatol Rep 2011; 13(3):175–81.
8. Lambova SN, Muller-Ladner U. The role of capillaroscopy in differentiation of primary and secondary Raynaud's phenomenon in rheumatic diseases: a review of the literature and two case reports. Rheumatol Int 2009;29(11):1263–71.
9. Gauhar UA, Gaffo AL, Alarcon GS. Pulmonary manifestations of rheumatoid arthritis. Semin Respir Crit Care Med 2007;28(4):430–40.
10. Raghu G, Collard HR, Egan JJ, et al. An official ATS/ERS/JRS/ALAT statement: idiopathic pulmonary fibrosis: evidence-based guidelines for diagnosis and management. Am J Respir Crit Care Med 2011;183(6):788–824.
11. Strange C, Highland KB. Interstitial lung disease in the patient who has connective tissue disease. Clin Chest Med 2004;25(3):549–59, vii.
12. Fischer A, Swigris JJ, du Bois RM, et al. Anti-synthetase syndrome in ANA and anti-Jo-1 negative

patients presenting with idiopathic interstitial pneumonia. Respir Med 2009;103(11):1719–24.

13. Fischer A, West SG, Swigris JJ, et al. Connective tissue disease-associated interstitial lung disease: a call for clarification. Chest 2010;138(2):251–6.

14. Popper MS, Bogdonoff ML, Hughes RL. Interstitial rheumatoid lung disease. A reassessment and review of the literature. Chest 1972;62(3):243–50.

15. Frank ST, Weg JG, Harkleroad LE, et al. Pulmonary dysfunction in rheumatoid disease. Chest 1973; 63(1):27–34.

16. Bjoraker JA, Ryu JH, Edwin MK, et al. Prognostic significance of histopathologic subsets in idiopathic pulmonary fibrosis. Am J Respir Crit Care Med 1998;157(1):199–203.

17. Chetta A, Aiello M, Foresi A, et al. Relationship between outcome measures of six-minute walk test and baseline lung function in patients with interstitial lung disease. Sarcoidosis Vasc Diffuse Lung Dis 2001;18(2):170–5.

18. Parker CM, Fitzpatrick MF, O'Donnell DE. Physiology of interstitial lung disease. In: Schwarz MI, King TE, editors. Interstitial lung disease. Shelton (CT): People's Medical Publishing House; 2011. p. 61–84.

19. Hughes JM, Lockwood DN, Jones HA, et al. DLCO/Q and diffusion limitation at rest and on exercise in patients with interstitial fibrosis. Respir Physiol 1991;83(2):155–66.

20. Harris-Eze AO, Sridhar G, Clemens RE, et al. Oxygen improves maximal exercise performance in interstitial lung disease. Am J Respir Crit Care Med 1994;150(6 Pt 1):1616–22.

21. Miller W. Diagnostic thoracic imaging. New York: McGraw-Hill; 2006. p. 68.

22. Stack BH, Grant IW. Rheumatoid interstitial lung disease. Br J Dis Chest 1965;59(4):202–11.

23. Kim EA, Lee KS, Johkoh T, et al. Interstitial lung diseases associated with collagen vascular diseases: radiologic and histopathologic findings. Radiographics 2002;22(Spec No):S151–65.

24. Tanaka N, Kim JS, Newell JD, et al. Rheumatoid arthritis-related lung diseases: CT findings. Radiology 2004;232(1):81–91.

25. Mori S, Cho I, Koga Y, et al. Comparison of pulmonary abnormalities on high-resolution computed tomography in patients with early versus long-standing rheumatoid arthritis. J Rheumatol 2008; 35(8):1513–21.

26. Kocheril SV, Appleton BE, Somers EC, et al. Comparison of disease progression and mortality of connective tissue disease-related interstitial lung disease and idiopathic interstitial pneumonia. Arthritis Rheum 2005;53(4):549–57.

27. Hunninghake GW, Zimmerman MB, Schwartz DA, et al. Utility of a lung biopsy for the diagnosis of idiopathic pulmonary fibrosis. Am J Respir Crit Care Med 2001;164(2):193–6.

28. Schmidt SL, Sundaram B, Flaherty KR. Diagnosing fibrotic lung disease: when is high-resolution computed tomography sufficient to make a diagnosis of idiopathic pulmonary fibrosis? Respirology 2009;14(7):934–9.

29. Hunninghake GW, Lynch DA, Galvin JR, et al. Radiologic findings are strongly associated with a pathologic diagnosis of usual interstitial pneumonia. Chest 2003;124(4):1215–23.

30. Flaherty KR, Toews GB, Travis WD, et al. Clinical significance of histological classification of idiopathic interstitial pneumonia. Eur Respir J 2002; 19(2):275–83.

31. Kim EJ, Collard HR, King TE Jr. Rheumatoid arthritis-associated interstitial lung disease: the relevance of histopathologic and radiographic pattern. Chest 2009;136(5):1397–405.

32. Kim TS, Lee KS, Chung MP, et al. Nonspecific interstitial pneumonia with fibrosis: high-resolution CT and pathologic findings. AJR Am J Roentgenol 1998;171(6):1645–50.

33. Kligerman SJ, Groshong S, Brown KK, et al. Nonspecific interstitial pneumonia: radiologic, clinical, and pathologic considerations. Radiographics 2009;29(1):73–87.

34. Travis WD, Hunninghake G, King TE Jr, et al. Idiopathic nonspecific interstitial pneumonia: report of an American Thoracic Society project. Am J Respir Crit Care Med 2008;177(12):1338–47.

35. Park JS, Lee KS, Kim JS, et al. Nonspecific interstitial pneumonia with fibrosis: radiographic and CT findings in seven patients. Radiology 1995;195(3): 645–8.

36. Lynch DA, Travis WD, Muller NL, et al. Idiopathic interstitial pneumonias: CT features. Radiology 2005;236(1):10–21.

37. Dawson JK, Fewins HE, Desmond J, et al. Predictors of progression of HRCT diagnosed fibrosing alveolitis in patients with rheumatoid arthritis. Ann Rheum Dis 2002;61(6):517–21.

38. Shin KM, Lee KS, Chung MP, et al. Prognostic determinants among clinical, thin-section CT, and histopathologic findings for fibrotic idiopathic interstitial pneumonias: tertiary hospital study. Radiology 2008;249(1):328–37.

39. Committee, TBCGS. Bronchoalveolar lavage constituents in healthy individuals, idiopathic pulmonary fibrosis, and selected comparison groups. The BAL Cooperative Group Steering Committee. Am Rev Respir Dis 1990;141(5 Pt 2):S169–202.

40. Strange C, Bolster MB, Roth MD, et al. Bronchoalveolar lavage and response to cyclophosphamide in scleroderma interstitial lung disease. Am J Respir Crit Care Med 2008;177(1):91–8.

41. Nagasawa Y, Takada I, Shimizu I, et al. Inflammatory cells in lung disease associated with rheumatoid arthritis. Intern Med 2009;48(14):1209–17.

42. Biederer J, Schnabel A, Muhle C, et al. Correlation between HRCT findings, pulmonary function tests and bronchoalveolar lavage cytology in interstitial lung disease associated with rheumatoid arthritis. Eur Radiol 2004;14(2):272–80.

43. Garcia JG, James HL, Zinkgraf S, et al. Lower respiratory tract abnormalities in rheumatoid interstitial lung disease. Potential role of neutrophils in lung injury. Am Rev Respir Dis 1987;136(4):811–7.

44. Komocsi A, Kumanovics G, Zibotics H, et al. Alveolitis may persist during treatment that sufficiently controls muscle inflammation in myositis. Rheumatol Int 2001;20(3):113–8.

45. Meyer KC, Raghu G. Bronchoalveolar lavage for the evaluation of interstitial lung disease: is it clinically useful? Eur Respir J 2011;38(4):761–9.

46. Kowal-Bielecka O, Kowal K, Highland KB, et al. Bronchoalveolar lavage fluid in scleroderma interstitial lung disease: technical aspects and clinical correlations: review of the literature. Semin Arthritis Rheum 2010;40(1):73–88.

47. Haslam PL, Baughman RP. Report of ERS Task Force: guidelines for measurement of acellular components and standardization of BAL. Eur Respir J 1999;14(2):245–8.

48. Baughman RP. Technical aspects of bronchoalveolar lavage: recommendations for a standard procedure. Semin Respir Crit Care Med 2007;28(5):475–85.

49. Costabel U, Guzman J, Bonella F, et al. Bronchoalveolar lavage in other interstitial lung diseases. Semin Respir Crit Care Med 2007;28(5):514–24.

50. Schnabel A, Richter C, Bauerfeind S, et al. Bronchoalveolar lavage cell profile in methotrexate induced pneumonitis. Thorax 1997;52(4):377–9.

51. Ramirez P, Valencia M, Torres A. Bronchoalveolar lavage to diagnose respiratory infections. Semin Respir Crit Care Med 2007;28(5):525–33.

52. American Thoracic Society, European Respiratory Society. American Thoracic Society/European Respiratory Society International Multidisciplinary Consensus Classification of the Idiopathic Interstitial Pneumonias. This joint statement of the American Thoracic Society (ATS), and the European Respiratory Society (ERS) was adopted by the ATS board of directors, June 2001 and by the ERS Executive Committee, June 2001. Am J Respir Crit Care Med 2002;165(2):277–304.

53. Lee HK, Kim DS, Yoo B, et al. Histopathologic pattern and clinical features of rheumatoid arthritis-associated interstitial lung disease. Chest 2005;127(6):2019–27.

54. Kim DS, Yoo B, Lee JS, et al. The major histopathologic pattern of pulmonary fibrosis in scleroderma is nonspecific interstitial pneumonia. Sarcoidosis Vasc Diffuse Lung Dis 2002;19(2):121–7.

55. Douglas WW, Tazelaar HD, Hartman TE, et al. Polymyositis-dermatomyositis-associated interstitial lung disease. Am J Respir Crit Care Med 2001;164(7):1182–5.

56. Kim DS. Interstitial lung disease in rheumatoid arthritis: recent advances. Curr Opin Pulm Med 2006;12(5):346–53.

57. Yousem SA, Colby TV, Carrington CB. Lung biopsy in rheumatoid arthritis. Am Rev Respir Dis 1985;131(5):770–7.

58. Riha RL, Duhig EE, Clarke BE, et al. Survival of patients with biopsy-proven usual interstitial pneumonia and nonspecific interstitial pneumonia. Eur Respir J 2002;19(6):1114–8.

59. Park JH, Kim DS, Park IN, et al. Prognosis of fibrotic interstitial pneumonia: idiopathic versus collagen vascular disease-related subtypes. Am J Respir Crit Care Med 2007;175(7):705–11.

60. Tansey D, Wells AU, Colby TV, et al. Variations in histological patterns of interstitial pneumonia between connective tissue disorders and their relationship to prognosis. Histopathology 2004;44(6):585–96.

61. Kim EJ, Elicker BM, Maldonado F, et al. Usual interstitial pneumonia in rheumatoid arthritis-associated interstitial lung disease. Eur Respir J 2010;35(6):1322–8.

62. Moghadam-Kia S, Werth VP. Prevention and treatment of systemic glucocorticoid side effects. Int J Dermatol 2010;49(3):239–48.

63. Bradley B, Branley HM, Egan JJ, et al. Interstitial lung disease guideline: the British Thoracic Society in collaboration with the Thoracic Society of Australia and New Zealand and the Irish Thoracic Society. Thorax 2008;63(Suppl 5):v1–58.

64. Clark M, Cooper B, Singh S, et al. A survey of nocturnal hypoxaemia and health related quality of life in patients with cryptogenic fibrosing alveolitis. Thorax 2001;56(6):482–6.

65. Nici L, Donner C, Wouters E, et al. American Thoracic Society/European Respiratory Society statement on pulmonary rehabilitation. Am J Respir Crit Care Med 2006;173(12):1390–413.

66. Laviolette L, Bourbeau J, Bernard S, et al. Assessing the impact of pulmonary rehabilitation on functional status in COPD. Thorax 2008;63(2):115–21.

67. Swigris JJ, Brown KK, Make BJ, et al. Pulmonary rehabilitation in idiopathic pulmonary fibrosis: a call for continued investigation. Respir Med 2008;102(12):1675–80.

68. Holland A, Hill C. Physical training for interstitial lung disease. Cochrane Database Syst Rev 2008;4:CD006322.

69. Garvey C. Interstitial lung disease and pulmonary rehabilitation. J Cardiopulm Rehabil Prev 2010;30(3):141–6.

70. Salhi B, Troosters T, Behaegel M, et al. Effects of pulmonary rehabilitation in patients with restrictive lung diseases. Chest 2010;137(2):273–9.

71. Ryerson CJ, Garvey C, Collard HR. Pulmonary rehabilitation for interstitial lung disease. Chest 2010;138(1):240–1 [author reply: 241–2].

72. Singer HK, Ruchinskas RA, Riley KC, et al. The psychological impact of end-stage lung disease. Chest 2001;120(4):1246–52.

73. Ponnuswamy A, Manikandan R, Sabetpour A, et al. Association between ischaemic heart disease and interstitial lung disease: a case-control study. Respir Med 2009;103(4):503–7.

74. Nathan SD, Basavaraj A, Reichner C, et al. Prevalence and impact of coronary artery disease in idiopathic pulmonary fibrosis. Respir Med 2010; 104(7):1035–41.

75. Villa-Forte A, Mandell BF. Cardiovascular disorders and rheumatic disease. Rev Esp Cardiol 2011; 64(9):809–17 [in Spanish].

76. Adzic TN, Pesut DP, Nagorni-Obradovic LM, et al. Clinical features of lung cancer in patients with connective tissue diseases: a 10-year hospital based study. Respir Med 2008;102(4):620–4.

77. Khurana R, Wolf R, Berney S, et al. Risk of development of lung cancer is increased in patients with rheumatoid arthritis: a large case control study in US veterans. J Rheumatol 2008;35(9):1704–8.

78. Lancaster LH, Mason WR, Parnell JA, et al. Obstructive sleep apnea is common in idiopathic pulmonary fibrosis. Chest 2009;136(3):772–8.

79. Mermigkis C, Stagaki E, Tryfon S, et al. How common is sleep-disordered breathing in patients with idiopathic pulmonary fibrosis? Sleep Breath 2010; 14(4):387–90.

80. Rasche K, Orth M. Sleep and breathing in idiopathic pulmonary fibrosis. J Physiol Pharmacol 2009;60(Suppl 5):13–4.

81. Sode BF, Dahl M, Nielsen SF, et al. Venous thromboembolism and risk of idiopathic interstitial pneumonia: a nationwide study. Am J Respir Crit Care Med 2010;181(10):1085–92.

82. Petri M. Update on anti-phospholipid antibodies in SLE: the Hopkins' Lupus Cohort. Lupus 2010; 19(4):419–23.

83. Tobin RW, Pope CE 2nd, Pellegrini CA, et al. Increased prevalence of gastroesophageal reflux in patients with idiopathic pulmonary fibrosis. Am J Respir Crit Care Med 1998;158(6):1804–8.

84. Raghu G, Freudenberger TD, Yang S, et al. High prevalence of abnormal acid gastro-oesophageal reflux in idiopathic pulmonary fibrosis. Eur Respir J 2006;27(1):136–42.

85. Raghu G, Yang ST, Spada C, et al. Sole treatment of acid gastroesophageal reflux in idiopathic pulmonary fibrosis: a case series. Chest 2006; 129(3):794–800.

86. Christmann RB, Wells AU, Capelozzi VL, et al. Gastroesophageal reflux incites interstitial lung disease in systemic sclerosis: clinical, radiologic, histopathologic, and treatment evidence. Semin Arthritis Rheum 2010;40(3):241–9.

87. de Souza RB, Borges CT, Capelozzi VL, et al. Centrilobular fibrosis: an underrecognized pattern in systemic sclerosis. Respiration 2009;77(4):389–97.

88. Patel NM, Lederer DJ, Borczuk AC, et al. Pulmonary hypertension in idiopathic pulmonary fibrosis. Chest 2007;132(3):998–1006.

89. Goldberg A. Pulmonary arterial hypertension in connective tissue diseases. Cardiol Rev 2010; 18(2):85–8.

90. Corte TJ, Wort SJ, Wells AU. Pulmonary hypertension in idiopathic pulmonary fibrosis: a review. Sarcoidosis Vasc Diffuse Lung Dis 2009;26(1): 7–19.

91. Mittoo S, Jacob T, Craig A, et al. Treatment of pulmonary hypertension in patients with connective tissue disease and interstitial lung disease. Can Respir J 2010;17(6):282–6.

92. Hassoun PM. Pulmonary arterial hypertension complicating connective tissue diseases. Semin Respir Crit Care Med 2009;30(4):429–39.

93. Saggar R, Khanna D, Furst DE, et al. Systemic sclerosis and bilateral lung transplantation: a single centre experience. Eur Respir J 2010;36(4): 893–900.

94. Gasper WJ, Sweet MP, Golden JA, et al. Lung transplantation in patients with connective tissue disorders and esophageal dysmotility. Dis Esophagus 2008;21(7):650–5.

95. Shitrit D, Amital A, Peled N, et al. Lung transplantation in patients with scleroderma: case series, review of the literature, and criteria for transplantation. Clin Transplant 2009;23(2):178–83.

96. O'Beirne S, Counihan IP, Keane MP. Interstitial lung disease and lung transplantation. Semin Respir Crit Care Med 2010;31(2):139–46.

97. Martinez FJ, Safrin S, Weycker D, et al. The clinical course of patients with idiopathic pulmonary fibrosis. Ann Intern Med 2005;142(12 Pt 1):963–7.

98. Mogulkoc N, Brutsche MH, Bishop PW, et al. Pulmonary function in idiopathic pulmonary fibrosis and referral for lung transplantation. Am J Respir Crit Care Med 2001;164(1):103–8.

99. Merlo CA, Orens JB. Candidate selection, overall results, and choosing the right operation. Semin Respir Crit Care Med 2010;31(2):99–107.

100. Aletaha D, Neogi T, Silman AJ, et al. 2010 Rheumatoid Arthritis Classification Criteria: an American College of Rheumatology/European League Against Rheumatism collaborative initiative. Arthritis Rheum 2010;62(9):2569–81.

101. Klareskog L, Catrina AI, Paget S. Rheumatoid arthritis. Lancet 2009;373(9664):659–72.

102. Gabriel SE, Michaud K. Epidemiological studies in incidence, prevalence, mortality, and comorbidity of the rheumatic diseases. Arthritis Res Ther 2009;11(3):229.

103. Spector TD. Rheumatoid arthritis. Rheum Dis Clin North Am 1990;16(3):513–37.

104. Mori S, Cho I, Koga Y, et al. A simultaneous onset of organizing pneumonia and rheumatoid arthritis, along with a review of the literature. Mod Rheumatol 2008;18(1):60–6.

105. Gochuico BR, Avila NA, Chow CK, et al. Progressive preclinical interstitial lung disease in rheumatoid arthritis. Arch Intern Med 2008;168(2):159–66.

106. Suzuki A, Ohosone Y, Obana M, et al. Cause of death in 81 autopsied patients with rheumatoid arthritis. J Rheumatol 1994;21(1):33–6.

107. Hakala M. Poor prognosis in patients with rheumatoid arthritis hospitalized for interstitial lung fibrosis. Chest 1988;93(1):114–8.

108. King TE, Kim EJ, Kinder BW. Connective tissue diseases. In: Schwarz MI, King TE, editors. Interstitial lung disease. Shelton (CT): People's Medical Publishing House; 2011. p. 689–764.

109. Christie GS. Pulmonary lesions in rheumatoid arthritis. Australas Ann Med 1954;3(1):49–58.

110. Dixon AS, Ball J. Honeycomb lung and chronic rheumatoid arthritis; a case report. Ann Rheum Dis 1957;16(2):241–5.

111. Ellman P, Ball RE. Rheumatoid disease with joint and pulmonary manifestations. Br Med J 1948; 2(4583):816–20.

112. Catterall M, Rowell NR. Respiratory function studies in patients with certain connective tissue diseases. Br J Dermatol 1965;77:221–5.

113. Dawson JK, Fewins HE, Desmond J, et al. Fibrosing alveolitis in patients with rheumatoid arthritis as assessed by high resolution computed tomography, chest radiography, and pulmonary function tests. Thorax 2001;56(8):622–7.

114. Gabbay E, Tarala R, Will R, et al. Interstitial lung disease in recent onset rheumatoid arthritis. Am J Respir Crit Care Med 1997;156(2 Pt 1):528–35.

115. Bilgici A, Ulusoy H, Kuru O, et al. Pulmonary involvement in rheumatoid arthritis. Rheumatol Int 2005;25(6):429–35.

116. Turesson C, O'Fallon WM, Crowson CS, et al. Occurrence of extraarticular disease manifestations is associated with excess mortality in a community based cohort of patients with rheumatoid arthritis. J Rheumatol 2002;29(1):62–7.

117. Cimmino MA, Salvarani C, Macchioni P, et al. Extraarticular manifestations in 587 Italian patients with rheumatoid arthritis. Rheumatol Int 2000;19(6): 213–7.

118. Brannan HM, Good CA, Divertie MB, et al. Pulmonary disease associated with rheumatoid arthritis. JAMA 1964;189:914–8.

119. Gizinski AM, Mascolo M, Loucks JL, et al. Rheumatoid arthritis (RA)-specific autoantibodies in patients with interstitial lung disease and absence of clinically apparent articular RA. Clin Rheumatol 2009;28(5):611–3.

120. Akira M, Sakatani M, Hara H. Thin-section CT findings in rheumatoid arthritis-associated lung disease: CT patterns and their courses. J Comput Assist Tomogr 1999;23(6):941–8.

121. Sumikawa H, Johkoh T, Ichikado K, et al. Nonspecific interstitial pneumonia: histologic correlation with high-resolution CT in 29 patients. Eur J Radiol 2009;70(1):35–40.

122. Hubbard R, Venn A. The impact of coexisting connective tissue disease on survival in patients with fibrosing alveolitis. Rheumatology (Oxford) 2002;41(6):676–9.

123. Cannon GW. Methotrexate pulmonary toxicity. Rheum Dis Clin North Am 1997;23(4):917–37.

124. Ito S, Sumida T. Interstitial lung disease associated with leflunomide. Intern Med 2004;43(12):1103–4.

125. Kamata Y, Nara H, Kamimura T, et al. Rheumatoid arthritis complicated with acute interstitial pneumonia induced by leflunomide as an adverse reaction. Intern Med 2004;43(12):1201–4.

126. Suissa S, Hudson M, Ernst P. Leflunomide use and the risk of interstitial lung disease in rheumatoid arthritis. Arthritis Rheum 2006;54(5):1435–9.

127. Huggett MT, Armstrong R. Adalimumab-associated pulmonary fibrosis. Rheumatology (Oxford) 2006; 45(10):1312–3.

128. Tournadre A, Ledoux-Eberst J, Poujol D, et al. Exacerbation of interstitial lung disease during etanercept therapy: two cases. Joint Bone Spine 2008;75(2):215–8.

129. Villeneuve E, St-Pierre A, Haraoui B. Interstitial pneumonitis associated with infliximab therapy. J Rheumatol 2006;33(6):1189–93.

130. Saag KG, Kolluri S, Koehnke RK, et al. Rheumatoid arthritis lung disease. Determinants of radiographic and physiologic abnormalities. Arthritis Rheum 1996;39(10):1711–9.

131. Kinder AJ, Hassell AB, Brand J, et al. The treatment of inflammatory arthritis with methotrexate in clinical practice: treatment duration and incidence of adverse drug reactions. Rheumatology (Oxford) 2005;44(1):61–6.

132. Imokawa S, Colby TV, Leslie KO, et al. Methotrexate pneumonitis: review of the literature and histopathological findings in nine patients. Eur Respir J 2000;15(2):373–81.

133. Chang HK, Park W, Ryu DS. Successful treatment of progressive rheumatoid interstitial lung disease with cyclosporine: a case report. J Korean Med Sci 2002;17(2):270–3.

134. Kelly C, Saravanan V. Treatment strategies for a rheumatoid arthritis patient with interstitial lung

disease. Expert Opin Pharmacother 2008;9(18): 3221–30.

135. Saketkoo LA, Espinoza LR. Experience of mycophe-nolate mofetil in 10 patients with autoimmune-related interstitial lung disease demonstrates promising effects. Am J Med Sci 2009;337(5):329–35.

136. Saketkoo LA, Espinoza LR. Rheumatoid arthritis interstitial lung disease: mycophenolate mofetil as an antifibrotic and disease-modifying antirheu-matic drug. Arch Intern Med 2008;168(15):1718–9.

137. Vassallo R, Matteson E, Thomas CF Jr. Clinical response of rheumatoid arthritis-associated pulmo-nary fibrosis to tumor necrosis factor-alpha inhibi-tion. Chest 2002;122(3):1093–6.

138. Hassoun P. Lung involvement in systemic sclerosis. Presse Med 2011;40(1 Pt 2):e3–17.

139. Castelino FV, Varga J. Interstitial lung disease in connective tissue diseases: evolving concepts of pathogenesis and management. Arthritis Res Ther 2010;12(4):213.

140. Steen VD, Medsger TA. Changes in causes of death in systemic sclerosis, 1972-2002. Ann Rheum Dis 2007;66(7):940–4.

141. Wells AU, Steen V, Valentini G. Pulmonary compli-cations: one of the most challenging complications of systemic sclerosis. Rheumatology (Oxford) 2009;48(Suppl 3):iii40–4.

142. De Santis M, Bosello S, La Torre G, et al. Functional, radiological and biological markers of alveolitis and infections of the lower respiratory tract in patients with systemic sclerosis. Respir Res 2005;6:96.

143. Highland KB, Garin MC, Brown KK. The spectrum of scleroderma lung disease. Semin Respir Crit Care Med 2007;28(4):418–29.

144. D'Angelo WA, Fries JF, Masi AT, et al. Pathologic observations in systemic sclerosis (scleroderma). A study of fifty-eight autopsy cases and fifty-eight matched controls. Am J Med 1969;46(3):428–40.

145. Ostojic P, Damjanov N. Different clinical features in patients with limited and diffuse cutaneous systemic sclerosis. Clin Rheumatol 2006;25(4):453–7.

146. Toya SP, Tzelepis GE. The many faces of sclero-derma sine scleroderma: a literature review focusing on cardiopulmonary complications. Rheu-matol Int 2009;29(8):861–8.

147. Wells AU, Hansell DM, Rubens MB, et al. Fibrosing alveolitis in systemic sclerosis: indices of lung func-tion in relation to extent of disease on computed tomography. Arthritis Rheum 1997;40(7):1229–36.

148. Steen V, Medsger TA Jr. Predictors of isolated pulmonary hypertension in patients with systemic sclerosis and limited cutaneous involvement. Arthritis Rheum 2003;48(2):516–22.

149. Bouros D, Wells AU, Nicholson AG, et al. Histopath-ologic subsets of fibrosing alveolitis in patients with systemic sclerosis and their relationship to outcome. Am J Respir Crit Care Med 2002;165(12):1581–6.

150. Plastiras SC, Karadimitrakis SP, Ziakas PD, et al. Scleroderma lung: initial forced vital capacity as predictor of pulmonary function decline. Arthritis Rheum 2006;55(4):598–602.

151. Assassi S, Del Junco D, Sutter K, et al. Clinical and genetic factors predictive of mortality in early systemic sclerosis. Arthritis Rheum 2009;61(10): 1403–11.

152. Steen VD, Conte C, Owens GR, et al. Severe restrictive lung disease in systemic sclerosis. Arthritis Rheum 1994;37(9):1283–9.

153. Assassi S, Sharif R, Lasky RE, et al. Predictors of interstitial lung disease in early systemic sclerosis: a prospective longitudinal study of the GENISOS cohort. Arthritis Res Ther 2010;12(5):R166.

154. Garin MC, Highland KB, Silver RM, et al. Limita-tions to the 6-minute walk test in interstitial lung disease and pulmonary hypertension in sclero-derma. J Rheumatol 2009;36(2):330–6.

155. Pignone A, Matucci-Cerinic M, Lombardi A, et al. High resolution computed tomography in systemic sclerosis. Real diagnostic utilities in the assess-ment of pulmonary involvement and comparison with other modalities of lung investigation. Clin Rheumatol 1992;11(4):465–72.

156. Desai SR, Veeraraghavan S, Hansell DM, et al. CT features of lung disease in patients with systemic sclerosis: comparison with idiopathic pulmonary fibrosis and nonspecific interstitial pneumonia. Radiology 2004;232(2):560–7.

157. Launay D, Remy-Jardin M, Michon-Pasturel U, et al. High resolution computed tomography in fibrosing alveolitis associated with systemic sclerosis. J Rheumatol 2006;33(9):1789–801.

158. Shah RM, Jimenez S, Wechsler R. Significance of ground-glass opacity on HRCT in long-term follow-up of patients with systemic sclerosis. J Thorac Imaging 2007;22(2):120–4.

159. Kim HG, Tashkin DP, Clements PJ, et al. A computer-aided diagnosis system for quantita-tive scoring of extent of lung fibrosis in sclero-derma patients. Clin Exp Rheumatol 2010;28(5 Suppl 62):S26–35.

160. Camiciottoli G, Orlandi I, Bartolucci M, et al. Lung CT densitometry in systemic sclerosis: correlation with lung function, exercise testing, and quality of life. Chest 2007;131(3):672–81.

161. Goh NS, Desai SR, Veeraraghavan S, et al. Intersti-tial lung disease in systemic sclerosis: a simple staging system. Am J Respir Crit Care Med 2008; 177(11):1248–54.

162. Strollo D, Goldin J. Imaging lung disease in systemic sclerosis. Curr Rheumatol Rep 2010; 12(2):156–61.

163. Ebert EC. Esophageal disease in progressive systemic sclerosis. Curr Treat Options Gastroenter-ol 2008;11(1):64–9.

164. Johnson DA, Drane WE, Curran J, et al. Pulmonary disease in progressive systemic sclerosis. A complication of gastroesophageal reflux and occult aspiration? Arch Intern Med 1989;149(3): 589–93.

165. Denis P, Ducrotte P, Pasquis P, et al. Esophageal motility and pulmonary function in progressive systemic sclerosis. Respiration 1981;42(1):21–4.

166. Lock G, Pfeifer M, Straub RH, et al. Association of esophageal dysfunction and pulmonary function impairment in systemic sclerosis. Am J Gastroenterol 1998;93(3):341–5.

167. Marie I, Dominique S, Levesque H, et al. Esophageal involvement and pulmonary manifestations in systemic sclerosis. Arthritis Rheum 2001;45(4): 346–54.

168. Steen VD, Medsger TA Jr. Case-control study of corticosteroids and other drugs that either precipitate or protect from the development of scleroderma renal crisis. Arthritis Rheum 1998;41(9): 1613 9.

169. Steen VD, Lanz JK Jr, Conte C, et al. Therapy for severe interstitial lung disease in systemic sclerosis. A retrospective study. Arthritis Rheum 1994; 37(9):1290–6.

170. Akesson A, Scheja A, Lundin A, et al. Improved pulmonary function in systemic sclerosis after treatment with cyclophosphamide. Arthritis Rheum 1994;37(5):729–35.

171. White B, Moore WC, Wigley FM, et al. Cyclophosphamide is associated with pulmonary function and survival benefit in patients with scleroderma and alveolitis. Ann Intern Med 2000;132(12):947–54.

172. Tashkin DP, Elashoff R, Clements PJ, et al. Cyclophosphamide versus placebo in scleroderma lung disease. N Engl J Med 2006;354(25):2655–66.

173. Martinez FJ, McCune WJ. Cyclophosphamide for scleroderma lung disease. N Engl J Med 2006; 354(25).2707–9.

174. Tashkin DP, Elashoff R, Clements PJ, et al. Effects of 1-year treatment with cyclophosphamide on outcomes at 2 years in scleroderma lung disease. Am J Respir Crit Care Med 2007;176(10):1026–34.

175. Wells AU, Latsi P, McCune WJ. Daily cyclophosphamide for scleroderma: are patients with the most to gain underrepresented in this trial? Am J Respir Crit Care Med 2007;176(10):952–3.

176. Hoyles RK, Ellis RW, Wellsbury J, et al. A multicenter, prospective, randomized, double-blind, placebo-controlled trial of corticosteroids and intravenous cyclophosphamide followed by oral azathioprine for the treatment of pulmonary fibrosis in scleroderma. Arthritis Rheum 2006; 54(12):3962–70.

177. Yiannopoulos G, Pastromas V, Antonopoulos I, et al. Combination of intravenous pulses of cyclophosphamide and methylprednizolone in patients with systemic sclerosis and interstitial lung disease. Rheumatol Int 2007;27(4):357–61.

178. Zamora AC, Wolters PJ, Collard HR, et al. Use of mycophenolate mofetil to treat scleroderma-associated interstitial lung disease. Respir Med 2008;102(1):150–5.

179. Gerbino AJ, Goss CH, Molitor JA. Effect of mycophenolate mofetil on pulmonary function in scleroderma-associated interstitial lung disease. Chest 2008;133(2):455–60.

180. Dheda K, Lalloo UG, Cassim B, et al. Experience with azathioprine in systemic sclerosis associated with interstitial lung disease. Clin Rheumatol 2004;23(4):306–9.

181. Berezne A, Ranque B, Valeyre D, et al. Therapeutic strategy combining intravenous cyclophosphamide followed by oral azathioprine to treat worsening interstitial lung disease associated with systemic sclerosis: a retrospective multicenter open-label study. J Rheumatol 2008;35(6):1064–72.

182. Seibold JR, Denton CP, Furst DE, et al. Randomized, prospective, placebo-controlled trial of bosentan in interstitial lung disease secondary to systemic sclerosis. Arthritis Rheum 2010;62(7): 2101–8.

183. Spiera RF, Gordon JK, Mersten JN, et al. Imatinib mesylate (Gleevec) in the treatment of diffuse cutaneous systemic sclerosis: results of a 1-year, phase IIa, single-arm, open-label clinical trial. Ann Rheum Dis 2010;70(6):1003–9.

184. Daniels CE, Lasky JA, Limper AH, et al. Imatinib treatment for idiopathic pulmonary fibrosis: randomized placebo-controlled trial results. Am J Respir Crit Care Med 2009;181(6):604–10.

185. Daoussis D, Liossis SN, Tsamandas AC, et al. Experience with rituximab in scleroderma: results from a 1-year, proof-of-principle study. Rheumatology (Oxford) 2010;49(2):271–80.

186. Tsukamoto H, Nagafuji K, Horiuchi T, et al. A phase I-II trial of autologous peripheral blood stem cell transplantation in the treatment of refractory autoimmune disease. Ann Rheum Dis 2006;65(4): 508–14.

187. Farge D, Nash R, Laar JM. Autologous stem cell transplantation for systemic sclerosis. Autoimmunity 2008;41(8):616–24.

188. Rosas V, Conte JV, Yang SC, et al. Lung transplantation and systemic sclerosis. Ann Transplant 2000; 5(3):38–43.

189. Bohan A, Peter JB. Polymyositis and dermatomyositis (first of two parts). N Engl J Med 1975;292(7):344–7.

190. Bohan A, Peter JB. Polymyositis and dermatomyositis (second of two parts). N Engl J Med 1975; 292(8):403–7.

191. Spiera R, Kagen L. Extramuscular manifestations in idiopathic inflammatory myopathies. Curr Opin Rheumatol 1998;10(6):556–61.

192. Frazier AR, Miller RD. Interstitial pneumonitis in association with polymyositis and dermatomyositis. Chest 1974;65(4):403–7.

193. Schwarz MI, Matthay RA, Sahn SA, et al. Interstitial lung disease in polymyositis and dermatomyositis: analysis of six cases and review of the literature. Medicine (Baltimore) 1976;55(1):89–104.

194. Cottin V, Thivolet-Bejui F, Reynaud-Gaubert M, et al. Interstitial lung disease in amyopathic dermatomyositis, dermatomyositis and polymyositis. Eur Respir J 2003;22(2):245–50.

195. Dalakas MC, Hohlfeld R. Polymyositis and dermatomyositis. Lancet 2003;362(9388):971–82.

196. Targoff IN, Miller FW, Medsger TA Jr, et al. Classification criteria for the idiopathic inflammatory myopathies. Curr Opin Rheumatol 1997;9(6):527–35.

197. Hall VC, Keeling JH, Davis MD. Periorbital edema as the presenting sign of dermatomyositis. Int J Dermatol 2003;42(6):466–7.

198. Mii S, Kobayashi R, Nakano T, et al. A histopathologic study of mechanic's hands associated with dermatomyositis: a report of five cases. Int J Dermatol 2009;48(11):1177–82.

199. Marie I, Hachulla E, Cherin P, et al. Interstitial lung disease in polymyositis and dermatomyositis. Arthritis Rheum 2002;47(6):614–22.

200. Danko K, Ponyi A, Constantin T, et al. Long-term survival of patients with idiopathic inflammatory myopathies according to clinical features: a longitudinal study of 162 cases. Medicine (Baltimore) 2004;83(1):35–42.

201. Hepper NG, Ferguson RH, Howard FM Jr. Three types of pulmonary involvement in polymyositis. Med Clin North Am 1964;48:1031–42.

202. Dickey BF, Myers AR. Pulmonary disease in polymyositis/dermatomyositis. Semin Arthritis Rheum 1984;14(1):60–76.

203. Braun NM, Arora NS, Rochester DF. Respiratory muscle and pulmonary function in polymyositis and other proximal myopathies. Thorax 1983;38(8):616–23.

204. Fathi M, Vikgren J, Boijsen M, et al. Interstitial lung disease in polymyositis and dermatomyositis: longitudinal evaluation by pulmonary function and radiology. Arthritis Rheum 2008;59(5):677–85.

205. Richards TJ, Eggebeen A, Gibson K, et al. Characterization and peripheral blood biomarker assessment of anti-Jo-1 antibody-positive interstitial lung disease. Arthritis Rheum 2009;60(7):2183–92.

206. Friedman AW, Targoff IN, Arnett FC. Interstitial lung disease with autoantibodies against aminoacyl-tRNA synthetases in the absence of clinically apparent myositis. Semin Arthritis Rheum 1996;26(1):459–67.

207. Ideura G, Hanaoka M, Koizumi T, et al. Interstitial lung disease associated with amyopathic dermatomyositis: review of 18 cases. Respir Med 2007;101(7):1406–11.

208. Fathi M, Dastmalchi M, Rasmussen E, et al. Interstitial lung disease, a common manifestation of newly diagnosed polymyositis and dermatomyositis. Ann Rheum Dis 2004;63(3):297–301.

209. Tanizawa K, Handa T, Nakashima R, et al. HRCT features of interstitial lung disease in dermatomyositis with anti-CADM-140 antibody. Respir Med 2011;105(9):1380–7.

210. Mukae H, Ishimoto H, Sakamoto N, et al. Clinical differences between interstitial lung disease associated with clinically amyopathic dermatomyositis and classic dermatomyositis. Chest 2009;136(5):1341–7.

211. Love LA, Leff RL, Fraser DD, et al. A new approach to the classification of idiopathic inflammatory myopathy: myositis-specific autoantibodies define useful homogeneous patient groups. Medicine (Baltimore) 1991;70(6):360–74.

212. Marguerie C, Bunn CC, Beynon HL, et al. Polymyositis, pulmonary fibrosis and autoantibodies to aminoacyl-tRNA synthetase enzymes. Q J Med 1990;77(282):1019–38.

213. Labirua A, Lundberg IE. Interstitial lung disease and idiopathic inflammatory myopathies: progress and pitfalls. Curr Opin Rheumatol 2010;22(6):633–8.

214. Sato S, Kuwana M, Hirakata M. Clinical characteristics of Japanese patients with anti-OJ (anti-isoleucyl-tRNA synthetase) autoantibodies. Rheumatology (Oxford) 2007;46(5):842–5.

215. Kalluri M, Sahn SA, Oddis CV, et al. Clinical profile of anti-PL-12 autoantibody. Cohort study and review of the literature. Chest 2009;135(6):1550–6.

216. La Corte R, Lo Mo Naco A, Locaputo A, et al. In patients with antisynthetase syndrome the occurrence of anti-Ro/SSA antibodies causes a more severe interstitial lung disease. Autoimmunity 2006;39(3):249–53.

217. Vancsa A, Csipo I, Nemeth J, et al. Characteristics of interstitial lung disease in SS-A positive/Jo-1 positive inflammatory myopathy patients. Rheumatol Int 2009;29(9):989–94.

218. Connors GR, Christopher-Stine L, Oddis CV, et al. Interstitial lung disease associated with the idiopathic inflammatory myopathies: what progress has been made in the past 35 years? Chest 2010;138(6):1464–74.

219. Ikezoe J, Johkoh T, Kohno N, et al. High-resolution CT findings of lung disease in patients with polymyositis and dermatomyositis. J Thorac Imaging 1996;11(4):250–9.

220. Mino M, Noma S, Taguchi Y, et al. Pulmonary involvement in polymyositis and dermatomyositis: sequential evaluation with CT. AJR Am J Roentgenol 1997;169(1):83–7.

221. Hayashi S, Tanaka M, Kobayashi H, et al. High-resolution computed tomography characterization

of interstitial lung diseases in polymyositis/dermatomyositis. J Rheumatol 2008;35(2):260–9.

222. Tazelaar HD, Viggiano RW, Pickersgill J, et al. Interstitial lung disease in polymyositis and dermatomyositis. Clinical features and prognosis as correlated with histologic findings. Am Rev Respir Dis 1990;141(3):727–33.

223. Webb DR, Currie GD. Pulmonary fibrosis masking polymyositis. Remission with corticosteroid therapy. JAMA 1972;222(9):1146–9.

224. Marie I, Mouthon L. Therapy of polymyositis and dermatomyositis. Autoimmun Rev 2011;11(1):6–13.

225. Nawata Y, Kurasawa K, Takabayashi K, et al. Corticosteroid resistant interstitial pneumonitis in dermatomyositis/polymyositis: prediction and treatment with cyclosporine. J Rheumatol 1999;26(7):1527–33.

226. Rowen AJ, Reichel J. Dermatomyositis with lung involvement, successfully treated with azathioprine. Respiration 1983;44(2):143–6.

227. Tanaka F, Origuchi T, Migita K, et al. Successful combined therapy of cyclophosphamide and cyclosporine for acute exacerbated interstitial pneumonia associated with dermatomyositis. Intern Med 2000; 39(5):428–30.

228. Yamasaki Y, Yamada H, Yamasaki M, et al. Intravenous cyclophosphamide therapy for progressive interstitial pneumonia in patients with polymyositis/dermatomyositis. Rheumatology (Oxford) 2007; 46(1):124–30.

229. Lateef O, Shakoor N, Balk RA. Methotrexate pulmonary toxicity. Expert Opin Drug Saf 2005;4(4): 723–30.

230. Gruhn WB, Diaz-Buxo JA. Cyclosporine treatment of steroid resistant interstitial pneumonitis associated with dermatomyositis/polymyositis. J Rheumatol 1987;14(5):1045–7.

231. Wilkes MR, Sereika SM, Fertig N, et al. Treatment of antisynthetase-associated interstitial lung disease with tacrolimus. Arthritis Rheum 2005;52(8). 2439–46.

232. Hervier B, Masseau A, Mussini JM, et al. Long-term efficacy of mycophenolate mofetil in a case of refractory antisynthetase syndrome. Joint Bone Spine 2009;76(5):575–6.

233. Suzuki Y, Hayakawa H, Miwa S, et al. Intravenous immunoglobulin therapy for refractory interstitial lung disease associated with polymyositis/dermatomyositis. Lung 2009;187(3):201–6.

234. Sem M, Molberg O, Lund MB, et al. Rituximab treatment of the anti-synthetase syndrome: a retrospective case series. Rheumatology (Oxford) 2009;48(8):968–71.

235. Rios Fernandez R, Callejas Rubio JL, Sanchez Cano D, et al. Rituximab in the treatment of dermatomyositis and other inflammatory myopathies. A report of 4 cases and review of the literature. Clin Exp Rheumatol 2009;27(6):1009–16.

236. Papiris SA, Tsonis IA, Moutsopoulos HM. Sjogren's syndrome. Semin Respir Crit Care Med 2007;28(4): 459–71.

237. Kokosi M, Riemer EC, Highland KB. Pulmonary involvement in Sjogren syndrome. Clin Chest Med 2010;31(3):489–500.

238. Hatron PY, Tillie-Leblond I, Launay D, et al. Pulmonary manifestations of Sjogren's syndrome. Presse Med 2011;40(1 Pt 2):e49–64.

239. Amarasena R, Bowman S. Sjogren's syndrome. Clin Med 2007;7(1):53–6.

240. Garcia-Carrasco M, Ramos-Casals M, Rosas J, et al. Primary Sjogren syndrome: clinical and immunologic disease patterns in a cohort of 400 patients. Medicine (Baltimore) 2002;81(4):270–80.

241. Vitali C, Bombardieri S, Jonsson R, et al. Classification criteria for Sjogren's syndrome: a revised version of the European criteria proposed by the American-European Consensus Group. Ann Rheum Dis 2002;61(6):554–8.

242. Davidson BK, Kelly CA, Griffiths ID. Ten year follow up of pulmonary function in patients with primary Sjogren's syndrome. Ann Rheum Dis 2000;59(9): 709–12.

243. Ramos-Casals M, Solans R, Rosas J, et al. Primary Sjogren syndrome in Spain: clinical and immunologic expression in 1010 patients. Medicine (Baltimore) 2008;87(4):210–9.

244. Segal I, Fink G, Machtey I, et al. Pulmonary function abnormalities in Sjogren's syndrome and the sicca complex. Thorax 1981;36(4):286–9.

245. Papathanasiou MP, Constantopoulos SH, Tsampoulas C, et al. Reappraisal of respiratory abnormalities in primary and secondary Sjogren's syndrome. A controlled study. Chest 1986;90(3): 370–4.

246. Constantopoulos SH, Drosos AA, Maddison PJ, et al. Xerotrachea and interstitial lung disease in primary Sjogren's syndrome. Respiration 1984; 46(3):310–4.

247. Parambil JG, Myers JL, Lindell RM, et al. Interstitial lung disease in primary Sjogren syndrome. Chest 2006;130(5):1489–95.

248. Papiris SA, Maniati M, Constantopoulos SH, et al. Lung involvement in primary Sjogren's syndrome is mainly related to the small airway disease. Ann Rheum Dis 1999;58(1):61–4.

249. Kelly C, Gardiner P, Pal B, et al. Lung function in primary Sjogren's syndrome: a cross sectional and longitudinal study. Thorax 1991;46(3):180–3.

250. Franquet T, Gimenez A, Monill JM, et al. Primary Sjogren's syndrome and associated lung disease: CT findings in 50 patients. AJR Am J Roentgenol 1997;169(3):655–8.

251. Koyama M, Johkoh T, Honda O, et al. Pulmonary involvement in primary Sjogren's syndrome: spectrum of pulmonary abnormalities and computed

tomography findings in 60 patients. J Thorac Imaging 2001;16(4):290–6.

252. Meyer CA, Pina JS, Taillon D, et al. Inspiratory and expiratory high-resolution CT findings in a patient with Sjogren's syndrome and cystic lung disease. AJR Am J Roentgenol 1997;168(1):101–3.

253. Voulgarelis M, Skopouli FN. Clinical, immunologic, and molecular factors predicting lymphoma development in Sjogren's syndrome patients. Clin Rev Allergy Immunol 2007;32(3):265–74.

254. Honda O, Johkoh T, Ichikado K, et al. Differential diagnosis of lymphocytic interstitial pneumonia and malignant lymphoma on high-resolution CT. AJR Am J Roentgenol 1999;173(1):71–4.

255. Franquet T, Diaz C, Domingo P, et al. Air trapping in primary Sjogren syndrome: correlation of expiratory CT with pulmonary function tests. J Comput Assist Tomogr 1999;23(2):169–73.

256. Ito I, Nagai S, Kitaichi M, et al. Pulmonary manifestations of primary Sjogren's syndrome: a clinical, radiologic, and pathologic study. Am J Respir Crit Care Med 2005;171(6):632–8.

257. Deheinzelin D, Capelozzi VL, Kairalla RA, et al. Interstitial lung disease in primary Sjogren's syndrome. Clinical-pathological evaluation and response to treatment. Am J Respir Crit Care Med 1996;154(3 Pt 1):794–9.

258. Isaksen K, Jonsson R, Omdal R. Anti-CD20 treatment in primary Sjogren's syndrome. Scand J Immunol 2008;68(6):554–64.

259. Seror R, Sordet C, Guillevin L, et al. Tolerance and efficacy of rituximab and changes in serum B cell biomarkers in patients with systemic complications of primary Sjogren's syndrome. Ann Rheum Dis 2007;66(3):351–7.

260. Kamen DL, Strange C. Pulmonary manifestations of systemic lupus erythematosus. Clin Chest Med 2010;31(3):479–88.

261. Tan EM, Cohen AS, Fries JF, et al. The 1982 revised criteria for the classification of systemic lupus erythematosus. Arthritis Rheum 1982; 25(11):1271–7.

262. Matthay RA, Schwarz MI, Petty TL, et al. Pulmonary manifestations of systemic lupus erythematosus: review of twelve cases of acute lupus pneumonitis. Medicine (Baltimore) 1975;54(5):397–409.

263. Torre O, Harari S. Pleural and pulmonary involvement in systemic lupus erythematosus. Presse Med 2011;40(1 Pt 2):e19–29.

264. Inoue T, Kanayama Y, Ohe A, et al. Immunopathologic studies of pneumonitis in systemic lupus erythematosus. Ann Intern Med 1979;91(1):30–4.

265. Matthay RA, Hudson LD, Petty TL. Acute lupus pneumonitis: response to azathioprine therapy. Chest 1973;63(1):117–20.

266. Schnabel A, Reuter M, Gross WL. Intravenous pulse cyclophosphamide in the treatment of interstitial lung disease due to collagen vascular diseases. Arthritis Rheum 1998;41(7):1215–20.

267. Zamora MR, Warner ML, Tuder R, et al. Diffuse alveolar hemorrhage and systemic lupus erythematosus. Clinical presentation, histology, survival, and outcome. Medicine (Baltimore) 1997;76(3):192–202.

268. Schwab EP, Schumacher HR Jr, Freundlich B, et al. Pulmonary alveolar hemorrhage in systemic lupus erythematosus. Semin Arthritis Rheum 1993;23(1): 8–15.

269. Santos-Ocampo AS, Mandell BF, Fessler BJ. Alveolar hemorrhage in systemic lupus erythematosus: presentation and management. Chest 2000;118(4): 1083–90.

270. Myers JL, Katzenstein AA. Microangiitis in lupus-induced pulmonary hemorrhage. Am J Clin Pathol 1986;85(5):552–6.

271. Erickson RW, Franklin WA, Emlen W. Treatment of hemorrhagic lupus pneumonitis with plasmapheresis. Semin Arthritis Rheum 1994;24(2):114–23.

272. Verzegnassi F, Marchetti F, Zennaro F, et al. Prompt efficacy of plasmapheresis in a patient with systemic lupus erythematosus and diffuse alveolar haemorrhage. Clin Exp Rheumatol 2010;28(3):445–6.

273. Canas C, Tobon GJ, Granados M, et al. Diffuse alveolar hemorrhage in Colombian patients with systemic lupus erythematosus. Clin Rheumatol 2007;26(11):1947–9.

274. Al Rashidi A, Alajmi M, Hegazi MO. Mycophenolate mofetil as a maintenance therapy for lupus-related diffuse alveolar hemorrhage. Lupus 2011;20(14): 1551–3.

275. Haupt HM, Moore GW, Hutchins GM. The lung in systemic lupus erythematosus. Analysis of the pathologic changes in 120 patients. Am J Med 1981;71(5):791–8.

276. Bankier AA, Kiener HP, Wiesmayr MN, et al. Discrete lung involvement in systemic lupus erythematosus: CT assessment. Radiology 1995;196(3): 835–40.

277. Boulware DW, Hedgpeth MT. Lupus pneumonitis and anti-SSA(Ro) antibodies. J Rheumatol 1989; 16(4):479–81.

278. Mochizuki T, Aotsuka S, Satoh T. Clinical and laboratory features of lupus patients with complicating pulmonary disease. Respir Med 1999;93(2):95–101.

279. Jacobsen S, Petersen J, Ullman S, et al. A multicentre study of 513 Danish patients with systemic lupus erythematosus. I. Disease manifestations and analyses of clinical subsets. Clin Rheumatol 1998;17(6):468–77.

280. de Lauretis A, Veeraraghavan S, Renzoni E. Review series: aspects of interstitial lung disease: connective tissue disease-associated interstitial lung disease: how does it differ from IPF? How should the clinical approach differ? Chron Respir Dis 2011;8(1):53–82.

281. Swigris JJ, Olson AL, Fischer A, et al. Mycopheno-late mofetil is safe, well tolerated, and preserves lung function in patients with connective tissue disease-related interstitial lung disease. Chest 2006;130(1):30–6.

282. Lim SW, Gillis D, Smith W, et al. Rituximab use in systemic lupus erythematosus pneumonitis and a review of current reports. Intern Med J 2006; 36(4):260–2.

283. Duskin A, Eisenberg RA. The role of antibodies in inflammatory arthritis. Immunol Rev 2010;233(1): 112–25.

284. Self SE. Autoantibody testing for autoimmune disease. Clin Chest Med 2010;31(3):415–22.

285. Peng S, Craft J. Anti-nuclear antibodies. In: Firestein GS, editor. Kelley's textbook of rheuma-tology. 8th edition. Philadelphia: Saunders Elsevier; 2008. p. 741–54.

Chronic Hypersensitivity Pneumonitis

Ulrich Costabel, MD[a],*, Francesco Bonella, MD[a], Josune Guzman, MD[b]

KEYWORDS

- Hypersensitivity pneumonitis • Farmer's lung
- Bird fancier's disease • HRCT • Histopathology • Prognosis

Hypersensitivity pneumonitis (HP), also known as extrinsic allergic alveolitis, is a syndrome caused by an exaggerated immune response to the inhalation of a variety of antigenic particles found in the environment. Because the resulting inflammatory response is not confined to the alveoli, which the term extrinsic allergic alveolitis implies, but also involves the terminal bronchiole, the term HP pneumonitis may be more correct.

The development of disease and the clinical presentation is influenced by several factors, such as the nature and the amount of the inhaled antigen; the intensity and frequency of exposure; and the host immune response, which is likely determined by a genetic background. Genetic susceptibility may explain why one individual develops disease, another individual with exactly the same exposure is only sensitized but remains healthy, and still another one will not even become sensitized.[1]

CAUSATIVE AGENTS

Farmer's lung, a term coined by Pepys and colleagues,[2] is the prototype of HP. In 1962, Pepys and coworkers were the first to associate HP with the development of serum precipitins to hay and mold extracts.[2] Since then, many agents have been identified as potential causes and the number is ever increasing. The antigens may be fungal, bacterial, protozoal, and animal (mostly bird) proteins, or low-molecular-weight chemical compounds (**Table 1**). HP may potentially arise in any work or home environment where bacteria and fungi grow or birds are kept. Moreover, the intake of certain drugs may cause HP as a noninhalational variant.

New Environments and Causes

A new type of domestic ultrasonic humidifier (misting fountain) has been described as the cause of cases of humidifier pneumonitis.[3] The patients were exposed to mist from fountain water contaminated with bacteria, molds, and yeasts. The contaminated water reservoir of a steam iron was the cause of HP in a woman who developed symptoms strictly associated with the use of the steam iron.[4] Several cases caused by exposure to dry sausage molds have been reported.[5–8] Wind instruments, saxophone and trombone, contaminated with mycobacterial or fungal species have caused disease.[9–11] A chiropodist developed HP caused by inhalational exposure to fungi in the foot skin and nails of her clients.[12] A larger series of patients with feather duvet lung, a rare subgroup of bird fancier's lung, has recently been published.[13]

This work was supported by Arbeitsgemeinschaft zur Förderung der Pneumologie an der Ruhrlandklinik (AFPR).

The authors have nothing to disclose.

[a] Department of Pneumology/Allergy, Ruhrlandklinik, University Hospital, Tueschener Weg 40, 45239 Essen, Germany

[b] Pathologisches Institut der Ruhr-Universität Bochum, BG-Kliniken Bergmannsheil, Buerkle-de-la-Camp-Platz 1, 44789 Bochum, Germany

* Corresponding author.

E-mail address: ulrich.costabel@ruhrlandklinik.uk-essen.de

Clin Chest Med 33 (2012) 151–163

doi:10.1016/j.ccm.2011.12.004

Table 1
Environmental exposure and antigens in various types of hypersensitivity pneumonitis

Disease	Exposure	Antigen
		Microorganisms
Farmer's lung	Moldy hay, grain	Saccharospora rectivirgula, Thermoactinomyces vulgaris, Aspergillus spp
Humidifier lung; air conditioner lung	Contaminated humidifiers and air conditioners	Amoebae, nematodes, yeasts, bacteria
Misting fountain HP	Contaminated water	Bacteria, molds, yeasts
Steam iron HP	Contaminated water reservo r	Sphingobacterium spiritivorum
Suberosis	Moldy cork	Penicillium spp
Sequoiosis	Moldy redwood dust	Graphium spp, Pullularia spp, Trichoderma spp
Woodworker's lung	Contaminated wood pulp or dust	Alternaria spp
Wood trimmer's lung	Contaminated wood trimmirgs	Rhizopus spp, Mucor spp
Maple-bark stripper's lung	Contaminated maple logs	Cryptostroma corticale
Domestic allergic alveolitis	Decayed wood	Molds
Sauna taker's lung	Contaminated sauna water	Aureobasidium spp
Basement lung	Contaminated basements	Cephalosporium spp, Penicillium spp
Hot tub lung	Mold on ceiling, tub water	Mycobacterium avium complex
Swimming pool lung	Mist from pool water, sprays, and fountains	Mycobacterium avium complex
Thatched roof lung	Dried grasses and leaves	Saccharomonospora viridis, T vulgaris, Aspergillus spp
Bagassosis	Moldy pressed sugar cane (bagasse)	Thermoactinomyces sacchari, T vulgaris
Mushroom worker's lung	Moldy compost and mushrooms	Saccharospora rectivirgula, T vulgaris, Aspergillus spp
Malt worker's lung	Contaminated barley	Aspergillus clavatus
Cheese washer's lung	Moldy cheese or cheese casirgs	Penicillium casei
Dry sausage worker's lung	Moldy sausage dust	Penicillium spp
Paprika slicer's lung	Moldy paprika pods	Mucor stolonifer
Compost lung	Compost	Aspergillus spp, T vulgaris
Wine maker's lung	Mold on grapes	Botrytis cinerea

Disease	Source	Agent
Tobacco grower's lung	Mold on tobacco	Aspergillus spp
Potato riddler's lung	Moldy hay around potatoes	Thermophilic actinomycetes, Aspergillus spp
Summer-type HP	Contaminated houses	Trychosporon cutaneum
Detergent lung, washing powder lung	Detergents (during processing or use)	Bacillus subtilis enzymes
Machine operator's lung	Contaminated metal-working fluid	Pseudomonas spp, nontuberculous mycobacteria, Aspergillus fumigatus
Stipatosis	Esparto dust	T actinomycetes
Peat moss HP	Contaminated peat moss	Monocillium spp, Penicillium citreonigum
Wind instrument lung	Contaminated saxophones, trombone	Molds, bacteria
Chiropodist's lung	Foot skin and nail dust	Fungi
		Animal proteins
Bird fancier's lung; pigeon breeder's lung	Parakeets, budgerigars, pigeons, parrots, cockatiels, chickens, turkeys, geese, ducks, love birds	Proteins in avian droppings, in serum and on feathers
Feather duvet lung	Feather beds, pillows, duvets	Avian proteins
Pituitary snuff taker's lung	Bovine and porcine pituitary powder	Pituitary proteins
Furrier's lung	Animal pelts	Animal fur dust
Animal handler's lung, laboratory worker's lung	Rats, gerbils	Proteins from urine, serum, pelts
Pearl oyster shell HP	Dust of shells	Pearl oyster proteins
Mollusk shell HP	Sea snail shell dust	Sea snail shell protein
Silk production HP	Dust from silkworm larvae and cocoons	Silkworm proteins
Miller's lung	Contaminated grain	Sitophilus granarius (ie, wheat weevil)
		Chemicals
Chemical worker's lung	Polyurethane foams, spray paints, elastomers, glues	Diisocyanates, trimellitic anhydride
Epoxy resin lung	Heated epoxy resin	Phthalic anhydride
		Unknown
Mummy handler's lung	Cloth wrappings of mummies	
Coffee worker's lung	Coffee-bean dust	
Tap water lung	Contaminated tap water	
Tea grower's lung	Tea plants	

EPIDEMIOLOGY

The more common forms of HP are farmer's lung, budgerigar (parakeet) keeper's lung (keeping of domestic birds), and pigeon breeder's lung in Europe, whereas summer-type HP is a disease limited to Japan. However, the prevalence of HP is difficult to determine, given that the disease is often unrecognized or misdiagnosed. Further, exposure conditions vary from country to country; even within a country, the climate, local customs, and local working conditions depend on the geographic areas. Farmer's lung is more prevalent in cold and wet regions. The introduction of modern techniques of haymaking and silage making has reduced the incidence of farmer's lung.

The estimates for the prevalence of farmer's lung range from 1% to 19% of exposed farmers[14–16]; from 6% to 20% of exposed pigeon breeders[17]; and for budgerigar's lung, from 0.5% to 7.5% of the at-risk population, which is 10% to 12% of the UK population who keep these birds in their homes.[18] The disease may arise in all age groups, including children. Clinical behavior in childhood is similar to adult disease.[19,20]

Smoking is less prevalent in patients with HP than in control populations.[16] Cigarette smoking seems to be protective against the development of HP. Nonsmokers exposed to antigens have significantly higher levels of specific immunoglobulin G (IgG) antibodies than smokers.[21] Cigarette smoking suppresses lymphocyte and macrophage function, thus, it may interfere with the alveolar macrophage capacity to take up, process, and present the inhaled antigen to lymphocytes. This activity may dampen the cellular immune response that is necessary to develop HP.

PATHOGENESIS

The pathogenesis of HP is complex, and many of the mechanisms involved are poorly understood. Particulate matters with an aerodynamic diameter smaller than 5 μm can reach the periphery of the lung and are capable of inducing HP. Most of the antigens are home or workplace related.

Several immune reactions seem to be involved. Early observations, especially the presence of circulating precipitins to the relevant sensitizing antigens,[2] supported the concept that the disease is mediated by the deposition of antigen/antibody complexes within the alveolar walls, which is compatible with a humoral, immune-complex–mediated reaction (type III hypersensitivity). However, several findings are not consistent with this hypothesis: (1) patients may develop disease but may lack serum precipitins[22]; (2) histopathology does not show vasculitis or prominent neutrophil infiltration; and (3) in animal models, passive serum transfer followed by aerosol exposure is not able to induce histologic changes of HP.[23]

There is more evidence for a cell mediated immune reaction (type IV hypersensitivity), such as the histology of lymphocytic interstitial infiltrates with granuloma formation and the bronchoalveolar lavage (BAL) findings with a significant lymphocytosis and signs of macrophage and lymphocyte activation.[24] Further, HP can be passively transferred with sensitized lymphocytes of the Th1-type followed by inhalational challenge.[25] There is evidence for overproduction of interferon-γ (Th1 cytokine) and amelioration by interleukin (IL)-10 of the severity of the disease from animal models and from BAL studies of patients with HP.[26] Overproduction of the Th1 cytokines, IL-12 and IL-18, by BAL macrophages from patients with HP has been reported.[27–29] Altered expression of tumor necrosis factor (TNF) superfamily receptors by alveolar macrophages is also seen.[30] Alveolar macrophages from patients with HP produce increased levels of soluble TNF receptors that may act as counter regulators of TNF.[31]

Although HP is typically defined as Th1 disease, chronic HP evolving to fibrosis seems to be characterized by a switch to a Th2-biased immune response. In this regard, BAL T cells from patients with chronic HP display a Th2 phenotype with an increase in CXCR4 (a Th2 chemokine receptor) and a decrease in CXCR3 (a Th1 chemokine receptor) expression.[32] Antigen-specific-stimulated cells from chronic HP produce higher levels of IL-4 and lower levels of interferon-γ compared with those from subacute HP.[32] Patients with chronic HP with a fibrotic histopathology showed a predominant Th2 response as evidenced by a higher ratio of TARC (a Th2 chemokine) to IP-10 (a Th1 chemokine) in comparison with those who had organizing pneumonia (OP) or nonspecific interstitial pneumonia (NSIP)–like histopathology.[33] A murine model of chronic HP confirmed that Th2-biased immune responses are important in the development of lung fibrosis in chronic HP.[34]

Although these studies have helped to understand the disease mechanisms, it is unknown why the disease develops only in a minority of exposed individuals. To explain this, it was postulated that for disease to occur, the presence of an inducing factor (inhaled antigen) and a promoting factor is necessary. An intrinsic promoting factor can be a genetic predisposition linked to the major histocompatibility complex. Differences in the TNF-α polymorphism were found in patients with pigeon breeder's disease and farmer's lung.[35,36] More recently, polymorphisms in the transporter associated with antigen processing (TAP) genes and in the low-molecular-weight proteasome LMP7 gene have been shown to be involved in the susceptibility to pigeon breeder's disease,[37,38] whereas polymorphisms in the TIMP-3 promoter region may protect against the development of HP.[39,40] Extrinsic promoting factors may be inhalation of insecticides, weed killers, or superimposed viral infections. In an animal model of farmer's lung with mice exposed to both the offending antigen and the parainfluenza 1 virus, the pulmonary inflammatory response was more enhanced and prolonged compared with antigen exposure only.[41] Despite all this progress, we still do not understand why some patients show resolution of disease and others progress to fibrosis even without further antigen exposure.

PATHOLOGY

The acute response within a few days is a nonspecific diffuse pneumonitis with infiltration of mononuclear cells and neutrophils of the bronchioles, alveoli, and the interstitium. With further continued or intermittent exposure, the subacute stage is characterized by a lymphocytic infiltration centered on the bronchioles. Within several weeks, noncaseating epithelioid cell granulomas may be formed and are seen in about 70% of histopathologic specimens. The characteristic histopathologic lesions of typical subacute HP are (1) cellular interstitial pneumonia (cellular NSIP), (2) cellular bronchiolitis, and (3) granulomatous inflammation. This histologic triad is seen in no more than 75% of patients with HP. Characteristically, the central regions of the secondary lobule are predominantly involved.[42]

With long-term exposure, chronic HP with progressive fibrosis and bronchiolitis obliterans may develop. Fibrosis may become extensive with honeycombing, so that in late chronic stages, histopathology may be similar to usual interstitial pneumonia (UIP). In general, histologic changes in chronic HP may not be different from the patterns found in other fibrotic lung disease. Several investigators have reported isolated UIP-like or fibrotic NSIP-like patterns.[43–48] A review of 10 cases of chronic HP identified 3 patterns of fibrosis: (1) predominantly peripheral fibrosis in a patchy pattern with architectural distortion and fibroblastic foci resembling UIP in 9 cases; (2) relatively homogeneous linear fibrosis resembling fibrotic NSIP in 4 cases; and (3) irregular predominantly peribronchiolar fibrosis in 3 cases, all of which also had UIP-like fibrosis. In all cases, granulomas or giant cells or areas of typical subacute HP were also present and helpful to arrive at the correct diagnosis.[49] Another study of 16 autopsy cases of chronic HP found that the fibrotic pattern closely resembled that in lungs with idiopathic pulmonary fibrosis (IPF)/UIP. Granulomas were not detected in any chronic HP case. Centrilobular fibrosis was the outstanding feature in all cases, often connecting to the perilobular areas in the appearance of bridging fibrosis, although considerable overlap with IPF/UIP was found.[50]

CLINICAL FEATURES

The spectrum of clinical presentation varies and is determined by the frequency and intensity of antigen exposure (**Table 2**). Acute, subacute, and chronic forms have been described. The term subclinical alveolitis has been coined for individuals being exposed to antigens and with a lymphocytic alveolitis on BAL but without clinical evidence of disease (no symptoms, normal chest radiographs and lung function test). These individuals are obviously sensitized to the offending antigen. Long-term follow-up studies of Canadian dairy farmers show that the BAL lymphocytosis persisted in these individuals and that no subject developed manifest farmer's lung disease.[51] The interval between sensitization by antigen inhalation and the clinical appearance of HP is unknown. It seems to be extremely variable and may range from many months to several years after the beginning of exposure.

Acute Form

This presentation is the most characteristic and specific presentation and is associated with intermittent, high-level exposure to the offending

Table 2	
Symptoms and signs in 116 patients with HP	
Feature	**Frequency (%)**
Dyspnea	98
Cough	91
Chills	34
Fever	19
Chest tightness	35
Weight loss	42
Body aches	24
Wheezing	31
Inspiratory crackles	87
Cyanosis	32
Clubbing	21

Data from Lacasse Y, Selman M, Costabel U, et al. Clinical diagnosis of hypersensitivity pneumonitis. Am J Respir Crit Care Med 2003;168:952–8.

antigen, typically in farmers working with moldy hay or in pigeon breeders when cleaning the pigeon loft. Symptoms occur approximately 4 to 12 hours after exposure. The disease onset is abrupt. Patients suffer a flulike syndrome (fever, chills, malaise, myalgia, headache) and respiratory symptoms (dry cough, dyspnea, tachypnea, chest tightness). The symptoms may occur at night once patients have gone to bed after a day with exposure. The clinical examination reveals bibasilar crackles and occasional cyanosis; finger clubbing is very unusual. These signs and symptoms peak between 6 and 24 hours and usually resolve spontaneously within a few days.[1]

Subacute Form

Occasionally, mild, acute episodes with fever may be seen in patients with a background of more chronic, progressive disease. This form would represent the subacute form, which may also become chronic and progress to fibrosis, after recurrent acute episodes. The patients with recurrent chronic bird fancier's lung tend to breed dozens of pigeons in a loft, whereas the patients with insidious chronic bird fancier's lung are exposed to smaller birds, usually budgerigars kept indoors.[52]

Chronic Form

The chronic form results from continuous, low-level exposure, usually to birds in the domestic environment (budgerigar/parakeet keepers). The onset of disease is insidious with slowly increasing dyspnea on exertion, usually dry cough, fatigue, and weight loss. The patients never relate their symptoms to the exposure to the birds. The

insidious onset of symptoms and lack of acute episodes lead the physician often to mistake the disease for other chronic interstitial lung diseases (ILD), such as IPF.

The clinical examination reveals bibasilar crackles. Digital clubbing may be seen in 20% to 50% of patients[1,52] as well as the manifestation of cor pulmonale. A rather unique clinical finding in chronic HP, in contrast to other chronic fibrotic lung disease, is the presence of inspiratory squeaks, which are caused by coexisting bronchiolitis in some patients. The frequency of important clinical and investigational characteristics seems to be determined by the histologic pattern in chronic HP (**Table 3**).[47]

INVESTIGATIONS
Chest Radiography

In acute HP, a transient, diffuse, ground-glass or airspace consolidation, associated with some micronodules, may be seen. The subacute forms may show micronodular and reticular shadowing. The chronic forms show a predominantly reticular pattern, with associated honeycombing. In contrast to IPF, the changes are diffuse and may show upper-zone predominance. Mild enlargement of the mediastinal lymph nodes can be observed occasionally. Pleural involvement is usually absent. The chest radiograph may be normal in up to 30% of patients and also in some patients with physiologically significant disease.

High-Resolution Computed Tomography

In acute and subacute HP, the characteristic findings on high-resolution computed tomography (HRCT) are patchy or diffuse ground-glass densities.

Table 3
Histologic pattern in chronic pigeon breeder's disease: correlation with clinical findings

	Typical HP Pattern n = 58	NSIP Pattern n = 22	UIP-like Pattern n = 10	P
Finger clubbing (%)	30/56 (53)	10/21 (48)	8/10 (80)	.26
BAL				
Lymphocytes (%)	65 ± 21	52 ± 23	36 ± 23	.0011
Macrophages (%)	34 ± 20	45 ± 23	59 ± 18	.0028
Eosinophils (%)	1 (0–9)	0 (0–13)	2 (0–13)	.11
Neutrophils (%)	0 (0–10)	1 (0–10)	1 (0–4)	.61
HRCT				
Inflammation (%)	30/40 (75)	11/16 (69)	1/7 (14)	<.007
Fibrosis (%)	10/40 (25)	5/16 (31)	6/7 (86)	<.007

Abbreviation: HRCT, high-resolution computed tomography.
Data from Gaxiola M, Buendia-Roldan I, Mejia M, et al. Morphologic diversity of chronic pigeon breeder's disease: clinical features and survival. Respir Med 2011;105:608–14.

Usually, there are small, centrilobular, ill-defined nodules of ground-glass densities, and evidence of mosaic perfusion (trapped air) caused by concomitant bronchiolitis. These micronodules may be found in those with acute, subacute, or chronic disease in decreasing frequency (**Fig. 1**). In the correct clinical context, they are strongly suggestive of HP.[53–57]

In chronic HP, there are signs of lung fibrosis, such as lobar volume loss, linear-reticular opacities, or honeycombing (**Fig. 2**). The distribution may be more prominent in the upper lobes or in the lower lobes. Usually, there is not the predominant subpleural involvement as in IPF. CT can be used to distinguish IPF from HP in many cases.[58] In most chronic cases, the presence of poorly defined centrilobular micronodules is suggestive of HP. In addition, emphysema can be seen in 20% of nonsmoking patients with chronic HP, particularly in farmer's lung.[54–56]

A study evaluated the role of HRCT in the differential diagnosis of chronic HP with IPF and idiopathic NSIP. In this study, a confident first-choice diagnosis at HRCT was made in 70 (53%) of 132 readings in patients with chronic HP, IPF, and NSIP and was correct in 94% of these readings.[59] These results are similar to those obtained in another study that included patients with IPF and HP. In that study, a first-choice diagnosis with a high level of confidence was made in 62% of the cases, and this diagnosis was correct in 90% of the observations.[58] The features that best differentiated chronic HP from IPF and NSIP at thin-section CT were the presence of lobular areas with decreased attenuation, centrilobular nodules, and a lack of lower-zone predominance of the abnormalities. NSIP can be differentiated from chronic HP mainly by the presence of relative subpleural sparing, absence of lobular areas with decreased attenuation, and lack of honeycombing.

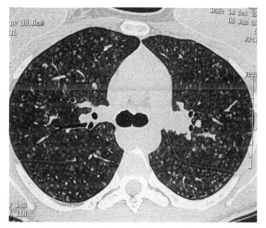

Fig. 1. HRCT of a patient with acute hypersensitivity pneumonitis.

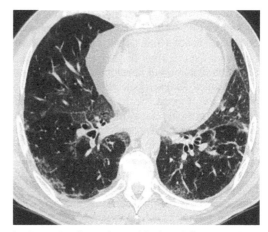

Fig. 2. HRCT of a patient with chronic hypersensitivity pneumonitis.

IPF can be differentiated from chronic HP by the basal predominance of honeycombing and the absence of relative subpleural sparing and centrilobular nodules. Cysts were also seen more commonly in patients with chronic HP than in those with IPF or NSIP and were only noticed in areas of ground-glass opacities. Importantly, honeycombing was seen in 64% of patients with chronic HP, which was similar to the frequency observed in the patients with IPF.[59]

Lung Function

The most frequent lung-function abnormalities are a restrictive ventilatory impairment or an impaired gas exchange (decreased diffusing capacity or increasing hypoxemia during exercise). In fact, these changes are consistent with the functional pattern of any ILD and are not specific for HP. During acute episodes and late in chronic progressive patients, hypoxemia at rest is observed. The most frequent functional abnormality is hypoxemia during exercise, with an elevated alveolar/arterial oxygen gradient greater than 10 mm Hg; the next frequent is a restrictive pattern. Only a few patients show obstruction of the peripheral airways. Some patients may develop bronchial hyperreactivity. The pulmonary function changes do not correlate with the magnitude of changes seen on the chest radiograph or HRCT scan.

Laboratory Tests

The presence of specific IgG antibodies (serum precipitins) to the inducing antigen is evidence of sensitization but not of disease. Between 30% and 60% of healthy farmers produce precipitating antibodies to the antigens they are exposed to. In budgerigar fanciers, only 3% of healthy exposed individuals produce precipitating antibodies, so that in this form of HP, the demonstration of precipitins against bird serum or droppings is much more specific for disease than findings of the precipitins in farmers. On the other hand, between 10% and 15% of patients do not develop serum precipitins, so a negative finding does not exclude the presence of the disease.[22,60,61] Despite these limitations, the precipitin assay is a useful additional laboratory test in the diagnostic assessment of HP, in particular to suggest a potential exposure that has not been recognized. Precipitins are usually assessed by radial diffusion (Ouchterlony) or by enzyme-linked immunosorbent assay techniques. Fenoglio and coworkers[62] assessed the diagnostic value of a relevant panel of antigens to detect serum precipitins in mold-induced HP. The predictive negative values varied from 81% to 88% and the predictive positive values from 71% to 75%. This finding was considered of help to diagnose mold-induced HP in a specific geographic region.[62]

In acute episodes, the white blood cell count shows increased leukocytes with a predominance of neutrophils. The C-reactive protein levels may also be elevated. In chronic forms, polyclonal increase of gamma globulins is a frequent finding. The rheumatoid factor may be positive in 50% of patients with pigeon HP.[63]

Bronchoalveolar Lavage

HP shows, by far, the most marked increase in BAL lymphocytes of all the interstitial diseases, usually with a relative predominance of CD8 T cells resulting in a low CD4/CD8 ratio. The total cell yield is very high, usually more than 20 million from a BAL of 100 mL total instillation. The lymphocyte count is usually greater than 50% of the total cells but may be less in the chronic fibrotic forms.[47,52,54] In addition, neutrophils, eosinophils, and mast cells may be mildly elevated.[24,64] A more specific finding is the increase in plasma cells. This cell type was found in a low percentage in 18 of 30 patients with bird keeper's disease; values ranged from 0.1% to 3.9% in this study.[65] Other morphologic features include signs of T-cell activation (folded nuclei, broad cytoplasm) and foamy macrophages.[66] A normal BAL cytology probably excludes acute or subacute extrinsic allergic alveolitis. On the other hand, BAL cannot differentiate between patients with overt disease and healthy subjects who have been exposed and sensitized.

In regard to the CD4/CD8 ratio, the different series reported in the literature show no consistent findings. Most studies show a significant decrease in the CD4/CD8 ratio, with mean values ranging between 0.5 and 1.0. Two studies found that CD4/CD8 ratios were borderline (1.3 and 1.5,

respectively). In Japan, a normal ratio of 2.0 has been reported for ventilation HP and even an increased mean ratio of 4.4 for farmer's lung.[67] The reasons for this discrepancy in reported CD4/CD8 ratios are unclear. Several explanations are possible and include different disease manifestations (acute vs chronic form), the timing of BAL investigations in relation to the last antigen exposure, and the type of antigen causing the disease. CD4/CD8 ratios are higher shortly after the last antigen exposure (within 24 hours) and lowest between 7 and 30 days after the last exposure.[68] In chronic HP, among patients exposed to avian antigens, the CD4/CD8 ratio is frequently increased, with a higher mean value relative to that found in subacute HP.[32]

Acute episodes of extrinsic allergic alveolitis are associated with an influx of neutrophils into the lungs, lasting for up to 1 week. After this period, the cellular profile of the BAL fluid returns to the significant increase in lymphocytes that was previously seen. In the follow-up, persistent BAL abnormalities may indicate that complete avoidance has not been achieved.

Provocation Tests

Inhalation provocation tests with the suspected antigen have been performed, but these tests are not standardized and are usually not needed. Natural workplace or home exposure seems a more reasonable way to provoke symptoms or deterioration of functional parameters in unclear cases.

DIAGNOSIS

Diagnosis should be suspected in every patient with unexplained cough and dyspnea on exertion, functional impairment (restriction or diffusion defect), and unclear fever, especially if exposure to potential antigens is known (workplace, domestic bird keeping, moldy walls in the home).

Diagnosis is based on 3 criteria:

- Proven or suspected exposure associated with exposure-related symptoms
- Proof of sensitization, which is possible by demonstration of serum precipitins or of lymphocytosis in the BAL fluid
- Demonstration of the consistent pattern of an ILD on chest radiography/HRCT or with pulmonary function test (restriction or diffusion defect)

A large, prospective, multicenter cohort study (116 patients with HP, 284 control subjects with other ILD) designed to develop a clinical prediction rule for the diagnosis of HP was able to determine simple clinical predictors. In this study, a logistic regression identified 6 significant predictors of HP: exposure to the known offending antigen, positive precipitating antibodies, recurrent episodes of symptoms, inspiratory crackles, symptoms 4 to 8 hours after exposure, and weight loss. If all 6 are present, the probability of having HP is 98%.[69]

Careful history taking is obligatory. The physician should have a specific expertise in the knowledge of exposure conditions and of the occupational and domestic environment, to be able to ask the relevant questions to detect potential sources of exposure. Important factors are hay feeding, bird keeping, feather duvet and pillows in the home, air conditioning or ventilators in the buildings, and formation of mold on room walls or in the cellars. Indirect contact with birds should also be sought, for example, visits to friends or relatives who keep birds in their home or cleaning the clothing of someone who is a bird keeper. Improvement on vacation or during hospitalization may also be a hint toward the diagnosis.

The most sensitive diagnostic test is BAL. In the authors' experience and based on literature review, a normal BAL excludes the diagnosis of HP. The characteristic finding is a lymphocytosis in the subacute and chronic forms and also in those cases without symptoms being sensitized only (subclinical alveolitis). It has been proposed that BAL lymphocytosis greater than 30% discriminates chronic HP showing UIP pattern on HRCT from IPF.[70]

HRCT is an extremely useful diagnostic test. Although it may be normal in some patients, the sensitivity is more than 95%, and the finding of a centrilobular micronodular ground-glass pattern and evidence of mosaic perfusion (trapped air) is characteristic of HP. The major differential diagnosis in this setting is (RB-ILD) respiratory bronchiolitis/ILD or pneumocystis carinii infection. Here, BAL can then facilitate the differentiation. lymphocytosis in HP, a predominance of smoker's macrophages in RB-ILD, and the demonstration of the organisms in pneumocystis carinii pneumonia.

Histopathologic evaluation of lung tissue is usually not necessary for the diagnosis of HP. If a biopsy is needed in unclear cases with low prot001 probability of HP, the preferred approach is surgical because transbronchial biopsy specimens are of limited diagnostic accuracy.

An important problem in the diagnosis of HP is the fact that in up to 20% to 30% of the patients in some series, the inciting antigen cannot be identified by exposure history or serologic testing. In these patients, the diagnosis is suspected based on histopathology, BAL findings, and HRCT characteristics.[71,72]

The differential diagnosis includes the wide spectrum of ILD. Frequent misdiagnosis is pneumonia in acute forms and chronic bronchitis in chronic forms with normal chest radiograph, which may occur in 20%. Chronic HP, especially the insidious form of bird fancier's lung, may closely mimic IPF or idiopathic fibrotic NSIP.[44]

NATURAL HISTORY AND PROGNOSIS

The prognosis of HP varies greatly and depends on the type and duration of antigen exposure, the dose of the inhaled antigen, and the clinical form of disease. Some patients may experience progression, even despite avoiding exposure and undergoing treatment. There is no good explanation for the mechanism behind this.

In general, acute HP seems to have a favorable prognosis. After acute attacks, complete remission is usually seen. Patients with recurrent attacks of farmer's lung tend to have emphysema more often than patients who experienced only a single attack and also have a significantly lower diffusing capacity.[73] No differences were observed in relation to fibrosis.[73]

In pigeon breeders, a long-term follow-up study of almost 20 years compared symptomatic with asymptomatic pigeon breeders. Symptomatic pigeon breeders had a 3- to 4-fold increase in the expected proportional decrease of FEV_1 and FVC with increasing age, whereas the group of asymptomatic pigeon breeders showed no difference compared with a healthy control population.[74] In bird breeder's lung, the prognosis was found to be excellent. If the duration of symptoms was less than 6 months, complete recovery and normalization of lung function was seen in every such patient.[75] Similar findings were reported in another study.[76] If, on the other hand, recognition of disease occurs late, in the chronic stage, with end-stage fibrosis and cor pulmonale, the prognosis is less favorable. These patients may experience a fatal outcome.[52]

In a Finish study, the estimated mortality rate of farmer's lung was 0.7% between 1980 and 1990.[77] Other earlier studies on farmer's lung showed a mortality rate between 9% and 17%, with a mean survival from onset of symptoms to death of 17 years.[77–80] In acute pigeon breeder's disease, mortality is low and was reported to be less than 1%.[81] In one study of a selective population of pigeon breeders from Mexico, who kept their birds as pets in their homes and had chronic disease, mortality was higher with approximately 25% within 5 years after the initial diagnosis.[82]

Acute exacerbations can occur not only in IPF but also in chronic HP.[83,84] A review of 100 consecutive patients with chronic bird farmer's lung showed that 14 patients developed an acute exacerbation, defined according to the criteria used in IPF, and 12 of them died of this episode. The 2-year frequency of an acute exacerbation was 11.5%.[84]

Lung cancer has been recognized with increased frequency in IPF. A recent study of 104 cases of chronic HP identified a similar prevalence of lung cancer (10.6%) as seen in IPF.[85]

Histopathologic Patterns and Survival

Recently, surgical lung biopsies from a cohort of Japanese patients with chronic bird fancier's lung were analyzed. The inflammatory and fibrotic lesions showed significant variation, with changes suggestive of OP, NSIP, or UIP. Patients with OP-like or cellular NSIP-like lesions tended to have presented with acute episodes, whereas patients with UIP-like lesions had an insidious onset. Patients with OP–like or cellular NSIP-like lesions had a more favorable outcome than those with fibrotic NSIP-like and UIP-like lesions.[44]

In another study, the median survival in patients with fibrotic HP was 7.1 years, which was significantly less than the survival in those without fibrosis. In an age-adjusted regression analysis, antigen class, symptom duration, and lung function had no effect on survival. Only the presence of pathologic fibrosis was predictive of increased mortality (hazard ratio 6.01).[86] A study of chronic pigeon breeder's disease showed that patients with UIP-like histology had the worst survival rate (hazard ratio 4.19), whereas those with an NSIP-like pattern showed the best survival (hazard ratio 0.18).[47] Similar results were reported by Churg and colleagues,[45] who found that 16 of the 18 patients with a UIP-like pattern died of the disease. Thus, the presence of histologic fibrosis, especially a UIP-like pattern, is associated with decreased survival.

HRCT Patterns and Survival

In chronic HP, CT findings of extensive reticular pattern, traction bronchiectasis, and honeycombing are closely related to the presence of histologic fibrosis.[46,72] CT findings of fibrosis are associated with reduced survival in patients with chronic HP and may serve as useful prognostic indicator.[44,46,57,71] One HRCT study compared 26 fibrotic and 43 nonfibrotic consecutive patients with HP and found that fibrotic patients had a markedly increased mortality (hazard ratio 4.6).[71]

MANAGEMENT

Avoidance of further antigen exposure is the first essential measure. This avoidance may be difficult in some patients who fear loss of employment or hesitate to remove a pet bird or give up a beloved hobby. Antigens may persist in rooms where birds have been kept for a long time. One patient suffered a relapse from the disease after taking off the curtains from a room 3 months after the bird had been given away. Indirect and occasional exposure in home of friends or relatives where birds are kept should also be avoided. Feather pillows and blankets should be removed. Outbreak of the disease has been observed in patients who have moved into a new home where birds were formerly kept.[87]

In farmers, dust masks with filters, appropriate ventilation, mechanization of the feeding process on farms, and alterations in forced-air ventilatory systems may be useful precautionary measures. Also, for farmers, it is prudent to recommend complete avoidance of further antigen exposure.

Corticosteroid therapy is usually recommended in patients who show functional impairment. Treatment continues until no further improvement in physiologic abnormalities is observed. The treatment schedule is similar to that in sarcoidosis and other ILD, 40 to 50 mg/d for 1 month, followed by a period of tapering during the next 2 to 3 months and a maintenance dose between 7.5 and 15.0 mg/d. There are no controlled treatment trials in subacute and chronic forms of the disease. There is one placebo-controlled study in acute farmer's lung from Finland.[88] Steroids were given over a period of 2 months, which induced a more rapid improvement in lung function. Five years later, no functional differences were observed, an outcome that is not surprising for acute HP. In chronic, progressive HP, immunosuppressants may be added as corticosteroid sparing agents, as done in other fibrotic ILD.[44]

Routine follow-up investigations should be narrower initially after diagnosis and during treatment (1–3 months is appropriate); later, the interval can be extended to every 6 to 12 months. If the course is favorable (ie, complete remission after avoidance of further exposure or corticosteroid treatment), then routine follow-up can be stopped after 2 to 3 years.

SUMMARY

HP is a complex syndrome caused by repeated inhalation of environmental and occupational antigens. The major exposures are against bird proteins and fungi. Although the acute and subacute forms have a favorable prognosis, usually with complete remission, chronic HP may become a relentlessly progressive fibrotic lung disorder with an increased mortality rate, even when avoiding exposure and undergoing treatment. There is no good explanation for the mechanism behind this. Chronic HP, especially the insidious form of bird fancier's lung, may closely mimic IPF or idiopathic fibrotic NSIP. Diagnosis may be difficult. Prompt recognition of the antigen is critical for diagnosis. Removal of antigen exposure is important for treatment. Histologic changes in chronic HP may not be different from the patterns found in other fibrotic lung diseases. The UIP-like or fibrotic NSIP-like pattern of histopathology can been seen in isolation. Fibrotic changes on the biopsy specimen or HRCT are markers of a poor prognosis.

REFERENCES

1. Selman M. Hypersensitivity pneumonitis. In: Schwarz MI, King TE, editors. Interstitial lung disease. Shelton (CT): People's Medical Publishing House-USA; 2011. p. 597–635.

2. Pepys J, Riddel R, Citron KM, et al. Precipitins against extracts of hay and moulds in the serum of patients with farmer's lung, aspergillosis, asthma, and sarcoidosis. Thorax 1962;17:366–74.

3. Koschel D, Stark W, Karmann F, et al. Extrinsic allergic alveolitis caused by misting fountains. Respir Med 2005;99:943–7.

4. Kampfer P, Engelhart S, Rolke M, et al. Extrinsic allergic alveolitis (hypersensitivity pneumonitis) caused by Sphingobacterium spiritivorum from the water reservoir of a steam iron. J Clin Microbiol 2005;43:4908–10.

5. Morell F, Cruz MJ, Gomez FP, et al. Chacinero's lung - hypersensitivity pneumonitis due to dry sausage dust. Scand J Work Environ Health 2011;37:349–56.

6. Dalphin JC, Francois J, Saugier B, et al. [A case of semi-delayed hypersensitivity to dry sausage dust]. Rev Mal Respir 1988;5:633–5 [in French].

7. Guillot M, Bertoletti L, Deygas N, et al. [Dry sausage mould hypersensitivity pneumonitis: three cases]. Rev Mal Respir 2008;25:596–600 [in French].

8. Rouzaud P, Soulat JM, Trela C, et al. Symptoms and serum precipitins in workers exposed to dry sausage mould: consequences of exposure to sausage mould. Int Arch Occup Environ Health 2001;74:371–4.

9. Metersky ML, Bean SB, Meyer JD, et al. Trombone player's lung: a probable new cause of hypersensitivity pneumonitis. Chest 2010;138:754–6.

10. Metzger F, Haccuria A, Reboux G, et al. Hypersensitivity pneumonitis due to molds in a saxophone player. Chest 2010;138:724–6.

11. Lodha S, Sharma OP. Hypersensitivity pneumonitis in a saxophone player. Chest 1988;93:1322.

12. Lingenfelser A, Sennekamp J. Fußpflege-Alveolitis als Berufskrankheit. Allergologie 2010;33:573–4 [in German].

13. Koschel D, Wittstruck H, Renck T, et al. Presenting features of feather duvet lung. Int Arch Allergy Immunol 2010;152:264–70.

14. Gruchow HW, Hoffmann RG, Marx JJ Jr, et al. Precipitating antibodies to farmer's lung antigens in a Wisconsin farming population. Am Rev Respir Dis 1981;124:411–5.

15. Terho EO, Heinonen OP, Lammi S, et al. Incidence of clinically confirmed farmer's lung in Finland and its relation to meteorological factors. Eur J Respir Dis Suppl 1987;152:47–56.

16. Depierre A, Dalphin JC, Pernet D, et al. Epidemiological study of farmer's lung in five districts of the French Doubs province. Thorax 1988;43:429–35.

17. Rodriguez de Castro F, Carrillo T, Castillo R, et al. Relationships between characteristics of exposure to pigeon antigens. Clinical manifestations and humoral immune response. Chest 1993;103:1059–63.

18. Hendrick DJ, Faux JA, Marshall R. Budgerigar-fancier's lung: the commonest variety of allergic alveolitis in Britain. Br Med J 1978;2:81–4.

19. Grech V, Vella C, Lenicker H. Pigeon breeder's lung in childhood: varied clinical picture at presentation. Pediatr Pulmonol 2000;30:145–8.

20. Ratjen F, Costabel U, Griese M, et al. Bronchoalveolar lavage fluid findings in children with hypersensitivity pneumonitis. Eur Respir J 2003;21: 144–8.

21. Baur X, Richter G, Pethran A, et al. Increased prevalence of IgG-induced sensitization and hypersensitivity pneumonitis (humidifier lung) in nonsmokers exposed to aerosols of a contaminated air conditioner. Respiration 1992;59:211–4.

22. Sennekamp J, Niese D, Stroehmann I, et al. Pigeon breeders' lung lacking detectable antibodies. Clin Allergy 1978;8:305–10.

23. Salvaggio JE, Robert A. Cooke memorial lecture. Hypersensitivity pneumonitis. J Allergy Clin Immunol 1987;79:558–71.

24. Costabel U. The alveolitis of hypersensitivity pneumonitis. Eur Respir J 1988;1:5–9.

25. Schuyler M, Gott K, Cherne A, et al. Th1 CD4+ cells adoptively transfer experimental hypersensitivity pneumonitis. Cell Immunol 1997;177:169–75.

26. Yamasaki H, Ando M, Brazer W, et al. Polarized type 1 cytokine profile in bronchoalveolar lavage T cells of patients with hypersensitivity pneumonitis. J Immunol 1999;163:3516–23.

27. Chen B, Tong Z, Nakamura S, et al. Production of IL-12, IL-18 and TNF-alpha by alveolar macrophages in hypersensitivity pneumonitis. Sarcoidosis Vasc Diffuse Lung Dis 2004;21:199–203.

28. Ye Q, Nakamura S, Sarria R, et al. Interleukin 12, interleukin 18, and tumor necrosis factor alpha release by alveolar macrophages: acute and chronic hypersensitivity pneumonitis. Ann Allergy Asthma Immunol 2009;102:149–54.

29. Mroz RM, Korniluk M, Stasiak-Barmuta A, et al. Increased levels of interleukin-12 and interleukin-18 in bronchoalveolar lavage fluid of patients with pulmonary sarcoidosis. J Physiol Pharmacol 2008; 59(Suppl 6):507–13.

30. Chen B, Tong Z, Ye Q, et al. Expression of tumour necrosis factor receptors by bronchoalveolar cells in hypersensitivity pneumonitis. Eur Respir J 2005; 25:1039–43.

31. Dai H, Guzman J, Chen B, et al. Production of soluble tumor necrosis factor receptors and tumor necrosis factor-alpha by alveolar macrophages in sarcoidosis and extrinsic allergic alveolitis. Chest 2005;127:251–6.

32. Barrera L, Mendoza F, Zuniga J, et al. Functional diversity of T-cell subpopulations in subacute and chronic hypersensitivity pneumonitis. Am J Respir Crit Care Med 2008;177:44–55.

33. Kishi M, Miyazaki Y, Jinta T, et al. Pathogenesis of cBFL in common with IPF? Correlation of IP-10/TARC ratio with histological patterns. Thorax 2008;63:810–6.

34. Mitaka K, Miyazaki Y, Yasui M, et al. Th2-biased immune responses are important in a murine model of chronic hypersensitivity pneumonitis. Int Arch Allergy Immunol 2011;154:264–74.

35. Camarena A, Juarez A, Mejia M, et al. Major histocompatibility complex and tumor necrosis factor-alpha polymorphisms in pigeon breeder's disease. Am J Respir Crit Care Med 2001;163:1528–33.

36. Schaaf BM, Seitzer U, Pravica V, et al. Tumor necrosis factor-alpha -308 promoter gene polymorphism and increased tumor necrosis factor serum bioactivity in farmer's lung patients. Am J Respir Crit Care Med 2001;163:379–82.

37. Aquino-Galvez A, Camarena A, Montano M, et al. Transporter associated with antigen processing (TAP) 1 gene polymorphisms in patients with hypersensitivity pneumonitis. Exp Mol Pathol 2008;84:173–7.

38. Camarena A, Aquino-Galvez A, Falfan-Valencia R, et al. PSMB8 (LMP7) but not PSMB9 (LMP2) gene polymorphisms are associated to pigeon breeder's hypersensitivity pneumonitis. Respir Med 2010; 104:889–94.

39. Hill MR, Briggs L, Montano MM, et al. Promoter variants in tissue inhibitor of metalloproteinase-3 (TIMP-3) protect against susceptibility in pigeon breeders' disease. Thorax 2004;59:586–90.

40. Janssen R, Kruit A, Grutters JC, et al. TIMP-3 promoter gene polymorphisms in BFL. Thorax 2005;60:974.

41. Cormier Y, Tremblay GM, Fournier M, et al. Long-term viral enhancement of lung response to Saccharopolyspora rectivirgula. Am J Respir Crit Care Med 1994;149:490–4.

42. Coleman A, Colby TV. Histologic diagnosis of extrinsic allergic alveolitis. Am J Surg Pathol 1988; 12:514–8.

43. Trahan S, Hanak V, Ryu JH, et al. Role of surgical lung biopsy in separating chronic hypersensitivity pneumonia from usual interstitial pneumonia/idiopathic pulmonary fibrosis: analysis of 31 biopsies from 15 patients. Chest 2008;134:126–32.

44. Ohtani Y, Saiki S, Kitaichi M, et al. Chronic bird fancier's lung: histopathological and clinical correlation. An application of the 2002 ATS/ERS consensus classification of the idiopathic interstitial pneumonias. Thorax 2005;60:665–71.

45. Churg A, Sin DD, Everett D, et al. Pathologic patterns and survival in chronic hypersensitivity pneumonitis. Am J Surg Pathol 2009;33:1765–70.

46. Lima MS, Coletta EN, Ferreira RG, et al. Subacute and chronic hypersensitivity pneumonitis: histopathological patterns and survival. Respir Med 2009; 103:508–15.

47. Gaxiola M, Buendia-Roldan I, Mejia M, et al. Morphologic diversity of chronic pigeon breeder's disease: clinical features and survival. Respir Med 2011;105:608–14.

48. Vourlekis JS, Schwarz MI, Cool CD, et al. Nonspecific interstitial pneumonitis as the sole histologic expression of hypersensitivity pneumonitis. Am J Med 2002;112:490–3.

49. Churg A, Muller NL, Flint J, et al. Chronic hypersensitivity pneumonitis. Am J Surg Pathol 2006;30: 201–8.

50. Akashi T, Takemura T, Ando N, et al. Histopathologic analysis of sixteen autopsy cases of chronic hypersensitivity pneumonitis and comparison with idiopathic pulmonary fibrosis/usual interstitial pneumonia. Am J Clin Pathol 2009;131:405–15.

51. Cormier Y, Letourneau L, Racine G. Significance of precipitins and asymptomatic lymphocytic alveolitis: a 20 year follow-up. Eur Respir J 2004;23: 523–5.

52. Ohtani Y, Saiki S, Sumi Y, et al. Clinical features of recurrent and insidious chronic bird fancier's lung. Ann Allergy Asthma Immunol 2003;90:604–10.

53. Adler BD, Padley SP, Muller NL, et al. Chronic hypersensitivity pneumonitis: high-resolution CT and radiographic features in 16 patients. Radiology 1992;185:91–5.

54. Remy-Jardin M, Remy J, Wallaert B, et al. Subacute and chronic bird breeder hypersensitivity pneumonitis: sequential evaluation with CT and correlation with lung function tests and bronchoalveolar lavage. Radiology 1993;189:111–8.

55. Erkinjuntti-Pekkanen R, Rytkonen H, Kokkarinen JI, et al. Long-term risk of emphysema in patients with farmer's lung and matched control farmers. Am J Respir Crit Care Med 1998;158:662–5.

56. Cormier Y, Brown M, Worthy S, et al. High-resolution computed tomographic characteristics in acute farmer's lung and in its follow-up. Eur Respir J 2000;16:56–60.

57. Tateishi T, Ohtani Y, Takemura T, et al. Serial high-resolution computed tomography findings of acute and chronic hypersensitivity pneumonitis induced by avian antigen. J Comput Assist Tomogr 2011; 35:272–9.

58. Lynch DA, Newell JD, Logan PM, et al. Can CT distinguish hypersensitivity pneumonitis from idiopathic pulmonary fibrosis? AJR Am J Roentgenol 1995;165:807–11.

59. Silva CIS, Muller NL, Lynch DA, et al. Chronic hypersensitivity pneumonitis: differentiation from idiopathic pulmonary fibrosis and nonspecific interstitial pneumonia by using thin-section CT. Radiology 2008;246:288–97.

60. Cormier Y, Belanger J. The fluctuant nature of precipitating antibodies in dairy farmers. Thorax 1989;44:469–73.

61. Erkinjuntti-Pekkanen R, Reiman M, Kokkarinen JI, et al. IgG antibodies, chronic bronchitis, and pulmonary function values in farmer's lung patients and matched controls. Allergy 1999;54:1181–7.

62. Fenoglio CM, Reboux G, Sudre B, et al. Diagnostic value of serum precipitins to mould antigens in active hypersensitivity pneumonitis. Eur Respir J 2007;29:706–12.

63. Aguilar Leon DE, Novelo Retana V, Martinez-Cordero E. Anti-avian antibodies and rheumatoid factor in pigeon hypersensitivity pneumonitis. Clin Exp Allergy 2003;33:226–32.

64. Semenzato G, Bjermer L, Costabel U, et al. Clinical guidelines and indications for bronchoalveolar lavage (BAL): extrinsic allergic alveolitis. Eur Respir J 1990;3:945–6, 961–9.

65. Drent M, Wagenaar S, van Velzen-Blad H, et al. Relationship between plasma cell levels and profile of bronchoalveolar lavage fluid in patients with subacute extrinsic allergic alveolitis. Thorax 1993;48:835–9.

66. Costabel U, Bross KJ, Ruhle KH, et al. Ia-like antigens on T-cells and their subpopulations in pulmonary sarcoidosis and in hypersensitivity pneumonitis. Analysis of bronchoalveolar and blood lymphocytes. Am Rev Respir Dis 1985;131:337–42.

67. Ando M, Konishi K, Yoneda R, et al. Difference in phenotypes of bronchoalveolar lavage lymphocytes in patients with summer-type hypersensitivity pneumonitis, farmer's lung, ventilation pneumonitis, and bird fancier's lung: report of a nationwide epidemiologic study in Japan. J Allergy Clin Immunol 1991; 87:1002–9.

68. Drent M, van Velzen-Blad H, Diamant M, et al. Bronchoalveolar lavage in extrinsic allergic alveolitis: effect of time elapsed since antigen exposure. Eur Respir J 1993;6:1276–81.

69. Lacasse Y, Selman M, Costabel U, et al. Clinical diagnosis of hypersensitivity pneumonitis. Am J Respir Crit Care Med 2003;168:952–8.

70. Ohshimo S, Bonella F, Cui A, et al. Significance of bronchoalveolar lavage for the diagnosis of idiopathic pulmonary fibrosis. Am J Respir Crit Care Med 2009;179:1043–7.

71. Hanak V, Golbin JM, Hartman TE, et al. High-resolution CT findings of parenchymal fibrosis correlate with prognosis in hypersensitivity pneumonitis. Chest 2008;134:133–8.

72. Sahin H, Brown KK, Curran-Everett D, et al. Chronic hypersensitivity pneumonitis: CT features comparison with pathologic evidence of fibrosis and survival. Radiology 2007;244:591–8.

73. Erkinjuntti-Pekkanen R, Kokkarinen JI, Tukiainen HO, et al. Long-term outcome of pulmonary function in farmer's lung: a 14 year follow-up with matched controls. Eur Respir J 1997;10:2046–50.

74. Schmidt CD, Jensen RL, Christensen LT, et al. Longitudinal pulmonary function changes in pigeon breeders. Chest 1988;93:359–63.

75. Allen DH, Williams GV, Woolcock AJ. Bird breeder's hypersensitivity pneumonitis: progress studies of lung function after cessation of exposure to the provoking antigen. Am Rev Respir Dis 1976;114:555–66.

76. de Gracia J, Morell F, Bofill JM, et al. Time of exposure as a prognostic factor in avian hypersensitivity pneumonitis. Respir Med 1989;83:139–43.

77. Kokkarinen J, Tukiainen H, Terho EO. Mortality due to farmer's lung in Finland. Chest 1994;106:509–12.

78. Barbee RA, Callies Q, Dickie HA, et al. The long-term prognosis in farmer's lung. Am Rev Respir Dis 1968;97:223–31.

79. Emanuel DA, Wenzel FJ, Bowerman CI, et al. Farmer's Lung: clinical, pathologic and immunologic study of twenty-four patients. Am J Med 1964;37:392–401.

80. Braun SR, doPico GA, Tsiatis A, et al. Farmer's lung disease: long-term clinical and physiologic outcome. Am Rev Respir Dis 1979;119:185–91.

81. Bourke SJ, Banham SW, Carter R, et al. Longitudinal course of extrinsic allergic alveolitis in pigeon breeders. Thorax 1989;44:415–8.

82. Perez-Padilla R, Salas J, Chapela R, et al. Mortality in Mexican patients with chronic pigeon breeder's lung compared with those with usual interstitial pneumonia. Am Rev Respir Dis 1993;148:49–53.

83. Olson AL, Huie TJ, Groshong SD, et al. Acute exacerbations of fibrotic hypersensitivity pneumonitis. Chest 2008;134:844–50.

84. Miyazaki Y, Tateishi T, Akashi T, et al. Clinical predictors and histologic appearance of acute exacerbations in chronic hypersensitivity pneumonitis. Chest 2008;134:1265–70.

85. Kuramochi J, Inase N, Miyazaki Y, et al. Lung cancer in chronic hypersensitivity pneumonitis. Respiration 2011;82:263–7.

86. Vourlekis JS, Schwarz MI, Cherniack RM, et al. The effect of pulmonary fibrosis on survival in patients with hypersensitivity pneumonitis. Am J Med 2004; 116:662–8.

87. Greinert U, Lepp U, Vollmer E, et al. Vogelhalterlunge ohne Vogelhaltung. Pneumologie 2000;54:179–83.

88. Kokkarinen JI, Tukiainen HO, Terho EO. Effect of corticosteroid treatment on the recovery of pulmonary function in farmer's lung. Am Rev Respir Dis 1992;145:3–5.

Smoking-Related Interstitial Lung Diseases

Robert Vassallo, MD[a,b], Jay H. Ryu, MD[a,*]

KEYWORDS

- Smoking • Interstitial lung disease
- Respiratory bronchiolitis
- Desquamative interstitial pneumonia • Fibrosis
- Pulmonary Langerhans cell histiocytosis
- Acute eosinophilic pneumonia

Cigarette smoke is a complex mixture of more than 4000 chemicals, many of which exert toxic effects on cellular function. In addition to chronic obstructive pulmonary disease (COPD) and cancer, cigarette smokers may develop certain diffuse interstitial and bronchiolar disorders (**Box 1**, **Table 1**).[1–4] These diffuse lung diseases are referred to as smoking-related interstitial lung diseases (ILDs), a term that recognizes the suspected causal association with cigarette smoking. Novel insights regarding the relationship between smoking and ILD are highlighted in this review.

SMOKING AND ILD

Cigarette smoking is now widely accepted as the primary cause of certain ILDs, namely, respiratory bronchiolitis–associated ILD (RB-ILD), desquamative interstitial pneumonia (DIP), and pulmonary Langerhans cell histiocytosis (PLCH).[1–5] Cigarette smoking is also a risk factor for the development of idiopathic pulmonary fibrosis (IPF)[14] and rheumatoid arthritis (RA)-associated ILD[15,24] and has been reported to cause some cases of acute eosinophilic pneumonia (AEP)[25] and pulmonary hemorrhage syndromes. Paradoxically, cigarette smoking may confer protection from developing some other ILDs such as hypersensitivity pneumonitis (HP).[26] The authors recently described a classification scheme (see **Box 1**) outlining these subgroups and their relationship with smoking.[27] This classification illustrates the highly complex effects of smoking on lung parenchyma and ILDs.

The group 1 diseases (see **Box 1**) include the 3 diffuse lung diseases widely regarded as true smoking-related ILDs. This designation is supported by several lines of clinical, epidemiologic, and investigative evidence showing a direct role for cigarette smoking as witnessed in the temporal relationship to disease onset and progression, resolution on smoking cessation, and recurrence on resumption of smoking.[6,28–31] Several case series have reported a history of smoking in the overwhelming majority of patients with group 1 diseases, with the prevalence being highest in RB-ILD,[4,32] followed by PLCH,[2,5] and least common in DIP.[4,7] The reported coexistence of all 3 lesions in the same patient,[6] the potential for disease remission with smoking cessation,[4] the recurrence of disease in transplanted lungs,[33,34] and the description of analogous lesions in mice exposed to high doses of cigarette smoke[29] provide support to the designation of RB-ILD, DIP, and PLCH as smoking-induced ILDs.

Supported by a Flight Attendant Medical Research Institute (FAMRI) award to R.V.

The authors have no conflict of interest.

All authors have directly contributed to the content of this manuscript and reviewed the final version.

[a] Division of Pulmonary and Critical Care Medicine, Mayo Clinic, Gonda 18 South, 200 First Street Southwest, Rochester, MN 55905, USA

[b] Department of Physiology and Biomedical Engineering, Mayo Clinic, Rochester, MN 55905, USA

* Corresponding author.

E-mail address: ryu.jay@mayo.edu

Clin Chest Med 33 (2012) 165–178

doi:10.1016/j.ccm.2011.11.004

Box 1
Proposed classification of smoking-related ILDs

Group 1: chronic ILDs that are very likely caused by cigarette smoking[4–8]

    Respiratory bronchiolitis–associated ILD

    Desquamative interstitial pneumonia

    Adult pulmonary Langerhans cell histiocytosis

Group 2: acute ILDs that may be precipitated by cigarette smoking[9–13]

    Acute eosinophilic pneumonia

    Pulmonary hemorrhage syndromes

Group 3: ILDs that are statistically more prevalent in smokers[14–18]

    Idiopathic pulmonary fibrosis

    Rheumatoid arthritis–associated ILD

Group 4: ILDs that are less prevalent in smokers[19–23]

    Hypersensitivity pneumonitis

    Sarcoidosis

Diseases allocated to group 2 (see **Box 1**) differ because the association with cigarette smoking is less robust than that for group 1 diseases. Cigarette smoking, particularly during the relatively early phase of initiation of smoking, seems to be an important precipitating factor in some but not all cases of group 2 diseases. The most relevant conditions in this category include AEP and certain pulmonary hemorrhage syndromes.[9–11,25,35] AEP deserves particular attention because several recent studies have implicated recent-onset exposure to cigarette smoke as a principal inducer of this disease in some patients diagnosed to have this disorder.[10,12,35–37] Of particular interest is the response of certain subjects with resolved AEP to a rechallenge with cigarette smoke exposure that triggers peripheral eosinophilia and other associated pathophysiologic abnormalities suggesting exposure to cigarette smoke to induce certain responses relevant to the development of acute diffuse lung disease in susceptible hosts.[10]

Diseases included in group 3 (see **Box 1**) are chronic diffuse lung diseases that are statistically more likely to develop in cigarette smokers.[16,17] For instance, cigarette smoking is known to increase the relative risk of RA-associated ILD, possibly by triggering RA-specific immune reactions to citrullinated proteins.[16,18,24] Similarly, smokers have a higher risk of developing IPF than nonsmokers.[17] The precise significance of these observations has been a topic of substantial debate, but there is limited evidence that smoking itself is directly fibrogenic to the lung.[38] It is not appropriate to consider smoking as an inducer of these diseases, but rather a disease modifier or potentially a cofactor that facilitates the development of profibrotic responses that lead to these diffuse fibrotic lung diseases.

Table 1
Key characteristics of group 1 chronic smoking–related diffuse lung diseases

	RB-ILD	DIP	PLCH
Association with Cigarette Smoking	95%	60%–90%	95%–97%
Clinical Features	Chronic cough and dyspnea, inspiratory crackles	Chronic cough and dyspnea, inspiratory crackles	Chronic cough and dyspnea. Pneumothorax in 15%
High-Resolution Computed Tomographic Findings	Centrilobular nodules and ground-glass opacities	Ground-glass and reticular opacities	Peribronchiolar nodules, cavitated nodules, and cysts with relative sparing of lung bases
Key Histologic Findings	Pigment-laden macrophages in the respiratory bronchioles and alveolar ducts	Diffuse alveolar filling with pigment-laden macrophages	Bronchiolocentric nodules, stellate lesions, CD1a-positive Langerhans cells
Response to Corticosteroids	Modest, variable	Modest, variable	Modest, variable

Abbreviations: DIP, desquamative interstitial pneumonia; PLCH, pulmonary Langerhans cell histiocytosis; RB-ILD, respiratory bronchiolitis–associated interstitial lung disease.

The fourth and final group consists of diseases that are less prevalent in smokers than nonsmokers and includes sarcoidosis and HP.[19–22] Cigarette smoking seems to provide certain protective effects that diminish the potential development of these granulomatous inflammatory lung diseases, possibly by inhibiting certain immunologic responses in the lung that are required for granuloma formation or the development of T-helper subtype 1 (T_H1)-polarized immune responses following exposure to inhaled antigens.[39,40] Epidemiologic studies demonstrate that levels of circulating IgG antibodies to pigeon antigens are higher among nonsmokers than smokers.[41] A similar study in farmers showed that nonsmokers and previous smokers had a higher prevalence of serum precipitin levels to various farmer's lung antigens compared with current smokers.[42] Lung macrophages from cigarette smokers also have lower levels of costimulatory molecules than controls.[40] Because costimulatory molecules play a critical role in shaping the immune response to inhaled antigens, it is possible that smokers are hyporesponsive to inhaled antigens by virtue of diminished antigen-presenting capacity in the lung. Cigarette smoking and nicotine have also been demonstrated to inhibit the production of the potent T_H1-polarizing cytokine interleukin (IL) 12.[39] It is conceivable that the diminished capacity of smokers' macrophages and dendritic cells to generate IL-12 may impede the development of hypersensitivity response to inhaled antigens and granuloma formation in the context of sarcoidosis. The observation that smoking is associated with a lower prevalence of sarcoidosis and HP should not be construed as an indication to promote smoking in patients with these diseases. On the contrary, the insight gained from dissecting mechanisms by which smoking suppresses T_H1 immunity, an essential driver of the immunopathogenic processes that characterize these diffuse lung diseases, is also relevant to the pathogenesis of smoking-related lung cancer and airway diseases, diseases that are more prevalent in smokers partly because of impaired T_H1 immunity.

The fact that some cases of RB-ILD or DIP may be induced by factors other than cigarette smoke exposure and that some patients with PLCH are nonsmokers had been interpreted as implying that these disease do not necessarily represent specific smoking-induced lung diseases. However, it is well recognized that several specific histopathologic entities can be induced by heterogeneous etiologies, potentially a reflection that the lung has only a limited number of ways of responding to various insults. For example, the lesion of usual interstitial pneumonia (UIP) may be induced by asbestos exposure and may be seen in patients

with chronic HP, as well as in the context of autoimmune diseases such as RA-associated ILD.[43,44] Cigarette smoking is the most well-defined etiologic factor associated with the development of RB-ILD, DIP, and PLCH; however, the histopathologic lesions of RB, DIP, and PLCH do not exclusively occur in smokers and may occasionally be idiopathic or encountered in the context of other exposures or causes.[5,7,8]

Defining the relationship between smoking and specific ILDs has important clinical implications. Smoking cessation is imperative for all the diseases listed under groups 1 to 3 in **Box 1**. Physicians use aggressive tobacco cessation strategies in these patients, and, for these patients, there is a low threshold for referral to nicotine dependence counselors. It is the authors' practice to explicitly refer to diseases in group 1 as smoking induced to underscore the importance of smoking cessation and encourage removal of all tobacco products from the vicinity of the patient, including second-hand tobacco smoke exposure. Similarly, all current smokers with diseases in groups 2 and 3 should be counseled regarding the emerging and compelling data implicating a direct pathogenic role for cigarette smoke exposure as a potential inducer or cofactor in disease induction and progression. Methods that should be considered in smoking cessation therapy include counseling and behavior therapy, nicotine replacement therapy, and pharmacotherapy, including the use of bupropion, varenicline, and clonidine in selected patients.[45]

MECHANISMS BY WHICH TOBACCO SMOKE MAY PROMOTE ILD

Even in smokers without clinically detectable lung disease, cigarette smoking induces inflammatory cell recruitment, consisting primarily of macrophages, neutrophils, and Langerhans cells (a subtype of the myeloid dendritic cell family expressing surface CD1a receptors), to small airways.[46,47] Although all smokers have some degree of inflammation in the airways, only a minority develop clinically significant diffuse lung disease. The relative rarity of smoking-related ILDs compared with the overall prevalence of cigarette smoking suggests that cigarette smoke is not the only factor responsible for the induction of these diseases and implies that additional factors (endogenous such as genetic factors or exogenous such as infectious pathogens or allergens) are required for the induction of disease.

A characteristic morphologic feature of all group 1 smoking-related ILDs is prominent bronchiolar inflammation.[6,48–50] In addition, group 1 diseases demonstrate increased macrophages in the interstitium and alveolar spaces.[48,49,51] Pigmented macrophage accumulation in small airways, interstitium, and distal air spaces is a key feature of many smoking-related ILDs. Specific mechanisms by which exaggerated macrophage accumulation occurs in group 1 diseases are not fully defined but likely involve exaggerated generation of macrophage recruiting and differentiating factors by airway epithelial cells, enhanced macrophage survival locally, and/or diminished apoptosis of recruited macrophages.[52] In these patients, lung epithelial cells have been demonstrated to aberrantly produce excessive granulocyte-macrophage colony-stimulating factor (GM-CSF), a cytokine that provides proliferative and activation signals to both macrophages and dendritic cells.[53,54] Cigarette smoke extracts have also been shown to induce transforming growth factor β (TGF-β) production by lung epithelial cells, a cytokine that is involved in Langerhans cell development, immune modulation, and fibrogenic responses in the airways.[55]

Cigarette smoking induces several abnormalities in immune and other lung cells that are likely relevant to the pathogenesis of smoking-related ILDs.[39,56,57] Certain constituents in cigarette smoke are known to activate epithelial cells, macrophages, neutrophils, and dendritic cells in vitro, promoting generation of chemokines and cytokines that lead to inflammation by promoting immune cell recruitment.[58,59] It is reasonable to speculate that smokers in whom ILD develops have an amplified inflammatory cascade associated with activation of multiple immune cell types that promote a vicious cycle of inflammatory cell recruitment. Whether failure of endogenous antiinflammatory mechanisms or additional exogenous insults such as viral infections have a role in promoting smoking-related ILDs is unknown but should be an important area of future research.

RB-ILD

Niewoehner and colleagues[60] described RB as a histopathologic finding of pigmented macrophage accumulation centering on respiratory bronchioles and neighboring alveoli, a finding that was ubiquitous in cigarette smokers. Subsequent case series described similar findings on lung biopsy specimens from cigarette smokers.[1,6,8] RB can thus be considered a histologic marker of smoking and must be distinguished from RB-ILD, a term coined by Myers and colleagues[50] to recognize the clinicopathologic ILD occurring in cigarette smokers in whom surgical lung biopsy revealed only RB. In patients with RB-ILD, the lesion of RB is not felt to be a mere indicator of exposure to smoking but rather constitutes the primary and only histopathologic lesion accountable for the observed diffuse lung disease. Following the original description by Myers and colleagues, other reports described with greater detail the clinical and radiologic features of RB-ILD as a specific interstitial and bronchiolar process occurring in smokers and defined by the presence of RB as the only definable pathologic abnormality present on lung biopsy.[1,8,61]

The true prevalence of RB-ILD is difficult to estimate because many patients with this disorder may be asymptomatic.[4] The duration of exposure to cigarette smoke need not be lengthy or severe, although many have substantial cumulative tobacco exposures.[1] Most patients present in the fourth and fifth decade of life, and there is no gender predilection.[3,4,32] A clinicopathologic syndrome indistinguishable from RB-ILD can occasionally be encountered following exposure to solder fumes,[8] diesel smoke, and fiberglass.[1]

RB-ILD usually presents in a nonspecific manner with chronic cough and exertional dyspnea; rarely, acute presentation may occur.[62] The physical examination reveals inspiratory crackles in approximately one-half of the patients, but digital clubbing is infrequent.[3,4,32] Pulmonary function testing yields various patterns including normal, obstructive, restrictive, or mixed abnormalities.[4,32] The severity of physiologic impairment, if present, is usually mild to moderate.[4]

Chest radiography reveals bilateral, fine reticular, or reticulonodular opacities in about 60% to 70% of patients but may appear normal in some patients.[4,8,32] The main findings on chest high-resolution computed tomography (HRCT) include bronchial wall thickening, fine centrilobular nodules, and patchy areas of ground-glass attenuation.[4,8,32] The ground-glass changes are typically bilateral and affect both upper and lower lung fields (Fig. 1).[51,63] Coexisting emphysematous changes are frequently noted but honeycombing, traction bronchiectasis, and parenchymal fibrosis are not.

The differential diagnosis of RB-ILD includes consideration of other bronchiolar diseases, including infectious bronchiolitis, follicular bronchiolitis, and diffuse aspiration bronchiolitis, and also ILDs characterized by ground-glass opacities, particularly HP and nonspecific interstitial pneumonia (NSIP). Although surgical lung biopsy is often required for a definitive diagnosis, in clinical practice, a provisional diagnosis may be established in many patients on the basis of epidemiologic, clinical, and radiologic features and reasonable exclusion of other potential

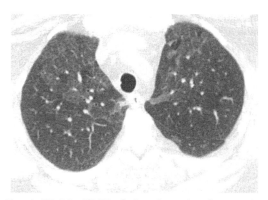

Fig. 1. RB-ILD. HRCT of the chest showing patchy areas of ground-glass attenuation in upper lung fields in a smoker with RB-ILD.

diagnoses.[8] Bronchoscopic lung biopsy has a low yield and bronchoalveolar lavage (BAL) findings are nonspecific in RB-ILD but may be diagnostically helpful in distinguishing RB-ILD from other conditions such as HP that are associated with more specific features.

The histopathologic findings required for the diagnosis of RB-ILD are those of RB and include the presence of yellow-brown–pigmented macrophages in the lumens of respiratory bronchioles, alveolar ducts, and peribronchiolar alveolar spaces without significant associated interstitial pneumonia.[4,64] At low power, these features are patchy and generally confined to peribronchiolar regions (bronchiolocentric distribution). Mild peribronchiolar fibrosis can be seen, but honeycombing is unusual.[8,63]

As in all group 1 diseases, smoking cessation is a key component of RB-ILD management. Smoking cessation may lead to improvement in radiologic abnormalities and lung function.[4,65] The degree of improvement following smoking cessation seems to be limited in some patients, and abnormalities may persist for years.[1,32] For patients with significant lung impairment, corticosteroids or other immunosuppressive medications have been used in an attempt to limit progression of lung disease; however, evidence of their effectiveness is lacking.[4,32] Most patients with RB-ILD have a relatively good prognosis, and mortality from RB-ILD is uncommon.[4,32] Although smoking cessation may lead to disease remission in some patients with RB-ILD, longitudinal studies have shown that some patients remain symptomatic for years after smoking cessation.[32]

DIP

DIP was originally believed to be a diffuse lung disease resulting from desquamation of alveolar epithelial cells into the alveolar space but later was recognized as a process of alveolar filling from macrophage accumulation.[66] DIP is associated with cigarette smoking in at least two-thirds of cases[4,7,61] but can also be seen in nonsmokers, particularly in the context of autoimmune diseases,[43] some infections,[67] and drug exposures.[67,68] It has been reported to occur in children as well as adults.[4]

The clinical presentation of DIP is nonspecific with dyspnea and cough, and physical examination reveals inspiratory crackles in approximately 60% and digital clubbing in 25% to 50% of patients.[4] Pulmonary function testing reveals restriction in one-third of cases, normal findings in 10% to 20%, and a mixed defect in the remainder.[4]

Chest radiography typically reveals patchy haziness or interstitial patterns with lower zone predominance.[4,69] The striking abnormality on HRCT is ground-glass opacities predominantly in the lower lung zones and often in a peripheral distribution (**Fig. 2**).[70] Irregular linear opacities are frequently present; however, honeycombing and significant architectural distortion are uncommon. In some instances, patients with DIP have been reported to develop HRCT findings suggestive of fibrotic NSIP (irregular linear opacities) on longitudinal follow-up.[3,71] Small parenchymal cysts and apical emphysematous changes may also be seen.[72]

On light microscopy, lung biopsies show characteristic filling of alveolar spaces with pigment-laden alveolar macrophages.[7] Although both RB-ILD and DIP are associated with the accumulation of pigment-laden macrophages in alveolar spaces, the distribution of abnormality is more bronchiolocentric and patchy in RB, whereas in DIP it tends to be more diffuse.[6] The extent of interstitial fibrosis, lymphoid follicles, and eosinophilic infiltration has been reported to be more

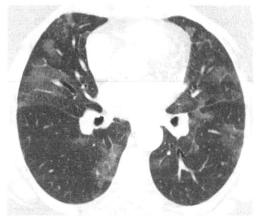

Fig. 2. DIP. HRCT of the chest showing more extensive ground-glass opacities in a smoker with DIP.

prevalent in DIP than RB-ILD.[7,61] Fibroblast foci are not seen, and the DIP lesion appears temporally uniform.[64] A definitive diagnosis of DIP usually requires surgical lung biopsy because it may be difficult to reliably differentiate DIP from NSIP or RB-ILD by clinical, radiologic, and bronchoscopic criteria.[6]

For those patients with DIP who are smokers, smoking cessation is an essential component of therapy. Prolonged remission of DIP after smoking cessation has been described, but, like all other smoking-related ILDs, the effect of smoking cessation on the natural history of DIP remains poorly characterized.[4,73] Although most patients with DIP have a relatively good prognosis with a better than 90% 5-year survival,[74] some patients progress to respiratory failure and premature death within 5 to 10 years after the diagnosis.[4,7] Patients with DIP are frequently treated with corticosteroids, but the effectiveness of steroid therapy is variable and has not been evaluated in a prospective study.[1] Other immunosuppressants such as azathioprine and methotrexate have been used in anecdotal cases.[75] Lung transplantation is an option for patients with progressive disease, but DIP can recur in the transplanted lung.[76,77]

PLCH

PLCH (also referred to as pulmonary Langerhans granulomatosis, pulmonary eosinophilic granuloma, or histiocytosis X) is induced by cigarette smoke exposure in most adult patients diagnosed to have this disorder and is characterized by accumulation of CD1a-expressing Langerhans cells in the lung and occasionally in other organ systems.[78,79] Adult PLCH forms part of the spectrum of histiocytic diseases, which ranges from relatively benign processes such as unifocal Langerhans cell histiocytosis (LCH) involving bone to disseminated multiorgan forms associated with significant morbidity and mortality.[80] Contrary to DIP and RB-ILD, which exclusively affect the lungs, approximately 15% of adult patients with PLCH may have disease outside the thoracic cavity.[5,81] PLCH represents approximately 5% of the total number of diffuse lung diseases diagnosed by lung biopsy.[81] PLCH tends to affect younger adults in their third and fourth decades.[5] PLCH seems to affect both men and women equally.

Approximately 95% of adults with PLCH are active or former smokers or have been exposed to substantial second-hand cigarette smoke.[2,49,81,82] Although the pathogenesis remains poorly understood, it is likely that cigarette smoke constituents activate epithelial cells and other cell types in the airways to produce cytokines that promote recruitment, activation, and retention of Langerhans cells in the subepithelial regions of the airways.[53,54,83] Cigarette smoke also induces the production of cytokines with profibrotic functions, such as TGF-β; in turn, TGF-β and other cytokines such as GM-CSF may further promote local expansion of Langerhans cells and facilitate the development of tissue remodeling and fibrosis as is evident in more advanced PLCH cases.[81] It is possible that certain cigarette smoke constituents are taken up by immune or other cells and result in direct immune cell activation in peribronchiolar regions. Activated Langerhans cells and macrophages in peribronchiolar regions are likely to then promote secondary recruitment of T cells, plasma cells, and eosinophils, resulting in the formation of eosinophilic granulomatous inflammation from which the descriptive term eosinophilic granuloma is derived.

As in other smoking-related ILDs, the clinical presentation tends to be nonspecific and includes dry cough and shortness of breath. About one-third of patients are asymptomatic.[5] Constitutional symptoms occur in approximately 20% to 30% of patients, whereas few patients (around 10%–15%) may present with a spontaneous pneumothorax, which can be recurrent.[5,85] Rarely, patients may present with symptoms related to extrapulmonary manifestation, such as skin, lymph node, or bony involvement.

Pulmonary function testing demonstrates variable results and may show obstructive, restrictive, mixed, or nonspecific abnormalities; pulmonary function testing may at times be completely normal.[5] Physiologic studies reveal limitations in the exercise capacity that can occur even with relatively normal resting ventilatory function. Exercise limitation correlates with markers of pulmonary vascular dysfunction, implying vascular involvement as an important cause of exercise limitation in these patients.[86]

The chest radiograph is usually abnormal and shows reticulonodular opacities more prominent in the middle and upper lung zones.[87] The HRCT of the chest often reveals characteristic abnormalities that include nodules and cysts in varying combinations bilaterally with relative sparing of the lung bases (**Fig. 3**). Nodules with or without cavitation predominate in early disease, whereas cystic changes predominate in more advanced disease.[87,88] A bronchoscopic or surgically obtained lung biopsy is recommended to confirm the diagnosis but is not always necessary. Bronchoscopy is diagnostically useful if elevated percentage of CD1a-positive cells is identified in the BAL fluid, with 5% or more being virtually diagnostic of PLCH.[89,90]

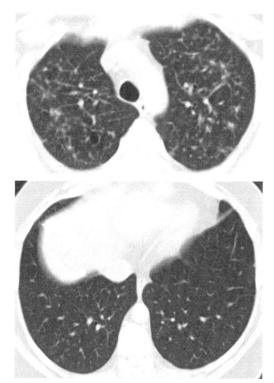

Fig. 3. PLCH. HRCT of the chest demonstrating a combination of nodular and cystic lesions in the upper lung fields and relative sparing of the lung bases in a smoker with PLCH.

Histologic features of early PLCH include loosely formed nodules of mixed inflammatory cells centered on small airways in a bronchiolocentric pattern.[48] These bronchiolocentric lesions of pulmonary LCH typically form stellate lesions with central scarring.[64] Langerhans cells are abundant in early lesions and may be identified by immunohistochemical staining for the CD1a or langerin cell surface antigens or by the identification of intracellular Birbeck granules (pentalaminar rod-shaped intracellular structures) by electron microscopy.[49,64,90,91] Eosinophilic infiltration is often encountered and may be quite extensive earlier in the course of the disease.[49,64,90,91] Varying degrees of parenchymal infiltration with macrophages, lymphocytes, and eosinophils are noted, and, in rare cases, extensive alveolar macrophage infiltration causes a pseudo-DIP reaction.[48] Some cases are associated with extensive vascular infiltration of inflammatory cells, resulting in a proliferative vasculopathy involving both arteries and veins.[92]

A critical component in the management of PLCH is smoking cessation. Smoking cessation often leads to stabilization of symptoms and radiologic abnormalities.[5,28,30,93] However, some individuals may show disease progression leading to respiratory failure despite smoking cessation.[5] There is no biomarker to predict which patient will improve and who will continue to get worse despite smoking cessation. For patients with severe disease, systemic pharmacotherapy is often considered in addition to smoking cessation. Corticosteroid therapy in the form of oral prednisone, 40 to 60 mg daily with slow tapering over months, has historically been used to treat patients with severe or progressive disease, but the data on therapeutic benefit of corticosteroids are limited.[81] Because of the perceived lack of effectiveness of corticosteroids, several other immunosuppressive agents, namely, vinblastine, chlorodeoxyadenosine (also known as 2-CDA),[94] cyclophosphamide, and methotrexate, have been used to treat progressive PLCH.[81] Chlorodeoxyadenosine has been successfully used in the management of multisystem LCH involving bone and skin, but its utility in the management of smoking-related PLCH is not well defined.[94,95] Whether immunosuppressive therapy is effective in the management of patients with progressive disease who continue to smoke is currently not known.

Management of PLCH also includes treating associated complications and sequelae, such as pneumothorax, pulmonary hypertension, and respiratory failure.[5,78,85,92] Pneumothorax is generally managed initially by chest tube drainage. Pleurodesis should be considered for most patients with spontaneous pneumothorax associated with PLCH because the recurrence rate of pneumothorax with conservative management only is approximately 60%.[85] Pulmonary hypertension is a complication that can be seen even in the absence of severe ventilatory impairment or hypoxemia In patients with PLCH and is present in nearly all patients with advanced disease.[81,92] The presence of pulmonary hypertension portends a poor prognosis.[81,92] The authors routinely perform a 2-dimensional echocardiogram in patients with PLCH at the time of diagnosis and later in the clinical course if dyspnea or the degree of hypoxemia seems out of proportion to the severity of ventilatory impairment on pulmonary function testing.[81] If the patient has echocardiographic evidence of pulmonary hypertension, a right heart catheterization should be performed to confirm the presence, determine the severity, and assess response to vasomodulator therapy. The use of vasomodulators such as the endothelin antagonist bosentan and the phosphodiesterase inhibitor sildenafil should be considered in patients with moderate to severe pulmonary hypertension.[96]

Overall, most patients with PLCH have a relatively good prognosis, particularly if complete smoking cessation is achieved. The overall median survival from time of diagnosis is approximately 13 years, with 5-year and 10-year survival rates of 75% and 64%, respectively.[81] Some individuals may progress to extensive pulmonary scarring and cystic changes leading to respiratory failure.[51,81] Lung transplantation is an option for patients with advanced PLCH. The overall survival of patients with PLCH with lung transplants is comparable to that of individuals with other indications for lung transplantation.[34,97] Recurrence of PLCH in the transplanted lung, even after smoking cessation, has been described in a few cases.[33,34,98]

ACUTE ILD ASSOCIATED WITH SMOKING

AEP is an acute respiratory illness characterized by bilateral lung opacities, hypoxemia, and pulmonary eosinophilia.[99] Although some cases of AEP are idiopathic, other cases have been linked to multiple etiologic factors including drugs,[100–103] toxin inhalation,[104] infections,[105,106] heavy metals,[104] and (more recently) cigarette smoke.[12,107,108] In 2004, 18 cases of AEP were documented among American military personnel deployed in the Iraq war.[25] The individuals affected were aged between 19 and 47 years; all were smokers, and 78% of them had begun smoking within 2 weeks to 2 months before the onset of illness.[25] Similar reports from Japan had previously described young adults with AEP occurring shortly after starting smoking.[9,10,35]

Very little is known regarding the pathogenesis of AEP. It is possible, although not proven, that acute cigarette smoke exposure coupled with other proallergic exposures may facilitate the generation of cytokines (eg, IL-5) that enable massive recruitment and activation of eosinophils in the lungs.[109,110] Eosinophilic infiltration may subsequently promote direct damage to the lung tissue by release of soluble factors in eosinophilic granules.

The presentation of AEP may be mistaken for community-acquired pneumonia or acute respiratory distress syndrome depending on the severity of the illness. After initial presentation, the illness may progress rapidly over a 7- to 14-day period to diffuse pulmonary opacities and respiratory failure. Chest radiography typically shows bilateral alveolar opacities and small pleural effusions (**Fig. 4**). Chest CT usually reveals patchy alveolar opacities of ground-glass and/or consolidative character, interlobular septal thickening, and pleural effusions.[111] Diagnosis rests on the identification of more than 20% eosinophils in the BAL fluid combined with the appropriate clinicoradiologic context.[112–114]

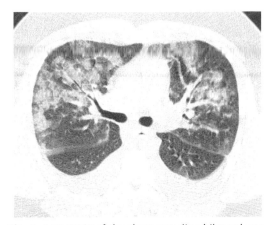

Fig. 4. AEP. HRCT of the chest revealing bilateral consolidative and ground-glass opacities as well as pleural effusions in a 22-year-old man with AEP. The patient had begun smoking cigarettes 3 weeks before this evaluation of progressive dyspnea.

The peripheral eosinophil count may be normal at presentation but is commonly elevated later in the clinical course.[112–114] Transbronchial lung biopsy is usually not required for diagnosis but when performed reveals marked eosinophilic infiltration in the interstitium and the alveoli.[115] The alveolar architecture is usually preserved.

Treatment consists of smoking cessation and corticosteroid therapy, for example, prednisone 40 to 60 mg/d, which usually results in relatively rapid improvement of respiratory insufficiency, pulmonary opacities, and pleural effusions.[25,116] The prognosis in cases that are appropriately treated is generally excellent, although few deaths have been reported caused by refractory respiratory failure.[25,116] After recovery, most patients have no long-term sequelae.[25,116]

Aside from AEP, cigarette smoking has also been implicated as an etiologic factor in acute pulmonary hemorrhage occurring in patients with Goodpasture syndrome, a pulmonary-renal syndrome associated with circulating anti–glomerular basement membrane (GBM) antibodies.[11,117] In a study of 51 patients with glomerulonephritis associated with anti-GBM antibodies, pulmonary hemorrhage occurred in all the cigarette smokers compared with only 20% of nonsmokers.[11] In addition, resumption of smoking was followed by recrudescence of pulmonary hemorrhage in 1 patient.[11]

SMOKING AND PULMONARY FIBROSIS

There are other diffuse fibrotic lung diseases that occur at a higher frequency in cigarette smokers than nonsmokers, but the cause-effect relationship is not well defined. For example, although there are several studies that have shown UIP, the histopathologic lesion in IPF, to be more common among smokers, there are limited data that cigarette smoking directly causes interstitial fibrosis.[14,17,118] It is conceivable that cigarette smoke might act as a cofactor along with some other unknown environmental or endogenous pro-fibrotic stimuli in susceptible individuals and promote interstitial fibrosis or possibly UIP. Smoking has also been reported to influence the clinical course associated with UIP.[119] A study on survival in patients with IPF showed that current smokers with IPF may have a survival advantage compared with those with IPF who quit smoking or never smoked. However, in multivariate analysis, this protective effect was lost, and both current and former smokers were observed to have a greater risk of death than those who never smoked.[119] The putative protective effect of smoking was also brought into question in a study of 249 patients with IPF in whom severity-adjusted survival was higher amongst those who never smoked.[118] This study demonstrated that severity-adjusted survival was higher in nonsmokers than either former smokers or the combined group of former and current smokers and showed that the presumed protective smoking effect is likely because of less severe disease at presentation in smokers or former smokers.

Some smokers manifest a combination of emphysema with fibrosis. In such patients, spirometric values may underestimate the degree of pulmonary dysfunction due to counteracting physiologic processes.[120,121] However, severe impairment of gas exchange will be evident, including a low diffusing capacity. These patients with combined pulmonary fibrosis and emphysema have a high prevalence of pulmonary hypertension and poor prognosis.[120,121]

Cigarette smokers are also at increased risk of developing RA, and individuals with established RA are at higher risk of developing ILD than nonsmokers with RA. A study of 336 patients with RA found that those with a more than 25 pack year smoking history were significantly more likely to have radiologic evidence of ILD (odds ratio [OR], 3.76; 95% confidence interval [CI], 1.59–8.88).[15] Cigarette smoking likely represents the principal preventable risk factor for RA-associated ILD.

The significance of interstitial opacities in smokers without clinically evident ILD is not well defined. Recently, Washko and colleagues[122] analyzed data from a large cohort of smokers included in the COPDGene study and reported interstitial radiographic abnormalities in 8% of this population. The presence of radiographic interstitial abnormalities correlated with less radiographic emphysema and a greater likelihood of spirometric restrictive impairment. The most frequently observed interstitial abnormalities on HRCT were centrilobular or peribronchial ground-glass opacities and subpleural reticular, nodular, or ground-glass opacities. Although histopathologic findings were not available for this study population, centrilobular nodules and ground-glass opacities most likely represent respiratory bronchiolitis, which is ubiquitous in smokers. It is tempting to speculate that the observed peripheral subpleural radiographic abnormality in older subjects is an early subclinical form of pulmonary fibrosis similar to that seen in IPF.[123]

ILDs THAT ARE LESS COMMON IN SMOKERS

HP is an allergic immune-mediated interstitial and small airway disease that may be induced by exposure to many different types of antigens in the environment. HP has been reported to occur less frequently among smokers than nonsmokers.[124] Potential mechanisms by which cigarette smoking may decrease the risk of HP in individuals exposed to antigens include inhibition of macrophage and dendritic cell costimulatory capacity, suppression of cytokines such as IL-12 by activated dendritic cells, and suppression of T-cell function.[40,125] However, HP can and does occur in smokers.[126] In one study that compared the clinical features of HP in smokers and nonsmokers, recurrence of symptoms following diagnosis and vital capacity measurements were worse in smokers.[126]

Sarcoidosis is another ILD that is less common in smokers than nonsmokers.[10] In a large case control study on etiologic factors in sarcoidosis, a history of cigarette smoking was less frequent among the 706 subjects with sarcoidosis than control subjects (OR, 0.62; 95% CI, 0.50–0.77).[127] Although smoking reduces the prevalence of sarcoidosis, it does not confer any benefit to patients with established sarcoidosis who may have a worse outcome than nonsmokers with sarcoidosis.[23]

SUMMARY

Substantial evidence implicates cigarette smoking as the principal etiologic factor responsible for the development of RB-ILD, DIP, and PLCH. Cigarette smoking is an important precipitant of AEP and pulmonary hemorrhage in patients with Goodpasture syndrome, and smokers are at higher risk of developing IPF and RA-associated ILD. It is important to recognize and continue to investigate the role of cigarette smoke in the pathogenesis and clinical course of these diverse diffuse lung diseases. Although relatively uncommon, these diseases are a significant health burden and frequently affect young adults in their most productive years. With the global increase in the prevalence of cigarette smoking, particularly in developing countries, it is likely that the burden of tobacco-related diseases, including smoking-related ILDs, will become heavier. Practitioners should use and recognize smoking cessation strategies as a critical component of therapy for these patients, with corticosteroids and other immune-modifying agents used as adjunctive treatments.

REFERENCES

1. Fraig M, Shreesha U, Savici D, et al. Respiratory bronchiolitis: a clinicopathologic study in current smokers, ex-smokers, and never-smokers. Am J Surg Pathol 2002;26(5):647–53.
2. Friedman PJ, Liebow AA, Sokoloff J. Eosinophilic granuloma of lung. Clinical aspects of primary histiocytosis in the adult. Medicine (Baltimore) 1981; 60(6):385–96.
3. Ryu JH, Colby TV, Hartman TE, et al. Smoking-related interstitial lung diseases: a concise review. Eur Respir J 2001;17(1):122–32.
4. Ryu JH, Myers JL, Capizzi SA, et al. Desquamative interstitial pneumonia and respiratory bronchiolitis-associated interstitial lung disease. Chest 2005; 127(1):178–84.
5. Vassallo R, Ryu JH, Schroeder DR, et al. Clinical outcomes of pulmonary Langerhans'-cell histiocytosis in adults. N Engl J Med 2002;346(7):484–90.
6. Vassallo R, Jensen EA, Colby TV, et al. The overlap between respiratory bronchiolitis and desquamative interstitial pneumonia in pulmonary Langerhans cell histiocytosis: high-resolution CT, histologic, and functional correlations. Chest 2003;124(4): 1199–205.
7. Craig PJ, Wells AU, Doffman S, et al. Desquamative interstitial pneumonia, respiratory bronchiolitis and their relationship to smoking. Histopathology 2004;45(3):275–82.
8. Moon J, du Bois RM, Colby TV, et al. Clinical significance of respiratory bronchiolitis on open lung biopsy and its relationship to smoking related interstitial lung disease. Thorax 1999;54(11): 1009–14.
9. Nakajima M, Matsushima T. Acute eosinophilic pneumonia following cigarette smoking. Intern Med 2000;39(10):759–60.
10. Watanabe K, Fujimura M, Kasahara K, et al. Acute eosinophilic pneumonia following cigarette smoking: a case report including cigarette-smoking challenge test. Intern Med 2002;41(11):1016–20.
11. Donaghy M, Rees AJ. Cigarette smoking and lung haemorrhage in glomerulonephritis caused by auto-antibodies to glomerular basement membrane. Lancet 1983;2(8364):1390–3.
12. Nakajima M, Manabe T, Niki Y, et al. A case of cigarette smoking-induced acute eosinophilic pneumonia showing tolerance. Chest 2000;118(5): 1517–8.
13. Kitahara Y, Matsumoto K, Taooka Y, et al. Cigarette smoking-induced acute eosinophilic pneumonia showing tolerance in broncho-alveolar lavage findings. Intern Med 2003;42(10):1016–21.
14. Miyake Y, Sasaki S, Yokoyama T, et al. Occupational and environmental factors and idiopathic pulmonary fibrosis in Japan. Ann Occup Hyg 2005;49(3):259–65.
15. Saag KG, Kolluri S, Koehnke RK, et al. Rheumatoid arthritis lung disease. Determinants of radiographic and physiologic abnormalities. Arthritis Rheum 1996;39(10):1711–9.
16. Wolfe F. The effect of smoking on clinical, laboratory, and radiographic status in rheumatoid arthritis. J Rheumatol 2000;27(3):630–7.
17. Baumgartner KB, Samet JM, Stidley CA, et al. Cigarette smoking: a risk factor for idiopathic pulmonary fibrosis. Am J Respir Crit Care Med 1997;155(1): 242–8.
18. Luukkainen R, Saltyshev M, Pakkasela R, et al. Relationship of rheumatoid factor to lung diffusion capacity in smoking and non-smoking patients with rheumatoid arthritis. Scand J Rheumatol 1995;24(2):119–20.
19. Valeyre D, Soler P, Clerici C, et al. Smoking and pulmonary sarcoidosis: effect of cigarette smoking on prevalence, clinical manifestations, alveolitis, and evolution of the disease. Thorax 1988;43(7): 516–24.
20. Hance AJ, Basset F, Saumon G, et al. Smoking and interstitial lung disease. The effect of cigarette smoking on the incidence of pulmonary histiocytosis X and sarcoidosis. Ann N Y Acad Sci 1986;465: 643–56.
21. Warren CP. Extrinsic allergic alveolitis: a disease commoner in non-smokers. Thorax 1977;32(5): 567–9.
22. Douglas JG, Middleton WG, Gaddie J, et al. Sarcoidosis: a disorder commoner in non-smokers? Thorax 1986;41(10):787–91.
23. Peros-Golubicic T, Ljubic S. Cigarette smoking and sarcoidosis. Acta Med Croatica 1995;49(4–5): 187–93.
24. Klareskog L, Stolt P, Lundberg K, et al. A new model for an etiology of rheumatoid arthritis: smoking

may trigger HLA-DR (shared epitope)-restricted immune reactions to autoantigens modified by citrullination. Arthritis Rheum 2006;54(1):38–46.

25. Shorr AF, Scoville SL, Cersovsky SB, et al. Acute eosinophilic pneumonia among US Military personnel deployed in or near Iraq. JAMA 2004; 292(24):2997–3005.

26. Girard M, Israel-Assayag E, Cormier Y. Pathogenesis of hypersensitivity pneumonitis. Curr Opin Allergy Clin Immunol 2004;4(2):93–8.

27. Patel RR, Ryu JH, Vassallo R. Cigarette smoking and diffuse lung disease. Drugs 2008;68(11): 1511–27.

28. Mogulkoc N, Veral A, Bishop PW, et al. Pulmonary Langerhans' cell histiocytosis: radiologic resolution following smoking cessation. Chest 1999;115(5): 1452–5.

29. Zeid NA, Muller HK. Tobacco smoke induced lung granulomas and tumors: association with pulmonary Langerhans cells. Pathology 1995; 27(3):247–54.

30. Negrin-Dastis S, Butenda D, Dorzee J, et al. Complete disappearance of lung abnormalities on high-resolution computed tomography: a case of histiocytosis X. Can Respir J 2007;14(4):235–7.

31. Bernstrand C, Cederlund K, Ashtrom L, et al. Smoking preceded pulmonary involvement in adults with Langerhans cell histiocytosis diagnosed in childhood. Acta Paediatr 2000;89(11): 1389–92.

32. Portnoy J, Veraldi KL, Schwarz MI, et al. Respiratory bronchiolitis-interstitial lung disease: long-term outcome. Chest 2007;131(3):664–71.

33. Etienne B, Bertocchi M, Gamondes JP, et al. Relapsing pulmonary Langerhans cell histiocytosis after lung transplantation. Am J Respir Crit Care Med 1998;157(1):288–91.

34. Dauriat G, Mal H, Thabut G, et al. Lung transplantation for pulmonary Langerhans' cell histiocytosis. a multicenter analysis. Transplantation 2006;81(5): 746–50.

35. Shiota Y, Kawai T, Matsumoto H, et al. Acute eosinophilic pneumonia following cigarette smoking. Intern Med 2000;39(10):830–3.

36. Alp H, Daum RS, Abrahams C, et al. Acute eosinophilic pneumonia: a cause of reversible, severe, noninfectious respiratory failure. J Pediatr 1998; 132(3 Pt 1):540–3.

37. Nakagome K, Kato J, Kubota S, et al. [Acute eosinophilic pneumonia induced by cigarette smoking]. Nihon Kokyuki Gakkai Zasshi 2000;38(2):113–6 [in Japanese].

38. Katzenstein AL, Mukhopadhyay S, Zanardi C, et al. Clinically occult interstitial fibrosis in smokers: classification and significance of a surprisingly common finding in lobectomy specimens. Hum Pathol 2010;41(3):316–25.

39. Vassallo R, Tamada K, Lau JS, et al. Cigarette smoke extract suppresses human dendritic cell function leading to preferential induction of Th-2 priming. J Immunol 2005;175(4):2684–91.

40. Israel-Assayag E, Dakhama A, Lavigne S, et al. Expression of costimulatory molecules on alveolar macrophages in hypersensitivity pneumonitis. Am J Respir Crit Care Med 1999;159(6):1830–4.

41. Anderson K, Morrison SM, Bourke S, et al. Effect of cigarette smoking on the specific antibody response in pigeon fanciers. Thorax 1988;43(10):798–800.

42. Cormier Y, Belanger J, Durand P. Factors influencing the development of serum precipitins to farmer's lung antigen in Quebec dairy farmers. Thorax 1985;40(2):138–42.

43. Hakala M, Paakko P, Huhti E, et al. Open lung biopsy of patients with rheumatoid arthritis. Clin Rheumatol 1990;9(4):452–60.

44. Churg A, Muller NL, Flint J, et al. Chronic hypersensitivity pneumonitis. Am J Surg Pathol 2006;30(2): 201–8.

45. Ranney L, Melvin C, Lux L, et al. Systematic review: smoking cessation intervention strategies for adults and adults in special populations. Ann Intern Med 2006;145(11):845–56.

46. Kuschner WG, D'Alessandro A, Wong H, et al. Dose-dependent cigarette smoking-related inflammatory responses in healthy adults. Eur Respir J 1996;9(10):1989–94.

47. Casolaro MA, Bernaudin JF, Saltini C, et al. Accumulation of Langerhans' cells on the epithelial surface of the lower respiratory tract in normal subjects in association with cigarette smoking. Am Rev Respir Dis 1988;137(2):406–11.

48. Colby TV, Lombard C. Histiocytosis X in the lung. Hum Pathol 1983;14(10):847–56.

49. Travis WD, Borok Z, Roum JH, et al. Pulmonary Langerhans cell granulomatosis (histiocytosis X). A clinicopathologic study of 48 cases. Am J Surg Pathol 1993;17(10):971–86.

50. Myers JL, Veal CF Jr, Shin MS, et al. Respiratory bronchiolitis causing interstitial lung disease. A clinicopathologic study of six cases. Am Rev Respir Dis 1987;135(4):880–4.

51. Remy-Jardin M, Remy J, Gosselin B, et al. Lung parenchymal changes secondary to cigarette smoking: pathologic-CT correlations. Radiology 1993;186(3):643–51.

52. Tomita K, Caramori G, Lim S, et al. Increased p21(CIP1/WAF1) and B cell lymphoma leukemia-x(L) expression and reduced apoptosis in alveolar macrophages from smokers. Am J Respir Crit Care Med 2002;166(5):724–31.

53. Tazi A, Bonay M, Bergeron A, et al. Role of granulocyte-macrophage colony stimulating factor (GM-CSF) in the pathogenesis of adult pulmonary histiocytosis X. Thorax 1996;51(6):611–4.

54. Tazi A, Bouchonnet F, Grandsaigne M, et al. Evidence that granulocyte macrophage-colony-stimulating factor regulates the distribution and differentiated state of dendritic cells/Langerhans cells in human lung and lung cancers. J Clin Invest 1993;91(2):566–76.

55. Wang RD, Wright JL, Churg A. Transforming growth factor-beta1 drives airway remodeling in cigarette smoke-exposed tracheal explants. Am J Respir Cell Mol Biol 2005;33(4):387–93.

56. D'Hulst AI, Vermaelen KY, Brusselle GG, et al. Time course of cigarette smoke-induced pulmonary inflammation in mice. Eur Respir J 2005;26(2): 204–13.

57. Lu LM, Zavitz CC, Chen B, et al. Cigarette smoke impairs NK cell-dependent tumor immune surveillance. J Immunol 2007;178(2):936–43.

58. Kode A, Yang SR, Rahman I. Differential effects of cigarette smoke on oxidative stress and proinflammatory cytokine release in primary human airway epithelial cells and in a variety of transformed alveolar epithelial cells. Respir Res 2006;7:132.

59. Yang SR, Chida AS, Bauter MR, et al. Cigarette smoke induces proinflammatory cytokine release by activation of NF-kappaB and posttranslational modifications of histone deacetylase in macrophages. Am J Physiol Lung Cell Mol Physiol 2006;291(1):L46–57.

60. Niewoehner DE, Kleinerman J, Rice DB. Pathologic changes in the peripheral airways of young cigarette smokers. N Engl J Med 1974;291(15): 755–8.

61. Yousem SA, Colby TV, Gaensler EA. Respiratory bronchiolitis-associated interstitial lung disease and its relationship to desquamative interstitial pneumonia. Mayo Clin Proc 1989;64(11):1373–80.

62. Mavridou D, Laws D. Respiratory bronchiolitis associated interstitial lung disease (RB-ILD): a case of an acute presentation. Thorax 2004; 59(10):910–1.

63. Hartman TE, Tazelaar HD, Swensen SJ, et al. Cigarette smoking: CT and pathologic findings of associated pulmonary diseases. Radiographics 1997; 17(2):377–90.

64. Aubry MC, Wright JL, Myers JL. The pathology of smoking-related lung diseases. Clin Chest Med 2000;21(1):11–35, vii.

65. Wells AU, Nicholson AG, Hansell DM, et al. Respiratory bronchiolitis-associated interstitial lung disease. Semin Respir Crit Care Med 2003; 24(5):585–94.

66. Liebow AA, Steer A, Billingsley JG. Desquamative interstitial pneumonia. Am J Med 1965;39:369–404.

67. Iskandar SB, McKinney LA, Shah L, et al. Desquamative interstitial pneumonia and hepatitis C virus infection: a rare association. South Med J 2004; 97(9):890–3.

68. Flores-Franco RA, Luevano-Flores E, Gaston-Ramirez C. Sirolimus-associated desquamative interstitial pneumonia. Respiration 2007;74(2); 237–8.

69. Hansell DM, Nicholson AG. Smoking-related diffuse parenchymal lung disease: HRCT-pathologic correlation. Semin Respir Crit Care Med 2003;24(4):377–92.

70. Heyneman LE, Ward S, Lynch DA, et al. Respiratory bronchiolitis, respiratory bronchiolitis-associated interstitial lung disease, and desquamative interstitial pneumonia: different entities or part of the spectrum of the same disease process? AJR Am J Roentgenol 1999;173(6):1617–22.

71. Hartman TE, Primack SL, Kang EY, et al. Disease progression in usual interstitial pneumonia compared with desquamative interstitial pneumonia. Assessment with serial CT [see comment]. Chest 1996;110(2):378–82.

72. Mueller-Mang C, Grosse C, Schmid K, et al. What every radiologist should know about idiopathic interstitial pneumonias. Radiographics 2007;27(3): 595–615.

73. Matsuo K, Tada S, Kataoka M, et al. Spontaneous remission of desquamative interstitial pneumonia. Intern Med 1997;36(10):728–31.

74. Bjoraker JA, Ryu JH, Edwin MK, et al. Prognostic significance of histopathologic subsets in idiopathic pulmonary fibrosis. Am J Respir Crit Care Med 1998;157(1):199–203.

75. Flusser G, Gurman G, Zirkin H, et al. Desquamative interstitial pneumonitis causing acute respiratory failure, responsive only to immunosuppressants. Respiration 1991;58(5–6):324–6.

76. Timmer SJ, Karamzadeh AM, Yung GL, et al. Predicting survival of lung transplantation candidates with idiopathic interstitial pneumonia: does PaO(2) predict survival? Chest 2002; 122(3):779–84.

77. Verleden GM, Sels F, Van Raemdonck D, et al. Possible recurrence of desquamative interstitial pneumonitis in a single lung transplant recipient. Eur Respir J 1998;11(4):971–4.

78. Vassallo R, Ryu JH, Colby TV, et al. Pulmonary Langerhans'-cell histiocytosis. N Engl J Med 2000;342(26):1969–78.

79. Tazi A. Adult pulmonary Langerhans' cell histiocytosis. Eur Respir J 2006;27(6):1272–85.

80. Favara BE, Feller AC, Pauli M, et al. Contemporary classification of histiocytic disorders. The WHO Committee On Histiocytic/Reticulum Cell Proliferations. Reclassification Working Group of the Histiocyte Society. Med Pediatr Oncol 1997;29(3): 157–66.

81. Chaowalit N, Pellikka PA, Decker PA, et al. Echocardiographic and clinical characteristics of pulmonary hypertension complicating pulmonary

Langerhans cell histiocytosis. Mayo Clin Proc 2004;79(10):1269–75.

82. Delobbe A, Durieu J, Duhamel A, et al. Determinants of survival in pulmonary Langerhans' cell granulomatosis (histiocytosis X). Groupe d'Etude en Pathologie Interstitielle de la Societe de Pathologie Thoracique du Nord. Eur Respir J 1996;9(10): 2002–6.

83. Aguayo SM, King TE Jr, Waldron JA Jr, et al. Increased pulmonary neuroendocrine cells with bombesin-like immunoreactivity in adult patients with eosinophilic granuloma. J Clin Invest 1990;86(3):838–44.

84. Asakura S, Colby TV, Limper AH. Tissue localization of transforming growth factor-beta1 in pulmonary eosinophilic granuloma. Am J Respir Crit Care Med 1996;154(5):1525–30.

85. Mendez JL, Nadrous HF, Vassallo R, et al. Pneumothorax in pulmonary Langerhans cell histiocytosis. Chest 2004;125(3):1028–32.

86. Crausman RS, Jennings CA, Tuder RM, et al. Pulmonary histiocytosis X: pulmonary function and exercise pathophysiology. Am J Respir Crit Care Med 1996;153(1):426–35.

87. Moore AD, Godwin JD, Muller NL, et al. Pulmonary histiocytosis X: comparison of radiographic and CT findings. Radiology 1989;172(1):249–54.

88. Brauner MW, Grenier P, Mouelhi MM, et al. Pulmonary histiocytosis X: evaluation with high-resolution CT. Radiology 1989;172(1):255–8.

89. Soler P, Chollet S, Jacque C, et al. Immunocytochemical characterization of pulmonary histiocytosis X cells in lung biopsies. Am J Pathol 1985; 118(3):439–51.

90. Chollet S, Soler P, Bernaudin JF, et al. [Exploratory bronchoalveolar lavage]. Presse Med 1984;13(24): 1503–8 [in French].

91. Yousem SA, Colby TV, Chen YY, et al. Pulmonary Langerhans' cell histiocytosis: molecular analysis of clonality. Am J Surg Pathol 2001;25(5). 630–6.

92. Fartoukh M, Humbert M, Capron F, et al. Severe pulmonary hypertension in histiocytosis X. Am J Respir Crit Care Med 2000;161(1):216–23.

93. Abbott GF, Rosado-de-Christenson ML, Franks TJ, et al. From the archives of the AFIP: pulmonary Langerhans cell histiocytosis. Radiographics 2001; 24(3):821–41.

94. Aerni MR, Aubry MC, Myers JL, et al. Complete remission of nodular pulmonary Langerhans cell histiocytosis lesions induced by 2-chlorodeoxyadenosine in a non-smoker. Respir Med 2008; 102(2):316–9.

95. Pardanani A, Phyliky RL, Li CY, et al. 2-Chlorodeoxyadenosine therapy for disseminated Langerhans cell histiocytosis. Mayo Clin Proc 2003;78(3):301–6.

96. Kiakouama L, Cottin V, Etienne-Mastroianni B, et al. Severe pulmonary hypertension in histiocytosis X:

long-term improvement with bosentan. Eur Respir J 2010;36(1):202–4.

97. Saleem I, Moss J, Egan JJ. Lung transplantation for rare pulmonary diseases. Sarcoidosis Vasc Diffuse Lung Dis 2005;22(Suppl 1):S85–90.

98. Gabbay E, Dark JH, Ashcroft T, et al. Recurrence of Langerhans' cell granulomatosis following lung transplantation. Thorax 1998;53(4):326–7.

99. Philit F, Etienne-Mastroianni B, Parrot A, et al. Idiopathic acute eosinophilic pneumonia: a study of 22 patients. Am J Respir Crit Care Med 2002;166(9): 1235–9.

100. Yokoyama A, Mizushima Y, Suzuki H, et al. Acute eosinophilic pneumonia induced by minocycline: prominent Kerley B lines as a feature of positive re-challenge test. Jpn J Med 1990;29(2): 195–8.

101. Barnes MT, Bascunana J, Garcia B, et al. Acute eosinophilic pneumonia associated with antidepressant agents. Pharm World Sci 1999;21(5): 241–2.

102. Noh H, Lee YK, Kan SW, et al. Acute eosinophilic pneumonia associated with amitriptyline in a hemodialysis patient. Yonsei Med J 2001;42(3):357–9.

103. McCormick M, Nelson T. Cocaine-induced fatal acute eosinophilic pneumonia: a case report. WMJ 2007;106(2):92–5.

104. Kawayama T, Fujiki R, Morimitsu Y, et al. Fatal idiopathic acute eosinophilic pneumonia with acute lung injury. Respirology 2002;7(4):373–5.

105. Takizawa H. Acute eosinophilic pneumonia: possible role of hyperreactivity of airway epithelial cells. Intern Med 2002;41(11):917.

106. Glazer CS, Cohen LB, Schwarz MI. Acute eosinophilic pneumonia in AIDS. Chest 2001;120(5): 1732–5.

107. Miki K, Miki M, Okano Y, et al. Cigarette smoke-induced acute eosinophilic pneumonia accompanied with neutrophilia in the blood. Intern Med 2002;41(11):993–6.

108. Al-Saieg N, Moammar O, Kartan R. Flavored cigar smoking induces acute eosinophilic pneumonia. Chest 2007;131(4):1234–7.

109. Rom WN, Weiden M, Garcia R, et al. Acute eosinophilic pneumonia in a New York City firefighter exposed to World Trade Center dust. Am J Respir Crit Care Med 2002;166(6):797–800.

110. Nakahara Y, Hayashi S, Fukuno Y, et al. Increased interleukin-5 levels in bronchoalveolar lavage fluid is a major factor for eosinophil accumulation in acute eosinophilic pneumonia. Respiration 2001; 68(4):389–95.

111. Daimon T, Johkoh T, Sumikawa H, et al. Acute eosinophilic pneumonia: thin-section CT findings in 29 patients. Eur J Radiol 2008;65(3):462–7.

112. Allen J. Acute eosinophilic pneumonia. Semin Respir Crit Care Med 2006;27(2):142–7.

113. King MA, Pope-Harman AL, Allen JN, et al. Acute eosinophilic pneumonia: radiologic and clinical features. Radiology 1997;203(3):715–9.

114. Allen JN, Pacht ER, Gadek JE, et al. Acute eosinophilic pneumonia as a reversible cause of noninfectious respiratory failure. N Engl J Med 1989; 321(9):569–74.

115. Tazelaar HD, Linz LJ, Colby TV, et al. Acute eosinophilic pneumonia: histopathologic findings in nine patients. Am J Respir Crit Care Med 1997;155(1): 296–302.

116. Uchiyama H, Suda T, Nakamura Y, et al. Alterations in smoking habits are associated with acute eosinophilic pneumonia. Chest 2008;133(5):1174–80.

117. Benz K, Amann K, Dittrich K, et al. Patient with antibody-negative relapse of Goodpasture syndrome. Clin Nephrol 2007;67(4):240–4.

118. Antoniou KM, Hansell DM, Rubens MB, et al. Idiopathic pulmonary fibrosis: outcome in relation to smoking status. Am J Respir Crit Care Med 2008; 177(2):190–4.

119. King TE Jr, Tooze JA, Schwarz MI, et al. Predicting survival in idiopathic pulmonary fibrosis: scoring system and survival model. Am J Respir Crit Care Med 2001;164(7):1171–81.

120. Cottin V, Le Pavec J, Prevot G, et al. Pulmonary hypertension in patients with combined pulmonary fibrosis and emphysema syndrome. Eur Respir J 2010;35(1):105–11.

121. Mejia M, Carrillo G, Rojas-Serrano J, et al. Idiopathic pulmonary fibrosis and emphysema: decreased survival associated with severe pulmonary arterial hypertension. Chest 2009;136(1):10–5.

122. Washko GR, Hunninghake GM, Fernandez IE, et al. Lung volumes and emphysema in smokers with interstitial lung abnormalities. N Engl J Med 2011; 364(10):897–906.

123. King TE Jr. Smoking and subclinical interstitial lung disease. N Engl J Med 2011;364(10):968–70.

124. Selman M. Hypersensitivity pneumonitis: a multifaceted deceiving disorder. Clin Chest Med 2004; 25(3):531–47, vi.

125. Arima K, Ando M, Ito K, et al. Effect of cigarette smoking on prevalence of summer-type hypersensitivity pneumonitis caused by Trichosporon cutaneum. Arch Environ Health 1992;47(4):274–8.

126. Ohtsuka Y, Munakata M, Tanimura K, et al. Smoking promotes insidious and chronic farmer's lung disease, and deteriorates the clinical outcome. Intern Med 1995;34(10):966–71.

127. Newman LS, Rose CS, Bresnitz EA, et al. A case control etiologic study of sarcoidosis: environmental and occupational risk factors. Am J Respir Crit Care Med 2004;170(12):1324–30.

Lung Transplantation for Interstitial Lung Disease

Timothy P.M. Whelan, MD

KEYWORDS

- Lung transplantation • Lung disease
- Parenchymal lung disease • Interstitial lung disease

There are more than 100 distinct interstitial or diffuse parenchymal lung diseases (DPLDs). These diseases are associated with underlying autoimmune disease, environmental/occupational exposures, and drug exposures. In addition, a large percentage of these disorders (approximately 30%–40%) are idiopathic. It is believed that previous prevalence estimates in the population have been grossly underestimated. Although DPLDs remain extremely rare in children, in adults the prevalence for parenchymal lung diseases is approximately 70 per 100,000 population.[1–3] Newer information indicates that the prevalence of the most common form of idiopathic interstitial pneumonia, idiopathic pulmonary fibrosis (IPF), is likely greater than previously expected. Clinical courses and prognoses across all types of DPLD are variable and dependent on the underlying subtype of lung disease. For IPF, there are no current medical therapies that clearly alter the progression of disease. In addition, the current literature consistently estimates the median survival for patients with newly diagnosed IPF is 3 to 5 years.[1,4–8] For IPF and the other DPLDs that progress despite best medical therapy, lung transplantation remains an appropriate treatment option for a select group of patients. Reitz and colleagues[9] performed the first successful heart and lung transplant at Stanford University in 1981. Subsequently, in 1983, Cooper and the Toronto Lung Transplant Group[10] successfully performed the first single lung transplant on a patient with IPF. During the past 25 years, the number of transplants performed worldwide has increased from the single digits per year to approximately 3000 per year (**Fig. 1**). The major indications for lung transplantation include chronic obstructive pulmonary disease, cystic fibrosis, and IPF. The proportion of transplants for IPF has consistently increased and this has been particularly true during the past decade. Worldwide, transplantation for IPF now approaches the proportion for non–α_1-antitrypsin deficiency chronic obstructive pulmonary disease transplants performed in 2008 (approximately 30% of all transplants).[11] In the United States, IPF and other DPLDs account for more than half of the lung transplants performed since 2008. This increase in the number of transplants contrasts with trends for idiopathic pulmonary arterial hypertension. With the advance of successful therapies for the treatment of pulmonary arterial hypertension, the number of transplants for this condition has significantly declined, accounting for approximately 2% of all transplants in 2008 compared with approximately 13% of transplants performed in 1990. This underscores the challenge that patients with IPF face: there is a lack of beneficial therapy for this devastating disease.

WHO SHOULD BE REFERRED AND LISTED FOR TRANSPLANT?

In 2006 the International Society for Heart and Lung Transplantation published a consensus report outlining appropriate guidelines for referral for transplantation.[12] The document also includes guidelines for actively placing an individual on a waiting list for transplant. The balance between

Division of Pulmonary, Allergy, Critical Care, and Sleep Medicine, Medical University of South Carolina, 96 Jonathan Lucas Street, CSB 812, MSC 630, Charleston, SC 29425, USA
E-mail address: whelant@musc.edu

Clin Chest Med 33 (2012) 179–189
doi:10.1016/j.ccm.2011.12.003
0272-5231/12/$ – see front matter © 2012 Elsevier Inc. All rights reserved.

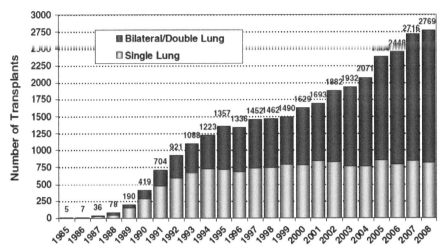

Fig. 1. Number of lung transplants and procedure type: 1985–2008. (*From* Christie JD, Edwards LB, Kucheryavaya AY, et al. The Registry of the International Society for Heart and Lung Transplantation: twenty-seventh official adult lung and heart-lung transplant report–2010. J Heart Lung Transplant 2010;29(10):1104–18; with permission.)

providing a short-term survival benefit must be weighed against the reality that donor lungs are a limited resource. Therefore, it is paramount that the appropriate transplant candidate be expected to have a reasonable opportunity to attain long-term survival. Assessment for potential long-term survival must include an appraisal of potential recipients' comorbidities. The 2006 guideline statement outlines several absolute and relative contraindications to performing lung transplantation (**Table 1**). In addition to medical considerations, lung transplant recipients must actively participate in the management of a complex medical regimen. Adherence to this treatment is central to good outcomes. As a result, a social support system that enhances adherence is beneficial, if not vital.

Transplantation centers agree that the moment of referral should allow the potential recipient adequate time to consider this treatment option. The initial transplantation discussion should not occur as a last-ditch effort at improving a patient's outcome. In this, or any, document, there are limitations in defining the appropriate time for referral and transplantation. Consideration of referral to a transplant center should include the referring physician's assessment of the individual's quality of life as well as overall life expectancy without a transplant. In addition, the potential recipient's desire to learn more about this treatment option is a factor in considering referral. The decision to actively list for transplant, alternatively, is based on organ allocation for a particular region, estimated risks and benefits based on the expertise of the individual

transplant center, and the personal assessments of the transplant recipient.

Choice of Procedure

There are 3 potential procedures for the interstitial lung disease recipient. These include heart and lung, single lung, and bilateral lung transplantation. Heart and lung transplantation was initially the procedure of choice during the 1980s and many centers continued this practice into the 1990s. After successful lung transplantation and the realization that the dilated right ventricle can remodel with good outcomes, heart and lung transplantation numbers have significantly declined. In 2008, there were 73 heart and lung transplants worldwide.[13] Currently, heart and lung transplant is only performed on those patients with significant left ventricular dysfunction or nonoperable congenital abnormalities.

The decision to perform single lung versus bilateral lung transplant remains controversial today. The only absolute criterion for the performance of bilateral lung transplant is suppurative lung disease. This is due to concerns that the native lung will soil the transplanted allograft in a chronically immunosuppressed host and lead to poor outcomes. In addition to this absolute indication, it is now common practice to perform bilateral lung transplant for patients with idiopathic pulmonary hypertension. This population is at high risk of developing primary graft dysfunction or early acute lung injury after transplantation. This risk is lower in patients who undergo bilateral lung transplantation.[14] For patients with very high pulmonary

Table 1
Absolute and relative contraindications to lung transplantation

Absolute Contraindications	Comment
Malignancy within past 2 years (excluding basal and squamous cell skin cancers)	Given effects of chronic immunosuppression on malignancy, a 5-year disease-free interval is prudent. Lung transplantation for bronchoalveolar cell carcinoma remains controversial
Untreatable advanced dysfunction of another major organ system	Coronary artery disease not amenable to intervention or associated with significant left ventricular dysfunction is an absolute contraindication but heart-lung transplant could be considered for select patients
Noncurable chronic extrapulmonary infection	Chronic active hepatitis B, hepatitis C, and HIV
Significant chest wall/spinal deformity	Abnormalities that preclude either safe removal of the native lung(s) or implantation of the donor lungs
Documented nonadherence or inability to follow through with medical therapy	Includes the need for a consistent and reliable social support system. In addition, untreatable psychiatric conditions that would impair the ability of the recipient to remain adherent are Included here
Substance addiction within the last 6 months	Alcohol, tobacco, illicit drug use
Relative Contraindications	**Comment**
Age >65 years old	There is an increased risk of worse long-term survival with higher age likely related to increased comorbidities at transplant[11]
Severely limited functional status	Decreased exercise tolerance has been associated with worse outcomes[84]
Colonization with highly resistant or virulent bacteria, fungi, or mycobacteria	Increased risk of perioperative sepsis as well as potential empyema and/or wound infections
Obesity with a body mass index >30 kg/m^2	Obesity has been cited in several studies to increase the risk of both long-term and short-term poor outcomes[85–89]
Mechanical ventilation	Increased perioperative mortality is associated with mechanical ventilation[11]
Other chronic comorbidities that have not resulted in end-stage organ damage	All medical conditions should be optimized before consideration for listing for transplant, including chronic management of diabetes, hypertension, gastroesophageal reflux, and coronary artery disease

Absolute contraindications are determined by individual transplant programs and the balance of the risks and benefits is determined by the individual transplant center. Similarly, the presence of several relative contraindications may significantly increase the risk of poor transplant outcome and preclude listing for transplant

Adapted from Orens JB, Estenne M, Arcasoy S et al. International guidelines for the selection of lung transplant candidates: 2006 update—a consensus report from the Pulmonary Scientific Council of the International Society for Heart and Lung Transplantation. J Heart Lung Transplant 2006;25(7):745–55; with permission.

vascular resistance before transplant, the right ventricle becomes acutely unloaded with the reanastamosis of the normal allograft pulmonary vasculature. High cardiac output ensues with high flow rates that may increase the risk of endothelial injury and subsequent pulmonary edema. This impact is likely attenuated by double the vascular volume of a bilateral transplant. For patients with DPLD, it is less clear that individuals with secondary pulmonary hypertension receive an absolute benefit from bilateral lung transplantation. Several investigators have come to differing conclusions regarding the benefits of a particular procedure type in this population.[14–16] Because there are no randomized controlled trials evaluating single lung versus bilateral lung transplantation for pulmonary fibrosis, there are inherent selection biases that confound any retrospective cohort. With this limitation, several recent analyses suggest that there may be a benefit to bilateral lung transplant in selected patients with IPF. It seems there is an increased risk of complications early with bilateral lung transplant but a longer-term potential survival benefit may ultimately prevail.[17–21]

Regardless of the rationale for the choice of procedure, recent data indicate that bilateral lung transplantation is increasing in frequency. In 2008, 71% of transplant procedures were bilateral lung transplants. During the same period, cystic fibrosis accounted for approximately 15% of transplants and idiopathic pulmonary hypertension less than 5%, and the frequency with which patients with an underlying diagnosis of IPF are transplanted is increasing. This suggests a trend toward increased bilateral transplantation in DPLD. One report evaluating waiting list mortality demonstrated a higher risk for those IPF patients listed for bilateral lung transplant as their only option.[22] The impact on the donor pool and, subsequently, the waiting list mortality from an increased number of bilateral lung transplant procedures remains unknown at this time.

Outcomes After Transplantation

The majority of information about outcomes after lung transplantation in DPLD comes from what is known about IPF recipients. Because the majority of DPLDs result in similar physiologic changes with restrictive lung disease and high risk for the development of secondary pulmonary hypertension, some generalizations across the disease type are accurate. More specific disease considerations are discussed later.

Survival after lung transplantation has consistently improved by era from 1988 through June of 2008.[23] The most striking improvements in outcome are during the perioperative period. These improvements are likely due to improved donor preservation, operative technique, and critical care management early after transplant. Currently, the median survival estimate for all recipients from 1994 through 2008 was 5.3 years. The 90-day survival rate was 88%. Although the impact has not been as great for long-term survival, this too is slowly improving. In the same era, unadjusted 10-year survival rates were 29%. Survival for patients with an underlying diagnosis of DPLD is generally consistent with these reported outcomes. The largest cohort of interstitial lung disease transplanted remains IPF and the median survival for this group is 4.3 years. For those patients with sarcoidosis, median survival was

5.1 years. These unadjusted survival rates need to be evaluated cautiously because additional recipient factors have an impact on survival after lung transplantation.

Early survival after transplantation is hampered by the development of primary graft dysfunction (PGD). PGD is the consequence of ischemia-reperfusion injury with resultant development of reactive oxygen species. Ultimately, this leads to acute lung injury and capillary leak.[24] PGD is based on clinical findings early after transplantation (Table 2). Several studies have identified pulmonary fibrosis and pulmonary hypertension as having strong associations with the development of this complication.[25–27]

PGD is the primary cause of death early after lung transplantation.[11] The severest form of PGD (grade 3 at 72 hours after transplant) affects long-term survival and pulmonary function and increases the risk for development of bronchiolitis obliterans syndrome (BOS).[28] In addition to the recipient risk factors, there are donor factors that increase the risk of development of this complication. Currently there are no recipient interventions to prevent its development. Further work into defining the best match for donor and recipient as well as the potential for conditioning of donor lungs may lead to improvements in the future.[29]

Patients are on lifelong immunosuppression and are typically treated with corticosteroids, a calcineurin inhibitor (tacrolimus or cyclosporine), and an antimetabolite (mycophenolate mofetil or azathioprine). Chronic immunosuppression places patients at risk for the development of comorbidities, including hypertension, diabetes, chronic kidney disease, and malignancy (Table 3). Notwithstanding

Table 2
Grading of primary graft dysfunction severity

Grade	PaO_2/FiO_2	Radiographic Infiltrates Consistent with Pulmonary Edema
0	>300	Absent
1	>300	Present
2	200–300	Present
3	<200	Present

Assessments are measured within 6 hours of reperfusion of the graft and out to 72 hours.

Values obtained at 72 hours seem to be the most predictive of subsequent outcome after transplant.

Adapted from Christie JD, Carby M, Bag R, et al. Report of the ISHLT Working Group on Primary Lung Graft Dysfunction part II: definition. A consensus statement of the International Society for Heart and Lung Transplantation. J Heart Lung Transplant 2005;24(10):1454–9; with permission.

Table 3 **Morbidity after lung transplant**		
Outcome	**≤1 Year**	**≤5 Years**
Hypertension	53%	84%
Renal dysfunction		
Creatinine <2.5 mg/dL	17%	23%
Creatinine >2.5 mg/dL	6%	8%
Chronic dialysis	1.6%	3%
Renal transplant	0.1%	0.5%
Hyperlipidemia	24%	57%
Diabetes	26%	38%
Bronchiolitis obliterans	9.6%	37%

Adapted from Christie JD, Edwards LB, Kucheryavaya AY, et al. The Registry of the International Society for Heart and Lung Transplantation: twenty-seventh official adult lung and heart-lung transplant report—2010. J Heart Lung Transplant 2010;29(10):1104–18; with permission.

the medical complexity, patients with DPLD who undergo lung transplantation garner a survival advantage from the procedure.[30–32] In addition, quality of life is significantly improved after transplantation in several studies.[33–36]

The main limitation to long-term survival after lung transplantation remains the development of BOS, or chronic rejection. BOS is defined by persistent airflow obstruction in comparison to a recipient's peak baseline values (**Table 4**). Complications that affect the allograft (acute rejection, anastamosis issues, disease recurrence, and

Table 4 **Criteria for grading of bronchiolitis obliterans syndrome**	
BOS 0	FEV_1 >90% of Baseline and $FEF_{25\%-75\%}$ >75% of Baseline
BOS 0p	FEV_1 81%–90% of baseline and/or $FEF_{25\%-75\%}$ <75% of baseline
BOS 1	FEV_1 66%–80% of baseline
BOS 2	FEV_1 51%–65% of baseline
BOS 3	FEV_1 50% or less of baseline

$FEF_{25\%-75\%}$, midexpiratory flow rate.

Baseline FEV_1 is based on the average of the 2 highest values obtained after transplant that are at least 3 weeks apart.

BOS grade is based on the subsequent average of 2 FEV_1 values that are obtained at least 3 weeks apart and compared with the baseline value.

Adapted from Estenne M, Maurer JR, Boehler A, et al. Bronchiolitis obliterans syndrome 2001: an update of the diagnostic criteria. J Heart Lung Transplant 2002; 21(3):297–310; with permission.

so forth) must be ruled out in addition to documenting a decline in pulmonary function. There are several probable and possible risk factors that set up the lung transplant recipient for the development of chronic small airways disease, including recurrent acute rejection, lymphocytic bronchiolitis, donor antigen-specific reactivity, and aspiration of gastroesophageal refluxate. Ultimately, chronic obstruction increases the risk of infection and sets the stage for respiratory failure. The rate of BOS varies in different series but has an estimated prevalence of approximately 45% at 5 years. Treatment interventions for this syndrome are limited but recent data suggest a role for the use of chronic azithromycin in these patients.[37–40]

DISEASE-SPECIFIC CONSIDERATIONS
Idiopathic Pulmonary Fibrosis

IPF remains a DPLD without a medical therapy of proved benefit and a consistently demonstrated median survival of 3 to 5 years. The increase in number of transplants for patients with IPF may be reflective of increasing incidence of IPF, increase in the awareness of this disease and subsequent increased diagnosis, and increased awareness of the severely poor prognosis associated with IPF or consistent with increasing trends to transplant older patients whom this disease most often afflicts. Regardless, this and other forms of pulmonary fibrosis are now the number one indication for lung transplantation in the United States, accounting for 52% of procedures performed in 2010 (United Network for Organ Sharing, personal communication, 2011). Worldwide, 29% of all procedures performed in 2008 were for an indication of IPF compared with 16% in 2000.[11]

The appropriate time for listing for transplantation must consider the potential survival benefit of the procedure. In the past decade there has been much work to define risk factors associated with worse outcomes in those with IPF before transplantation. Although the overall prognosis is grim, disease course remains variable for individual patients. As a result, identifying patients who are at particularly high risk is most appropriate when considering listing for lung transplantation.

Studies have focused on baseline characteristics as well as the change in study values over time to identify the group of patients at high risk for short-term mortality and, therefore, who are appropriate candidates for lung transplantation. Most of these publications are based on small series of retrospective data that have not been prospectively validated. Nonetheless, several clinical indicators (**Box 1**) are worth discussion because they likely portend a worse outcome and herald the need for lung transplantation.

CT scan fibrosis scoring has consistently correlated with risk for death. In several studies, the extent of the fibrosis is an independent predictor of outcome.[41–43] The extent of honeycomb change and reticulation is scored based on the percentage involvement of the lung parenchyma. Although these findings are consistent in the literature when interpreted by a thoracic radiologist, the lack of consistently trained radiologists limits its use in routine clinical practice. Nonetheless, extensive reticulation and/or honeycombing should raise the suspicion for future poor outcome.

Unlike the CT scan fibrosis score, baseline pulmonary function tests seem less helpful than serial measurements. This is borne out in both retrospective and prospective cohorts.[44,45] Martinez and colleagues[45] demonstrated that IPF patients enrolled in a clinical trial seemed at equal risk for subsequent decline regardless of their baseline pulmonary function. Despite the lack of risk assessment from a single measurement, there are consistent data that indicate repeated measures of pulmonary function that demonstrate decline in the FVC are predictive of worse outcomes.[44,46] Several studies have used 10% declines in FVC as a definition of significant decline to identify high-risk patients; however, a recent report suggests that smaller declines in FVC can also be clinically significant.[47] At this time, the absolute threshold for the decline in FVC to identify the highest-risk patient population remains unclear; however, any decline in FVC should warrant careful re-evaluation for a change in a patient's clinical status.

Assessment of a patient's exercise tolerance is also of independent value. Evidence of oxygen desaturation on 6-minute walk testing has demonstrated an increased risk for poor outcome in several studies.[48–50] These studies consistently demonstrate an increased risk for those who desaturate below 89% during a 6-minute walk test on room air. In addition, overall walk distance seems independently associated with future outcome.[51,52] In 2 separate cohorts of IPF patients, one awaiting lung transplantation and another evaluated at a referral center, similar poor 6-minute walk performance was associated with worse outcomes. One found a walk distance of less than 207 m associated with a 4-fold increased risk of death over the subsequent 6 months. The other found a walk distance of less than 212 m placed those individuals at high risk for mortality over the next 18 months. Consistent with the findings of pulmonary function testing, changes in exercise tolerance over time also seem predictive of outcome. Using data from a large randomized controlled trial, declines in 6-minute walk distance of greater than 50 m over 24 weeks were associated with a 4-fold increased risk of death during the next year.[53] These data indicate that poor exercise tolerance or falling exercise tolerance over time is indicative of a high-risk patient for mortality without transplantation.

Unfortunately, there remains a subset of patients who develop acute respiratory deterioration that suggests a less predictable course for patients with IPF. When the cause for the acute decline is unknown, this is termed, *acute exacerbation of IPF*.[54] Outcomes from different series seem variable but an exacerbation can be the defining event leading to frank respiratory failure. As a result, when there are no identifiable absolute contraindications to transplant, it is reasonable to refer all patients diagnosed with IPF to a transplant center.

The average IPF patient is diagnosed in the seventh decade. At this time, there is no absolute upper age limit for lung transplantation. Worldwide data demonstrate an increase in the number of lung transplants for those over age 65, accounting for 5% of all lung transplants performed in 2008. The International Society for Heart and Lung Transplantation Registry data indicate that those who are over age 65 suffer from worse long-term outcomes (median survival 3.3 years) compared with those who are under age 50 (median survival 6.3 years).[11] Although these survival outcomes are also affected by confounders because they are not adjusted, IPF patients are on average older and, therefore, may have worse outcomes than average. This fact does not preclude a potential survival benefit or quality-of-life improvement but is assessed by the transplant center for each individual patient with IPF.

Sarcoidosis

Sarcoidosis has a highly variable clinical course that is often extended over decades with the possibility of spontaneous remissions. Determining the right time for transplantation is challenging and characteristics associated with high risk for mortality come from limited data sources.[55–57] Patients who are African American, have higher mean pulmonary artery pressure, or require supplemental oxygen were found at increased risk of death while on the United Network for Organ Sharing (United States) waiting list. In addition, patients from a single-center cohort with right atrial pressure greater than 15 mm Hg had significantly increased risk of death while on the waiting list. Sarcoidosis accounted for approximately 3% of all transplants between 1995 and 2009.[11] Outcomes after transplantation are consistent with those for other indications although there is an increased risk of early mortality.[58,59] This may be reflective of the increased rates of pulmonary hypertension. Shorr and colleagues[58] also identified that African American patients are at higher risk of perioperative death. Despite this, the most recent data indicate a 5-year median survival after transplant. For those patients who fail to respond to conventional therapy and develop advanced lung disease, lung transplantation remains a viable therapeutic option.

Special considerations for those with sarcoidosis include its systemic nature. A thorough evaluation of sarcoidosis patients to ensure there is no clinically significant end organ damage is relevant to the preoperative evaluation of these patients. In addition, mycetomas are a common complication of cavitary lung disease and these can have an impact on transplant candidacy as well as management.[60] One unique feature of sarcoidosis after transplant is its common recurrence in the transplanted lung.[59,61–64] The reported prevalence of recurrent disease ranges from 20% to 80%. The granulomas are of recipient origin and disease recurrence typically is of little clinical significance after transplantation. Because patients are living longer after transplant, it remains to be seen if there are any longer-term complications from recurrence of disease.

Scleroderma Lung Disease and Connective Tissue Disease–Associated DPLD

The number of lung transplants performed for underlying connective tissue disease remains low, accounting for less than 1% of all lung

transplants in 2008.[11] Systemic sclerosis, rheumatoid arthritis, and undifferentiated connective tissue disease are associated with DPLD. The majority of data outlining outcomes after lung transplantation are from patients with systemic sclerosis. With the advent of angiotensin-converting enzyme inhibitors, renal crisis is no longer the main cause of death and this has been replaced with respiratory failure due to fibrosis and/or pulmonary hypertension.[65] As with sarcoidosis, connective tissue diseases are systemic, and careful consideration of comorbidities that hamper transplant outcome is imperative. One salient feature of systemic sclerosis is esophageal dysmotility. Several reports have associated chronic allograft dysfunction or BOS with gastroesophageal reflux.[66,67] Esophageal dysmotility may not only increase reflux episodes but also preclude fundoplication that has been associated with improvements in lung function in selected patients.[68,69] Gastroparesis is a common complication after lung transplantation as well.[70] Combining esophageal dysmotility and gastroparesis can lead to significant aspiration events that lead to graft dysfunction and loss. Guidelines that specifically outline criteria for acceptable esophageal function in systemic sclerosis remain elusive. Individual transplant programs assess this feature of disease on a case-by-case basis. Although the data are limited on outcomes for patients with systemic sclerosis, selected patients seem to have similar outcomes as patients with IPF and idiopathic pulmonary hyertension.[71–74] These series are limited by their small size and further data to define outcomes in this patient population are needed.

Lymphangioleiomyomatosis

Lymphangioleiomyomatosis (LAM) remains a rare indication for lung transplantation accounting for 1% of all transplants performed between 1995 and 2009. Initial reports suggested a far worse natural history for LAM than is currently known.[75] Despite this, there is a subset of patients who decline over time and develop significant morbidity associated with the disease.[76] For this group, transplant is a reasonable therapeutic option. From a single-center cohort, perioperative complications included significant blood loss with the removal of the explanted lungs and chylous effusions[77]; however, these findings did not preclude good long-term outcomes.[78] An additional evaluation of the US transplant registry demonstrated outcomes with statistically significantly better 5-year survival (65%) compared with other indications for lung transplant.[79] In addition to mortality data, there is now information that demonstrates an improved quality of life for those who have undergone lung transplantation compared with those who have severe advanced disease due to LAM.[34]

A novel intervention for patients with LAM deserves special mention. Sirolimus has been studied in a cohort of patients with moderate obstructive lung disease and found to reduce the decline in forced expiratory volume in 1 second (FEV1) over time.[80] This medication may be used more frequently in the future in patients with LAM; however, once the decision to list for transplant has been made, this medication should be avoided. Sirolimus has a prolonged half-life in those who are on a stable dose. It has been associated with the development of bronchial wound dehiscence in a previous randomized trial evaluating its safety and efficacy after lung transplantation.[81] This potentially fatal complication precludes the use of sirolimus in the perioperative period of lung transplantation.

Pulmonary Langerhans Cell Histiocytosis

Pulmonary Langerhans cell histiocytosis (PLCH) accounts for less than 0.5% of all lung transplants. Patients with this disorder typically have significant pulmonary hypertension. Lung transplant outcomes seem compatible with those for other patients with idiopathic pulmonary hypertension although recurrence of disease does occur in the allograft at a high rate (20% in one series).[82] The greatest risk factor for disease recurrence was a past history of systemic disease. The recurrence of disease was not reported to have an impact on survival; however, conclusions regarding the impact of disease recurrence are limited due to the small numbers and short follow-up. PLCH has also been associated with malignancy in several reports. Vassallo and colleagues[83] attempted to determine the risk for development of malignancy in their cohort, and a relationship could not be ruled in or ruled out. These past reports suggest it is prudent to carefully prescreen potential lung transplant recipients for malignancy. Given the small numbers of transplants and the reported outcomes to date, lung transplantation remains an appropriate therapeutic option for patients with advance disease due to PLCH.

SUMMARY

For selected DPLD patients who fail to respond to medical therapy and demonstrate declines in function that place them at increased risk for mortality, lung transplantation should be considered. Lung transplantation remains a complex medical intervention that requires a dedicated recipient and medical team. Despite the challenges, lung transplantation affords appropriate patients a reasonable chance at increased survival and improved quality of life. Lung transplantation remains an appropriate therapeutic option for selected patients with DPLD.

REFERENCES

1. Daniels CE, Lasky JA, Limper AH, et al. Imatinib treatment for idiopathic pulmonary fibrosis: randomized placebo-controlled trial results. Am J Respir Crit Care Med 2010;181(6):604–10.
2. Raghu G, Weycker D, Edelsberg J, et al. Incidence and prevalence of idiopathic pulmonary fibrosis. Am J Respir Crit Care Med 2006;174(7):810–6.
3. Coultas DB, Zumwalt RE, Black WC, et al. The epidemiology of interstitial lung diseases. Am J Respir Crit Care Med 1994;150(4):967–72.
4. Araki T, Katsura H, Sawabe M, et al. A clinical study of idiopathic pulmonary fibrosis based on autopsy studies in elderly patients. Intern Med 2003;42(6):483–9.
5. Bjoraker JA, Ryu JH, Edwin MK, et al. Prognostic significance of histopathologic subsets in idiopathic pulmonary fibrosis. Am J Respir Crit Care Med 1998;157(1):199–203.
6. Collard HR, Ryu JH, Douglas WW, et al. Combined corticosteroid and cyclophosphamide therapy does not alter survival in idiopathic pulmonary fibrosis. Chest 2004;125(6):2169–74.
7. Daniil ZD, Gilchrist FC, Nicholson AG, et al. A histologic pattern of nonspecific interstitial pneumonia is associated with a better prognosis than usual interstitial pneumonia in patients with cryptogenic fibrosing alveolitis. Am J Respir Crit Care Med 1999;160(3):899–905.
8. Nathan SD, Shlobin OA, Weir N, et al. Long-term course and prognosis of idiopathic pulmonary fibrosis in the new millennium. Chest 2011;140(1):221–9.
9. Reitz BA, Wallwork JL, Hunt SA, et al. Heart-lung transplantation: successful therapy for patients with pulmonary vascular disease. N Engl J Med 1982;306(10):557–64.
10. Unilateral lung transplantation for pulmonary fibrosis. Toronto Lung Transplant Group. N Engl J Med 1986;314(18):1140–5.
11. Christie JD, Edwards LB, Kucheryavaya AY, et al. The Registry of the International Society for Heart and Lung Transplantation: twenty-seventh official adult lung and heart-lung transplant report—2010. J Heart Lung Transplant 2010;29(10):1104–18.
12. Orens JB, Estenne M, Arcasoy S, et al. International guidelines for the selection of lung transplant candidates: 2006 update—a consensus report from the Pulmonary Scientific Council of the International

Society for Heart and Lung Transplantation. J Heart Lung Transplant 2006;25(7):745–55.

13. Christie JD, Edwards LB, Aurora P, et al. The registry of The International Society for Heart and Lung Transplantation: twenty-sixth official adult lung and heart-lung transplantation report—2009. J Heart Lung Transplant 2009;28(10):1031–49.

14. Conte JV, Borja MJ, Patel CB, et al. Lung transplantation for primary and secondary pulmonary hypertension. Ann Thorac Surg 2001;72(5):1673–9 [discussion: 1679–80].

15. Whelan TP, Dunitz JM, Kelly RF, et al. Effect of preoperative pulmonary artery pressure on early survival after lung transplantation for idiopathic pulmonary fibrosis. J Heart Lung Transplant 2005; 24(9):1269–74.

16. Huerd SS, Hodges TN, Grover FL, et al. Secondary pulmonary hypertension does not adversely affect outcome after single lung transplantation. J Thorac Cardiovasc Surg 2000;119(3):458–65.

17. Weiss ES, Allen JG, Merlo CA, et al. Survival after single versus bilateral lung transplantation for high-risk patients with pulmonary fibrosis. Ann Thorac Surg 2009;88(5):1616–25 [discussion: 1625–26].

18. Thabut G, Christie JD, Ravaud P, et al. Survival after bilateral versus single-lung transplantation for idiopathic pulmonary fibrosis. Ann Intern Med 2009; 151(11):767–74.

19. Neurohr C, Huppmann P, Thum D, et al. Potential functional and survival benefit of double over single lung transplantation for selected patients with idiopathic pulmonary fibrosis. Transpl Int 2010;23(9):887–96.

20. Algar FJ, Espinosa D, Moreno P, et al. Results of lung transplantation in idiopathic pulmonary fibrosis patients. Transplant Proc 2010;42(8):3211–3.

21. Force SD, Kilgo P, Neujahr DC, et al. Bilateral lung transplantation offers better long-term survival, compared with single-lung transplantation, for younger patients with idiopathic pulmonary fibrosis. Ann Thorac Surg 2011;91(1):244–9.

22. Nathan SD, Shlobin OA, Ahmad S, et al. Comparison of wait times and mortality for idiopathic pulmonary fibrosis patients listed for single or bilateral lung transplantation. J Heart Lung Transplant 2010; 29(10):1165–71.

23. 2009 Annual Report of the U.S. Organ procurement and transplantation network and the scientific registry of transplant recipients: transplant data 1999–2008. Rockville (MD): U.S. Department of Health and Human Services, Health Resources and Services Administration, Healthcare Systems Bureau, Division of Transplantation.

24. de Perrot M, Liu M, Waddell TK, et al. Ischemia-reperfusion-induced lung injury. Am J Respir Crit Care Med 2003;167(4):490–511.

25. Fang A, Studer S, Kawut SM, et al. Elevated pulmonary artery pressure is a risk factor for primary graft dysfunction following lung transplantation for idiopathic pulmonary fibrosis. Chest 2011;139(4): 782–7.

26. Lee JC, Christie JD, Keshavjee S. Primary graft dysfunction: definition, risk factors, short- and long-term outcomes. Semin Respir Crit Care Med 2010;31(2):161–71.

27. Barr ML, Kawut SM, Whelan TP, et al. Report of the ISHLT working group on primary lung graft dysfunction part IV: recipient-related risk factors and markers. J Heart Lung Transplant 2005;24(10):1468–82.

28. Whitson BA, Prekker ME, Herrington CS, et al. Primary graft dysfunction and long-term pulmonary function after lung transplantation. J Heart Lung Transplant 2007;26(10):1004–11.

29. Cypel M, Yeung JC, Liu M, et al. Normothermic ex vivo lung perfusion in clinical lung transplantation. N Engl J Med 2011;364(15):1431–40.

30. Thabut G, Mal H, Castier Y, et al. Survival benefit of lung transplantation for patients with idiopathic pulmonary fibrosis. J Thorac Cardiovasc Surg 2003;126(2):469–75.

31. Titman A, Rogers CA, Bonser RS, et al. Disease-specific survival benefit of lung transplantation in adults: a national cohort study. Am J Transplant 2009;9(7):1640–9.

32. Kotloff RM. Does lung transplantation confer a survival benefit? Curr Opin Organ Transplant 2009;14(5):499–503.

33. Kugler C, Fischer S, Gottlieb J, et al. Health-related quality of life in two hundred-eighty lung transplant recipients. J Heart Lung Transplant 2005;24(12): 2262–8.

34. Maurer JR, Ryu J, Beck G, et al. Lung transplantation in the management of patients with lymphangioleiomyomatosis: baseline data from the NHLBI LAM Registry. J Heart Lung Transplant 2007;26(12): 1293–9.

35. Santana MJ, Feeny D, Jackson K, et al. Improvement in health-related quality of life after lung transplantation. Can Respir J 2009;16(5):153–8.

36. Kugler C, Tegtbur U, Gottlieb J, et al. Health-related quality of life in long-term survivors after heart and lung transplantation: a prospective cohort study. Transplantation 2010;90(4):451–7.

37. Gerhardt SG, McDyer JF, Girgis RE, et al. Maintenance azithromycin therapy for bronchiolitis obliterans syndrome: results of a pilot study. Am J Respir Crit Care Med 2003;168(1):121–5.

38. Verleden GM, Dupont LJ. Azithromycin therapy for patients with bronchiolitis obliterans syndrome after lung transplantation. Transplantation 2004;77(9): 1465–7.

39. Yates B, Murphy DM, Forrest IA, et al. Azithromycin reverses airflow obstruction in established bronchiolitis obliterans syndrome. Am J Respir Crit Care Med 2005;172(6):772–5.

40. Vos R, Vanaudenaerde BM, Verleden SE, et al. A randomized placebo-controlled trial of azithromycin to prevent bronchiolitis obliterans syndrome after lung transplantation. Eur Respir J 2011; 37(1):164–72. [Epub 2010 Jun 18].

41. Lynch DA, Godwin JD, Safrin S, et al. High-resolution computed tomography in idiopathic pulmonary fibrosis: diagnosis and prognosis. Am J Respir Crit Care Med 2005;172(4):488–93.

42. Mogulkoc N, Brutsche MH, Bishop PW, et al. Pulmonary function in idiopathic pulmonary fibrosis and referral for lung transplantation. Am J Respir Crit Care Med 2001;164(1):103–8.

43. Gay SE, Kazerooni EA, Toews GB, et al. Idiopathic pulmonary fibrosis: predicting response to therapy and survival. Am J Respir Crit Care Med 1998; 157(4 Pt 1):1063–72.

44. Latsi PI, du Bois RM, Nicholson AG, et al. Fibrotic idiopathic interstitial pneumonia: the prognostic value of longitudinal functional trends. Am J Respir Crit Care Med 2003;168(5):531–7.

45. Martinez FJ, Safrin S, Weycker D, et al. The clinical course of patients with idiopathic pulmonary fibrosis. Ann Intern Med 2005;142(12 Pt 1):963–7.

46. Collard HR, King TE Jr, Bartelson BB, et al. Changes in clinical and physiologic variables predict survival in idiopathic pulmonary fibrosis. Am J Respir Crit Care Med 2003;168(5):538–42.

47. Zappala CJ, Latsi PI, Nicholson AG, et al. Marginal decline in forced vital capacity is associated with a poor outcome in idiopathic pulmonary fibrosis. Eur Respir J 2010;35(4):830–6.

48. Hallstrand TS, Boitano LJ, Johnson WC, et al. The timed walk test as a measure of severity and survival in idiopathic pulmonary fibrosis. Eur Respir J 2005; 25(1):96–103.

49. Lama VN, Flaherty KR, Toews GB, et al. Prognostic value of desaturation during a 6-minute walk test in idiopathic interstitial pneumonia. Am J Respir Crit Care Med 2003;168(9):1084–90.

50. Lettieri CJ, Nathan SD, Browning RF, et al. The distance-saturation product predicts mortality in idiopathic pulmonary fibrosis. Respir Med 2006; 100(10):1734–41.

51. Lederer DJ, Arcasoy SM, Wilt JS, et al. Six-minute-walk distance predicts waiting list survival in idiopathic pulmonary fibrosis. Am J Respir Crit Care Med 2006;174(6):659–64.

52. Caminati A, Bianchi A, Cassandro R, et al. Walking distance on 6-MWT is a prognostic factor in idiopathic pulmonary fibrosis. Respir Med 2009;103(1): 117–23.

53. Du Bois R, Albera C, Costabel U, et al. 6-Minute Walk Test Distance (6MWD) is a reliable, valid, and responsive outcome measure that predicts mortality in patients with IPF. Am J Respir Crit Care Med 2010; 181:A6026.

54. Collard HR, Moore BB, Flaherty KR, et al. Acute exacerbations of idiopathic pulmonary fibrosis. Am J Respir Crit Care Med 2007;176(7):636–43.

55. Arcasoy SM, Christie JD, Pochettino A, et al. Characteristics and outcomes of patients with sarcoidosis listed for lung transplantation. Chest 2001; 120(3):873–80.

56. Shorr AF, Davies DB, Nathan SD. Outcomes for patients with sarcoidosis awaiting lung transplantation. Chest 2002;122(1):233–8.

57. Shorr AF, Davies DB, Nathan SD. Predicting mortality in patients with sarcoidosis awaiting lung transplantation. Chest 2003;124(3):922–8.

58. Shorr AF, Helman DL, Davies DB, et al. Sarcoidosis, race, and short-term outcomes following lung transplantation. Chest 2004;125(3):990–6.

59. Milman N, Burton C, Andersen CB, et al. Lung transplantation for end-stage pulmonary sarcoidosis: outcome in a series of seven consecutive patients. Sarcoidosis Vasc Diffuse Lung Dis 2005;22(3):222–8.

60. Hadjiliadis D, Sporn TA, Perfect JR, et al. Outcome of lung transplantation in patients with mycetomas. Chest 2002;121(1):128–34.

61. Milman N, Andersen CB, Burton CM, et al. Recurrent sarcoid granulomas in a transplanted lung derive from recipient immune cells. Eur Respir J 2005; 26(3):549–52.

62. Ionescu DN, Hunt JL, Lomago D, et al. Recurrent sarcoidosis in lung transplant allografts: granulomas are of recipient origin. Diagn Mol Pathol 2005;14(3): 140–5.

63. Yeatman M, McNeil K, Smith JA, et al. Lung Transplantation in patients with systemic diseases: an eleven-year experience at Papworth Hospital. J Heart Lung Transplant 1996;15(2):144–9.

64. Johnson BA, Duncan SR, Ohori NP, et al. Recurrence of sarcoidosis in pulmonary allograft recipients. Am Rev Respir Dis 1993;148(5):1373–7.

65. Steen VD, Medsger TA. Changes in causes of death in systemic sclerosis, 1972-2002. Ann Rheum Dis 2007;66(7):940–4.

66. D'Ovidio F, Mura M, Tsang M, et al. Bile acid aspiration and the development of bronchiolitis obliterans after lung transplantation. J Thorac Cardiovasc Surg 2005;129(5):1144–52.

67. Murthy SC, Nowicki ER, Mason DP, et al. Pretransplant gastroesophageal reflux compromises early outcomes after lung transplantation. J Thorac Cardiovasc Surg 2011;142(1):47–52.e3.

68. Palmer SM, Miralles AP, Howell DN, et al. Gastroesophageal reflux as a reversible cause of allograft dysfunction after lung transplantation. Chest 2000; 118(4):1214–7.

69. Hartwig MG, Anderson DJ, Onaitis MW, et al. Fundoplication after lung transplantation prevents the allograft dysfunction associated with reflux. Ann Thorac Surg 2011;92(2):462–8 [discussion: 468–9].

70. Berkowitz N, Schulman LL, McGregor C, et al. Gastroparesis after lung transplantation. Potential role in postoperative respiratory complications. Chest 1995;108(6):1602–7.

71. Rosas V, Conte JV, Yang SC, et al. Lung transplantation and systemic sclerosis. Ann Transplant 2000; 5(3):38–43.

72. Schachna L, Medsger TA Jr, Dauber JH, et al. Lung transplantation in scleroderma compared with idiopathic pulmonary fibrosis and idiopathic pulmonary arterial hypertension. Arthritis Rheum 2006;54(12): 3954–61.

73. Shitrit D, Amital A, Peled N, et al. Lung transplantation in patients with scleroderma: case series, review of the literature, and criteria for transplantation. Clin Transplant 2009;23(2):178–83.

74. Saggar R, Khanna D, Furst DE, et al. Systemic sclerosis and bilateral lung transplantation: a single centre experience. Eur Respir J 2010;36(4):893–900.

75. Taylor JR, Ryu J, Colby TV, et al. Lymphangioleiomyomatosis. Clinical course in 32 patients. N Engl J Med 1990;323(18):1254–60.

76. Kitaichi M, Nishimura K, Itoh H, et al. Pulmonary lymphangioleiomyomatosis: a report of 46 patients including a clinicopathologic study of prognostic factors. Am J Respir Crit Care Med 1995;151(2 Pt 1): 527–33.

77. Pechet TT, Meyers BF, Guthrie TJ, et al. Lung transplantation for lymphangioleiomyomatosis. J Heart Lung Transplant 2004;23(3):301–8.

78. Boehler A, Speich R, Russi EW, et al. Lung transplantation for lymphangioleiomyomatosis. N Engl J Med 1996;335(17):1275–80.

79. Kpodonu J, Massad MG, Chaer RA, et al. The US experience with lung transplantation for pulmonary lymphangioleiomyomatosis. J Heart Lung Transplant 2005;24(9):1247–53.

80. McCormack FX, Inoue Y, Moss J, et al. Efficacy and safety of sirolimus in lymphangioleiomyomatosis. N Engl J Med 2011;364(17):1595–606.

81. Groetzner J, Kur F, Spelsberg F, et al. Airway anastomosis complications in de novo lung transplantation with sirolimus-based immunosuppression. J Heart Lung Transplant 2004;23(5):632–8.

82. Dauriat G, Mal H, Thabut G, et al. Lung transplantation for pulmonary langerhans' cell histiocytosis: a multicenter analysis. Transplantation 2006;81(5): 746–50.

83. Vassallo R, Ryu JH, Schroeder DR, et al. Clinical outcomes of pulmonary Langerhans'-cell histiocytosis in adults. N Engl J Med 2002;346(7):484–90.

84. Sager JS, Kotloff RM, Ahya VN, et al. Association of clinical risk factors with functional status following lung transplantation. Am J Transplant 2006;6(9): 2191–201.

85. Kanasky WF, Anton SD, Rodrigue JR, et al. Impact of body weight on long-term survival after lung transplantation. Chest 2002;121(2):401–6.

86. Madill J, Gutierrez C, Grossman J, et al. Nutritional assessment of the lung transplant patient: body mass index as a predictor of 90-day mortality following transplantation. J Heart Lung Transplant 2001;20(3):288–96.

87. Gonzalez-Castro A, Llorca J, Suberviola B, et al. Influence of nutritional status in lung transplant recipients. Transplant Proc 2006;38(8):2539–40.

88. Lederer DJ, Wilt JS, D'Ovidio F, et al. Obesity and underweight are associated with an increased risk of death after lung transplantation. Am J Respir Crit Care Med 2009;180(9):887–95.

89. Allen JG, Arnaoutakis GJ, Weiss ES, et al. The impact of recipient body mass index on survival after lung transplantation. J Heart Lung Transplant 2010;29(9):1026–33.

Index

Note: Page numbers of article titles are in **boldface** type.

Clin Chest Med 33 (2012) 191–197
doi:10.1016/S0272-5231(12)00014-7
0272-5231/12/$ – see front matter © 2012 Elsevier Inc. All rights reserved.

chestmed.theclinics.com

Printed and bound by CPI Group (UK) Ltd, Croydon, CR0 4YY

03/10/2024

01040361-0001